Cognitive-Behavioral Group Therapy for Social Phobia

TREATMENT MANUALS FOR PRACTITIONERS
David H. Barlow, *Editor*

Recent Volumes

COGNITIVE-BEHAVIORAL GROUP THERAPY FOR SOCIAL PHOBIA:
BASIC MECHANISMS AND CLINICAL STRATEGIES
Richard G. Heimberg and Robert E. Becker

REDUCING CHILD MALTREATMENT:
A GUIDEBOOK FOR PARENT SERVICES
John R. Lutzker and Kathryn M. Bigelow

SEXUAL DYSFUNCTION: A GUIDE FOR ASSESSMENT
AND TREATMENT, SECOND EDITION
John P. Wincze and Michael P. Carey

BRIEF THERAPY FOR COUPLES:
HELPING PARTNERS HELP THEMSELVES
W. Kim Halford

TREATING SUICIDAL BEHAVIOR:
AN EFFECTIVE, TIME-LIMITED APPROACH
M. David Rudd, Thomas Joiner, and M. Hasan Rajab

COGNITIVE-BEHAVIORAL TREATMENT OF IRRITABLE
BOWEL SYNDROME: THE BRAIN–GUT CONNECTION
Brenda B. Toner, Zindel V. Segal, Shelagh D. Emmott, and David Myran

MULTISYSTEMIC TREATMENT OF ANTISOCIAL
BEHAVIOR IN CHILDREN AND ADOLESCENTS
Scott W. Henggeler, Sonja K. Schoenwald, Charles M. Borduin,
Melisa D. Rowland, and Phillippe B. Cunningham

TREATING THE TRAUMA OF RAPE:
COGNITIVE-BEHAVIORAL THERAPY FOR PTSD
Edna B. Foa and Barbara Olasov Rothbaum

Cognitive-Behavioral Group Therapy for Social Phobia

Basic Mechanisms and Clinical Strategies

RICHARD G. HEIMBERG
ROBERT E. BECKER

Series Editor's Note by David H. Barlow

THE GUILFORD PRESS
New York   London

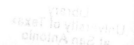

© 2002 The Guilford Press
A Division of Guilford Publications, Inc.
72 Spring Street, New York, NY 10012
www.guilford.com

Printed in the United States of America

This book is printed on acid-free paper.

Last digit is print number: 9   8   7   6   5   4   3   2   1

Library of Congress Cataloging-in-Publication Data

Heimberg, Richard G.
  Cognitive-behavioral group therapy for social phobia : basic
mechanisms and clinical strategies / Richard G. Heimberg, Robert E.
Becker.
       p. cm. — (Treatment manuals for practitioners)
Includes bibliographical references and index.
  ISBN 1-57230-770-6 (hardcover : alk. paper)
  1. Cognitive therapy. 2. Behavior therapy. 3. Group psychotherapy.
4. Phobias—Treatment. I. Becker, Robert E. II. Title. III. Series.
  RC489.C63 H455 2002
  616.89′142—dc21

                                                    2002003487

To my father,
Murray Heimberg
—R. G. H.

About the Authors

Richard G. Heimberg, PhD, is Professor and Director of the Clinical Psychology Training Program, as well as Director of the Adult Anxiety Clinic, at Temple University. Dr. Heimberg is well known for his efforts to develop and evaluate cognitive-behavioral treatments for social anxiety. He has published more than 200 articles and chapters on social phobia, the anxiety disorders, and related topics. In addition, he is coeditor or coauthor of *Social Phobia: Diagnosis, Assessment, and Treatment; Managing Social Anxiety: A Cognitive-Behavioral Therapy Approach*; and the forthcoming *Generalized Anxiety Disorder: Advances in Research and Practice*. Dr. Heimberg served as president of the Association for Advancement of Behavior Therapy, and was recently named one of the four most influential psychological researchers in anxiety in a survey of members of the Anxiety Disorders Association of America. He is a founding fellow of the Academy of Cognitive Therapy and the recipient of the Academy's inaugural Award for Significant and Enduring Contribution to Cognitive Therapy.

Robert E. Becker, PhD, received his doctoral degree in clinical psychology from the University at Albany, State University of New York. He was an Associate Professor of Psychiatry at Albany Medical College and then an Associate Professor of Psychiatry at the Medical College of Pennsylvania. Dr. Becker has authored or coauthored 32 publications, many focused on social skills training and social phobia. He has served as Principal Investigator or Co-Principal Investigator on several National Institute of Mental Health research grants. Currently he is president of Psychological Services Group, Inc., which provides psychological services to several hospitals in the Delaware Valley area of Pennsylvania.

Series Editor's Note

Everyone in the field of mental health has been sensitized to the issue of stigma. Equally troublesome is the tendency to trivialize psychological disorders as annoying traits that, with a little effort and desire on the part of the individual, can be overcome. Few disorders are as universally trivialized or ridiculed as severe social anxiety. In our own center we have treated children and adolescents who retreat to a bathroom stall to hide during lunch hour so as not to have to sit at a table with other kids; they have been doing this for years. Because these children bring little attention to themselves, they are often ignored or dismissed as going through a "shy" phase that they will outgrow. But we have seen many adults who never outgrew their social anxiety, and in fact had been so ridiculed and even brutalized by their peers during their teenage years that they now meet criteria for posttraumatic stress disorder. In our society there are few individuals who suffer more than the chronically and severely socially anxious adult.

For the past 20 years, Richard Heimberg and his colleagues have been in the forefront in developing efficient and effective brief psychological treatments for these problems, and they have succeeded admirably. It is safe to say that, since their development in our center in Albany in the 1980s, these treatments have been more widely utilized around the world for this serious condition than have any other existing treatments for severe social anxiety and social phobia. Now for the first time this treatment protocol, along with the conceptual and empirical foundations for its development, are available in this book, and its appearance is very timely indeed. Although medications are now available with proven effectiveness for this disorder, surveys of individuals consistently reveal that they would prefer a psychological treatment through which they actually learn new skills that they can take with them; and outcome data do indicate that these interventions have enduring effects. The appearance of this treatment protocol should allow clinicians everywhere to fulfill these wishes and desires.

DAVID H. BARLOW, PhD

Preface

Social phobia is a disorder of human functioning that, at its most severe, can totally disrupt the person's ability to interact with or even be around other human beings. As we demonstrate in the pages to come, it is associated with unfulfilled dreams, loneliness, depression, and even an increased risk of suicidal thinking. The economic and emotional burden of social phobia and the opportunities lost by persons with social phobia is unfathomable. However, until recent times, social phobia was also the Rodney Dangerfield of the anxiety disorders: It just did not get any respect. Unlike panic disorder, agoraphobia, or the specific phobias, social phobia has only recently become familiar to the general public. In fact, it was only 17 short years ago that Liebowitz, Gorman, Fyer, and Klein (1985, p. 729) referred to social phobia as the "neglected anxiety disorder."

The situation in the world of social phobia has changed from its humble and uncelebrated emergence in the third edition of the *Diagnostic and Statistical Manual of Mental Disorders* (American Psychiatric Association [APA], 1980). Most recently, social phobia has been recognized by pharmaceutical companies, which have been spurred on by reports of the substantial prevalence of social phobia and the degree of distress and impairment experienced by afflicted persons. Pharmacological treatment is not the focus of this book, but the involvement of pharmaceutical companies will have a number of far-reaching effects. These include increased public awareness, facilitated by direct-to-consumer advertising campaigns, and increased awareness by primary care physicians, as well as psychiatrists, who will be briefed by pharmaceutical company representatives. All this is to the good, and we can only hope that it will result in increased access to, and utilization of, a range of empirically supported and efficacious treatment alternatives by persons with social phobia. One side effect for which we must remain vigilant, however, is the increasingly prevalent notion that social phobia is a genetic disorder or disease that is best treated by biological interventions. Regardless of what we may someday know about the biological underpinnings of social phobia, we know that psychosocial treatments, especially cognitive-behavioral therapy, can be highly effective in the treatment of social phobia.

With this book, we hope to accomplish several goals. First, in Chapters 1 and 2, we introduce you to social phobia, allowing you get to know it "up close and personal." We address such questions as, "What is social phobia?," "How common is it?," "What causes it?," and "How does it affect the individual?" Although definitive answers to some of these questions are not available, we give you the best guesses based on the current research literature. In Chapter 1, we present the diagnosis of social phobia, trace the way in which the diagnosis has changed over the course of history, and examine the prevalence and nature of social phobia among men and women in the United States and around the world. We also investigate the different possible contributors to the development of social phobia, considering genetic and temperamental, as well as environmental, inputs. In Chapter 2, we take a close look at subtypes of social phobia and how social phobia relates to avoidant personality disorder, an issue that has been controversial for 20 years. We also examine the comorbidity of social phobia with other psychiatric disorders (both Axis I and Axis II) and the broad range of impairments that are associated with social phobia.

Second, we present the research that has provided the underpinnings for our thinking about the nature of social phobia and what it takes to treat it successfully. In Chapters 3 and 4, we review and discuss the many exciting research studies that have examined aspects of the way persons with social phobia think and process information. To us, as cognitive-behavioral therapists and researchers, these studies provide a rich and fertile field in which our conceptions of social phobia and its treatment can take root and grow. In Chapter 5, we present a theoretical model of social phobia that has been guided by this research and that has guided much of our own work. This cognitive-behavioral model addresses how social phobia develops and how, once developed, it may persist over time despite the pain that it brings to the person's life. This model has guided and been guided by our efforts to develop cognitive-behavioral approaches to the treatment of social phobia.

Third, in Chapter 6, we provide an overview of the psychometric assessment of social phobia, considering both self-report and clinician-administered measures and also including behavioral assessment, cognitive assessment, and assessment of related concerns such as depression, general anxiety, disability, and quality of life.

Fourth, in Part II of this book, we present in fine detail our method for the treatment of social phobia. The treatment package, which has come to be known as cognitive-behavioral group treatment for social phobia, or simply CBGT, was originally developed in 1982, when we first began to treat individuals with social phobia at the Center for Stress and Anxiety Disorders of the University at Albany, State University of New York. It is a growing, changing, and developing protocol that we continue to study at the Adult Anxiety Clinic of Temple University, and, in reality, it will never be "finished." Although many researchers have studied CBGT (or closely related cognitive-behavioral protocols) and although it has been administered to persons with social phobia the world over, this is the first time that our treatment manual has been set down in published form.

Part II gives you the information you will need to conduct CBGT. CBGT is an extensive and complex collection of procedures. It should not be conducted by persons without experience in the treatment of social phobia unless under the supervision of someone who is sophisticated both with the phenomenology of social phobia and the techniques, procedures, and theory of cognitive-behavioral treatment. Training and/or supervision experiences may be arranged through the Adult Anxiety Clinic of Temple University.

The chapters in Part II instruct the reader in the conduct of CBGT, beginning with Chapter 7. It provides an overview of CBGT and describes the session structure, goals, and basic techniques. It also raises a number of issues to be considered when putting a group together—issues such as group size and composition, therapist qualifications, and the setting in which the group should be conducted. Chapter 8 describes the procedures for interviewing and screening potential group members and preparing them to begin treatment. Chapters 9 and 10 provide detailed step-by-step instructions for the conduct of the first two sessions, during which structured exercises are employed to teach clients a number of new concepts central to CBGT. Chapter 11 describes the procedures involved in the staging of in-session exposures, that is, re-creations of personally relevant anxiety-provoking events in the group session. In-session exposures are the procedural hub around which much of CBGT revolves, and Chapter 11 includes not only instructions for their conduct but also numerous examples of in-session exposures for commonly feared situations and variations on standard procedure that are called for in more unique situations. Chapter 12 describes the use of cognitive restructuring procedures during group sessions. Cognitive restructuring procedures are presented in a step-by-step sequence, from the selection of a target situation to the processing of automatic thoughts about the situation to the conduct of the in-session exposure and, finally, to the processing of the outcome of the in-session exposure in the most adaptive fashion. Chapter 12 also contains extensive dialogue between therapists and clients as they do battle with irrational thoughts. Chapter 13 describes cognitive and behavioral procedures for use in homework assignments that clients complete between group sessions. Chapter 14 discusses apportionment of session time and describes issues specific to the final session of CBGT and problems that may arise in the conduct of CBGT that all cognitive-behavioral therapists should consider. It also provides a list of other materials that provide additional information about CBGT.

Throughout Part II, we refer you to specific sections of the Client Workbook (entitled *Managing Social Anxiety: A Cognitive-Behavioral Therapy Approach*

(Hope, Heimberg, Juster, & Turk, 2000). It is primarily intended for use with clients with social phobia who are treated in individual cognitive-behavioral therapy. However, it contains a great deal of material that may be usefully integrated into the conduct of social phobia group sessions. An accompanying therapist guide (Hope, Turk, & Heimberg) is in press. Wherever appropriate, we have brought the CBGT recording and monitoring forms in this book in line with those in the Client Workbook, so that the integration of the Client Workbook can be as seamless as possible. However, the Client Workbook is not required for the conduct of CBGT. The Client Workbook and therapist guide can be obtained from The Psychological Corporation (1-800-872-1726; www.psychcorp.com/catalogs/paipc/psy107dpri.htm).

We wish you the best in your efforts with CBGT. We welcome your comments on the manual and feedback about specific portions of it. We also hope you will let us know how you are doing with CBGT or other treatments for social phobia. Good luck!

RICHARD G. HEIMBERG
ROBERT E. BECKER

Acknowledgments

David H. Barlow, PhD, currently director of clinical training in the Department of Psychology of Boston University and director of the Center for Anxiety and Related Disorders at Boston University, first encouraged me to take on the treatment of socially anxious persons shortly after he joined me on the faculty of the University at Albany. Dave and Edward Blanchard, PhD, made the resources of their Center for Stress and Anxiety Disorders available to me for many years. James Vermilyea, PhD, Karen Goldfinger, PhD, Linda Zollo, PhD, Charles Kennedy, PhD, and Cynthia Dodge, PhD, were the first of my graduate students to devote their efforts to research on social phobia and its treatment. Many aspects of CBGT exist because these students "forced" me to listen to their ideas. Debra A. Hope, PhD, now professor of psychology and director of clinical psychology training at the University of Nebraska–Lincoln, came along shortly after and devoted her graduate career to research on social phobia. She has had more influence on the shape of CBGT than any other colleague or student and continues to be an outstanding colleague and collaborator and an even better friend. Ronald M. Rapee, PhD, professor of psychology at Macquarie University in Sydney, Australia, collaborated with me in the development of the theoretical model of social phobia presented here in Chapter 5 during my sabbatical stay in Sydney some years ago and has been a good friend and colleague since our days together in Albany. Craig S. Holt, PhD, associate director of the Social Phobia Program for 2 years, whose different points of view always stimulated productive debate, and Monroe A. Bruch, PhD, my colleague for many years at Albany, also had a large influence on the development of the treatment. Harlan Juster, who followed Craig Holt as associate director, basically ran the place for 5 years. Postdoctoral fellow Cynthia L. Turk, PhD, who contributed much to Chapters 5 and 6 of this book, has been a mainstay of the program at Temple University, as was David Fresco, PhD. Postdoctoral fellows Julie Lerner, PsyD, and Deborah Roth, PhD, also made meaningful contributions in their too-short stays with us. Special thanks are also due to Drs. Hope, Turk, Roth, and Fresco for their comments on an earlier draft of the manuscript. Stacey Slavkin, PhD, Cheryl Winning, PhD, Mark Mahone, PhD, Susan Orsillo, PhD, Annette Payne, PhD, Debra Salzman, PhD, Jill Mattia, PhD, Janet Klosko, PhD, Elissa Brown, PhD, Steve Safren, PhD, Emily Gonzalez, PhD, Greg Makris, PhD, Trevor Hart, PhD, Douglas Mennin, PhD, MacAndrew Jack, PhD, Anna Leung, Andrea Gifford, Meredith Coles, Brigette Erwin, Erin Scott, Winnie Eng, and countless others (graduate students at the time) ran groups under supervision and, in the process, contributed to the ongoing development of CBGT. Karen Law, office manager and administrative coordinator of the Social Phobia Program at the Center for Stress and Anxiety Disorders at the University at Albany for many years, and Ismael Alvarez, who holds the same position at Temple, have contributed to every activity I undertake. Without their good work, nothing would ever happen, and this book is no exception. Thanks, Karen and Ismael. Barbara Watkins, Senior Editor at The Guilford Press, provided a great deal of support, guidance, and patience in helping me bring the book to market. Finally, I tip my hat to the people who have received treatment in the Social Phobia Programs in Albany and Philadelphia. They have shown us their spirit, and it is because of them that we keep going.

RICHARD G. HEIMBERG

Contents

I. UNDERSTANDING THE NATURE OF SOCIAL PHOBIA

1. The Diagnosis and Etiology of Social Phobia   3

The Diagnosis of Social Phobia   4
The Etiology of Social Phobia   18

2. Subtypes of Social Phobia, Comorbidity, and Impairment   29

Subtypes of Social Phobia   29
Generalized Social Phobia and Avoidant Personality Disorder   34
Comorbidity of Social Phobia with Other Psychiatric Disorders   40
Personal Characteristics and Functional Impairment   47

3. Cognitive Function in Social Phobia   53

Negative Cognitive Content   53
Errors of Judgment and Interpretation   58

4. Dysfunctional Cognitive Processes in Social Phobia   73

Attentional Bias toward Social Threat   74
Memory Bias for Threatening Social Information   86
Perspective Taking in Social Phobic Imagery and Recall   90

5. A Cognitive-Behavioral Formulation of Social Phobia   93
with Ronald M. Rapee and Cynthia L. Turk

The Client   94
Confronting Feared Social Situations   98
After the Situation Concluded   105
Comment   105

6. Assessment of Social Phobia   107
   with Cynthia L. Turk

   Self-Report Assessment   108
   Clinician-Administered Measures   115
   Cognitive Assessment   119
   Behavioral Assessment Tests   123
   Adjunctive Measures   124

   II. COGNITIVE-BEHAVIORAL GROUP THERAPY
   FOR SOCIAL PHOBIA: A TREATMENT MANUAL

7. An Overview of Cognitive-Behavioral Group Therapy   129
   for Social Phobia

   The Treatment Orientation Interview   130
   Sessions 1 and 2   131
   Sessions 3 through 11   131
   Session 12   132
   Setting Up the Group   132

8. The Treatment Orientation Interview   136

   Clients for Whom Cognitive-Behavioral Group Therapy May Not
       Be Appropriate   137
   Discussion of the Specifics of the Client's Social Phobia   141
   The Individualized Fear and Avoidance Hierarchy   142
   The Subjective Units of Discomfort Scale (SUDS)   143
   Contracting about Specific Targets for Treatment   143
   Introduction to Group Procedures   146
   The Advantages of Group Treatment   146
   Ground Rules   147
   Preparing the Client to Begin Group Treatment Sessions   148

9. Session 1   149

   Introductions   150
   Ground Rules for Group Membership   151
   Sharing of Individual Problems and Goals   154
   Presentation of the Cognitive-Behavioral Model of Social Phobia   155
   Discussion of the Components of Treatment   163
   Assessment of Expectancy for Treatment Outcome   164
   Initial Training in Cognitive Restructuring   165
   Homework Assignment for Session 1: Monitoring and
       Recording Automatic Thoughts   173

10. Session 2   176

   Assessment of Fear of Negative Evaluation   176
   Review of Session 1 Homework Assignment   177
   Identification of Thinking Errors in Automatic Thoughts   177
   Disputing Automatic Thoughts and Developing Rational Responses   189
   Homework Assignment for Session 2: Cognitive Restructuring Practice   195
   Preparation for Initiation of In-Session Exposures   197

11. In-Session Exposures   199

Rationale for In-Session Exposures   199
Preparation for an In-Session Exposure   202
Incorporating Feared Outcomes   206
SUDS Recording   208
First Exposures   209
Choosing Role Players and Combined Exposures   210
In-Session Exposures versus Social Skills Training   211
Do In-Session Exposures Make Clients Anxious?   212
Examples of Common In-Session Exposures   213
In-Session Exposures for Specific Brief Behaviors   221

12. Integrating Cognitive Restructuring Procedures   227
    with In-Session Exposures

Before an In-Session Exposure   227
During an In-Session Exposure: SUDS Ratings and
    Rational Responses   250
After an In-Session Exposure: The Cognitive Debriefing   251
Behavioral Experiments   258
Cognitive Restructuring from Beginning to End   261
Group Involvement in Cognitive Restructuring   268

13. Homework Procedures   270

Before Attempting a Homework Assignment   271
The Behavioral Assignment   272
After the Assignment Is Completed   273
Summary of Homework Procedures   276
Sample Homework Tasks   276
Homework Review and Assignment   281

14. Sessions 3–12: Putting It All Together and Troubleshooting   283
    Cognitive-Behavioral Group Therapy

Reviewing Homework and Introducing In-Session Exposures
    in Session 3   284
Partitioning Session Time   285
Session 12: Consolidation of Gains and Looking to the Future   286
Termination Issues   289
Posttreatment Assessment   289
Additional Sessions   290
Session Planning in Cognitive-Behavioral Group Therapy   291
Troubleshooting Cognitive-Behavioral Group Therapy   291
Additional Source Materials for Cognitive-Behavioral Group Therapy   299

References   303

Index   327

I

UNDERSTANDING THE NATURE OF SOCIAL PHOBIA

1

The Diagnosis and Etiology
of Social Phobia

Heather was a 30-year-old night-shift nurse. As part of her job, she had to present each of the patients on her unit and any procedures they had required since the end of the previous shift to the doctors during morning rounds. However, she was very frightened by the prospect of speaking in front of others and being the center of their attention. To control her anxiety, she would go to the controlled substances cabinet and inject herself with morphine. Unfortunately, she soon became addicted. Her drug-taking behavior was detected, leading to her arrest and the loss of her professional license (Mennin, Heimberg, & Holt, 2000).

Jim was a 36-year-old unmarried man. He worked as a night watchman in a warehouse because this job required little social interaction. He was anxious in most any social situation, especially those involving women. He found that he could interact with women only after drinking heavily, and he had been involved in two relationships with alcoholic women who abused him. He spent most of his time alone, drunk, or depressed (Hope & Heimberg, 1990).

Maureen was a divorced mother in her 40s with three children. When her marriage deteriorated, she had to find work outside the home to support herself and her children. Quite the extravert, she did very well in a sales position and was soon earning a six-figure income. Her success led her employers to request that she train other agency employees in her sales techniques. At that point, in the absence of other visible means of support for herself or her children, she quit her job for fear of public speaking, and she remained unemployed for an extended period of time.

3

Jan was a 23-year-old single woman. She wanted nothing more than to be married and raise a family. However, she became highly anxious whenever she had to eat or drink in front of others. Her hands would shake, and she feared that she would humiliate herself by spilling her food. As a result, she was afraid that men she might date would believe there was something wrong with her. Despite above-average physical appearance and social skills, she had never dated.

These four very different people have something in common. They all have a problem known as social phobia, and it has taken a severe toll on their lives. But what is social phobia? This is not an easy question. Social phobia has been with us for years, with descriptions of afflicted individuals noted as early as Hippocrates. The famous French hypnotist Pierre Janet also made reference to *phobie des situations sociales* as early as 1903 (Heckelman & Schneier, 1995). However, most current thinking about social phobia dates from the writings of British psychiatrist Isaac Marks (Marks, 1970; Marks & Gelder, 1966), and his efforts led to its inclusion in the third edition of the *Diagnostic and Statistical Manual of Mental Disorders* (DSM-III; American Psychiatric Association [APA], 1980).

The Diagnosis of Social Phobia

DSM-III gave the problem of clinically significant social or performance anxiety a name and, along with it, an official existence. It now had a description and a set of criteria by which a mental health professional could make a proper diagnosis. As one might guess, this event marked the beginning of serious research on social phobia, and the amount of research in this area has steadily increased. However, the authors of DSM-III did not know as much about social phobia as we know now, and later editions of this manual (DSM-III-R: APA, 1987; DSM-IV: APA, 1994) have broadened its definition.

DSM-III (p. 228) defined social phobia as a "persistent, irrational fear of, and compelling desire to avoid, a situation in which the individual is exposed to possible scrutiny by others and fears that he or she may act in a way that will be humiliating or embarrassing." It was further stated that the individual experienced significant distress because of his or her social phobia, that the person recognized that the fear was excessive or unreasonable, and that the fear was not the result of another mental disorder.

Social phobia was conceptualized as something akin to a specific phobia of humiliation, embarrassment, or scrutiny by others. Examples of social phobias included fears of speaking or performing in public, of using public rest rooms, of eating in public, and of writing in the presence of others. Individuals were thought to have only one social phobia. Persons who experienced anxiety in the presence of others in a broad range of situations (people such as Jim, the night watchman) were not classified as having social phobia in DSM-III but instead were assigned the diagnosis of avoidant personality disorder (APD). Incorrectly, social phobia was not thought to be incapacitating unless it was extremely severe, although it was stated that considerable inconvenience might result from the need to avoid the phobic situation.

Several statements about social phobia in DSM-III were not based on empirical data and have been shown in the fullness of time to have been ill advised. In several later studies (e.g., Holt, Heimberg, Hope, & Liebowitz, 1992b; S. Turner, Beidel, Dancu, & Keys, 1986a), persons with social phobia reported fears of multiple situations, rather than a single social fear, as stated in DSM-III. Although DSM-III suggested that social phobia was rarely incapacitating, studies of the functional impairment experienced by persons with social phobia further suggested that it was a major negative force in their lives (Safren, Heimberg, Brown, & Holle, 1997a; Schneier, Johnson, Hornig, Liebowitz, & Weissman, 1992; Schneier et al., 1994; Wittchen & Beloch, 1996). Liebowitz and colleagues (1985) also expressed concern that the separation of clinically severe social anxiety into two separate diagnostic categories (social phobia and APD) and the placement of interpersonal anxiety on Axis II would discourage research into the treatment of this disorder.

Several revisions were made to the diagnostic criteria in DSM-III-R. The rule that social phobia could not be diagnosed in the presence of APD was removed, and the two diagnoses could be simultaneously applied. In addition, the criteria for social phobia were expanded to include broadly based interpersonal anxiety, and the notion of subtypes of social phobia was introduced. Specifically, DSM-III-R (p. 243, emphasis in original) added the following language: "**Specify generalized type** if the phobic situation includes most social situations, and also consider the additional diagnosis of Avoidant Personality Disorder." These changes have had a dramatic impact on the definition of social phobia, on determining who receives this diagnosis, and on the frequency with which it is applied. The importance of these changes is discussed more completely later in this chapter and in Chapter 2.

The criteria for social phobia included in DSM-IV are essentially unchanged from those in DSM-III-R, although several additions were made to accommodate the diagnosis of children with social phobia. Also, it was in DSM-IV that the term *social anxiety disorder* was first introduced. The new name was put forth to underscore the pervasiveness of anxiety symptoms and the broad impairments that may be experienced by persons who receive the diagnosis. Elsewhere, we (Liebowitz, Heimberg, Fresco, Travers, & Stein, 2000) have endorsed the use of the term "social anxiety disorder." However, the new name has just started to be broadly adopted, and most of the existing research addresses social phobia rather than social anxiety disorder; we do the same. DSM-IV criteria are presented in Table 1.1.

TABLE 1.1. DSM-IV Diagnostic Criteria for Social Phobia (Social Anxiety Disorder; 300.23)

A. A marked and persistent fear of one or more social or performance situations in which the person is exposed to unfamiliar people or to possible scrutiny by others. The individual fears that he or she will act in a way (or show anxiety symptoms) that will be humiliating or embarrassing. **Note:** In children, there must be evidence of the capacity for age-appropriate social relationships with familiar people and the anxiety must occur in peer settings, not just in interactions with adults.

B. Exposure to the feared social situation almost invariably provokes anxiety, which may take the form of a situationally bound or situationally predisposed Panic Attack. **Note:** In children, the anxiety may be expressed by crying, tantrums, freezing, or shrinking from social situations with unfamiliar people.

C. The person recognizes that the fear is excessive or unreasonable. **Note:** In children, this feature may be absent.

D. The feared social or performance situations are avoided or else are endured with intense anxiety or distress.

E. The avoidance, anxious anticipation, or distress in the feared social or performance situation(s) interferes significantly with the person's normal routine, occupational (academic) functioning, or social activities or relationships, or there is marked distress about having the phobia.

F. In individuals under age 18 years, the duration is at least 6 months.

G. The fear or avoidance is not due to the direct physiological effects of a substance (e.g., a drug of abuse, a medication) or a general medical condition and is not better accounted for by another mental disorder (e.g., Panic Disorder With or Without Agoraphobia, Separation Anxiety Disorder, Body Dysmorphic Disorder, a Pervasive Developmental Disorder, or Schizoid Personality Disorder).

H. If a general medical condition or another mental disorder is present, the fear in Criterion A is unrelated to it, e.g., the fear is not of Stuttering, trembling in Parkinson's disease, or exhibiting abnormal eating behavior in Anorexia Nervosa or Bulimia Nervosa.

Specify if:

Generalized: if the fears include most social situations (also consider the additional diagnosis of Avoidant Personality Disorder).

Note. From the *Diagnostic and Statistical Manual of Mental Disorders* (4th ed., pp. 416–417), by the American Psychiatric Association, 1994, Washington, DC: Author. Copyright 1994 by the American Psychiatric Association. Reprinted by permission.

Social Phobia and Shyness: Same or Different?

Beyond the formalities of diagnostic criteria, social phobia is similar to states that are much more familiar to everyday people and to other conditions that have themselves been the focus of considerable research. These include social anxiety, social-evaluative anxiety, heterosocial anxiety, heterosexual anxiety, interpersonal anxiety, embarrassability, dating anxiety, communication apprehension, public speaking anxiety, speech anxiety, stage fright, performance anxiety, audience anxiety, and, most notably, shyness (Leary, 1983b; Rapee, 1995). These conditions have often been the focus of the attention of social and personality psychologists, whereas social phobia has generally been the province of clinicians. Are these different names for the same thing, or do they represent different conditions? We consider this question in the context of social phobia and shyness.

Theorists such as Rapee (1995) and Leary (1983b) suggest that differences between social phobia and shyness are quantitative rather than qualitative. To them, social phobia is a more severe version of the social discomfort of shyness. If social phobia and shyness are, in fact, different variations on a theme, we may learn a lot about social phobia by getting to know more about persons who call themselves shy.

In early research on this topic, two groups of researchers compared persons with DSM-III-defined social phobia with shy college students in order to see how they might differ. S. Turner, Beidel, and Larkin (1986b) examined the physiological and cognitive responses of clients with social phobia and shy and nonshy college students after they had participated in three behavioral tests (conversation with a same-sex stranger, conversation with an opposite-sex stranger, brief impromptu speech). Although the individuals with social phobia and the shy students were routinely more anxious than the nonshy students, they differed minimally from each other. Nyman and Heimberg (1985) compared the responses of persons with DSM-III social phobia with those of age- and gender-matched normal controls, shy college students, and nonshy students to a series of questionnaires, visualizations of social interactions, and a social interaction role-play test. Individuals with social phobia and shy students routinely appeared more anxious than participants in either comparison group, and their behavior and thought processes were significantly more disrupted. On a number of measures, however, individuals with social phobia appeared more anxious and impaired than the shy students.

S. Turner, Beidel, and Townsley (1990), after a review of the literature, compared social phobia and shyness on six dimensions: somatic features, cognitive characteristics, behavioral responses, daily functioning, clinical course, and circumstances surrounding onset. Although there were many similarities, they concluded that social phobia and shyness differ on the latter four of these dimensions. Compared with shy persons, persons with social phobia engage in more extensive avoidance behavior, experience more profound impairment in daily functioning, are more likely to suffer on a chronic basis, and are more likely to report a conditioning event as the trigger for their anxiety. The question of differences in onset requires further research attention. Differences in avoidance, impairment, and chronicity may be a consequence of more severe symptoms experienced by persons with social phobia. These differences, as well as the findings of S. Turner et al. (1986b) and Nyman and Heimberg (1985), are consistent with the notion of a continuum of social anxiety ranging from mild and fleeting social discomfort to shyness to social phobia (Rapee, 1995).[1]

How Common Is Social Phobia?

Like the answer to What is social phobia? the answer to this question can be elusive, and the examination of the data on the prevalence of social phobia can be an exercise in confusion. There appear to be at least four reasons for this state of affairs.

First, prevalence—the percentage of cases of a disorder that appear in the population during a given time interval—must be a function of how the disorder is defined, and the definition of social phobia changed rather dramatically from DSM-III to DSM-III-R and DSM-IV. The inclusion of patients with generalized social fears in DSM-III-R and DSM-IV definitions of social phobia should serve to make it much more common than DSM-III-defined social phobia, as these patients should not have received a diagnosis of social phobia using DSM-III criteria. Most studies of subtypes of social phobia in clinical samples suggest that generalized social phobia is more common than the discrete situational fears described in DSM-III (see Heimberg, Holt, Schneier, Spitzer, & Liebowitz, 1993). However, as many as two-thirds of persons in the community who have social phobia may have the nongeneralized form of the disorder (Wittchen, Stein, & Kessler, 1999; but see Kessler, Stein, & Berglund, 1998).

Second, prevalence rates can be reported for virtually any time frame but are most commonly reported for 1 month, 6 months, 12 months, or a lifetime. All things being equal, the longer the time interval, the higher the prevalence estimate. Different investigators have reported prevalence rates for different time frames, making it difficult to compare findings across studies.

Third, studies vary rather dramatically in the number of social or performance situations probed. Prevalence rates will appear higher if the interviewer asks the person about fear in a greater number of situations (Stein, Walker, & Forde, 1994). Furthermore, prevalence rates will differ between studies if the specific situations probed in each study are not similar in relevance to social phobia or in their anxiety-evoking potential.

Fourth, the various studies that have addressed the prevalence of social phobia have not been entirely faithful to the diagnostic criteria for social phobia that were current at the time. The differences among studies in reported prevalence rates for the broad range of mental disorders and their potential implications for health care policy and research have been recently debated (Frances, 1998; Regier et al., 1998; Spitzer, 1998).

In the following sections, we first describe studies of the prevalence of DSM-III social phobia, followed by studies of the prevalence of DSM-III-R and DSM-IV social phobia. In each case, we describe the major studies, their prevalence time frames, the situations they probed, and the ways in which their definition of social phobia differed from that in DSM.

PREVALENCE OF DSM-III SOCIAL PHOBIA IN THE COMMUNITY

The Epidemiologic Catchment Area Study. The first, and still the largest, study of the prevalence of mental disorders in the community was the Epidemiologic Catchment Area (ECA) Study conducted by the National Institute of Mental Health during the early 1980s. This massive study was conducted in five major sites around the United States (New Haven, Connecticut; Baltimore, Maryland; St. Louis, Missouri; Durham, North Carolina; Los Angeles, California). The details of methodology have been described in several papers, including Eaton et al. (1984), Eaton and Kessler (1985), and Regier et al. (1984). Lay interviewers administered the Diagnostic Interview Schedule (DIS; Robins, Helzer, Croughan, & Ratcliff, 1981) to a total of 18,572 persons across the five sites, and many of these individuals were interviewed again 1 year later. However, the version of the DIS employed in New Haven did not include the items necessary for the diagnosis of social phobia (see the following), eliminating New Haven participants from current consideration, for a total sample from the four remaining sites of 13,537.

The DIS provides the data necessary for the determination of DSM-III diagnoses. It is suitable for administration by nonclinicians because it is highly structured and clinician judgment is not required for diagnosis. However, as suggested in the earlier discussion, it is not entirely faithful to the DSM-III diagnosis of social phobia. First, it provides diagnoses without reference to DSM-III's system of hierarchical exclusionary rules. That is, DSM-III states that some diagnoses should not be given if one set of symptoms is better accounted for by another mental disorder, but the DIS may provide diagnoses without reference to these exclusions. Thus social phobia may be diagnosed in the presence of schizophrenia, affective disorders, or other disorders that were determined to preempt social phobia in DSM-III. Second, only three social situations are examined in the DIS interview: (1) eating in front of other people, either people one knows or in public, (2) speaking in front of a small group of people one knows, and (3) speaking to strangers or meeting new people. Reactions to the infinite number of other potentially feared social situations are not assessed. Third, the DIS differs from DSM-III in the definition of phobic response to these situations. Whereas DSM-III requires that there be significant distress as a result of the fear, whether or not it interferes with the person's life, the more conservative DIS requires that the fear cause much interference with life and activities. Walker and Stein (1995) suggest that the latter two factors should lead the DIS to seriously underestimate the prevalence of DSM-III social phobia. However, the decision to forego hierarchical exclusionary rules may bias the DIS toward overestimation, leaving matters a little less than clear.

ECA Prevalence of Social Phobia. Myers et al. (1984) reported the 6-month prevalence of selected psychiatric disorders based on first interviews administered in New Haven, Baltimore, and St. Louis. Six-month prevalence of social phobia (for Baltimore and St. Louis only) ranged from 1.2% to 2.2%. Several other investigators have also examined the ECA database and reported prevalence figures for social phobia (Bourdon et al., 1988; Davidson, Hughes, George, & Blazer, 1993; Schneier et al., 1992). By far, the most thorough report is that of Schneier et al. (1992). These researchers decided to reclassify individuals who received diagnoses of both social phobia and schizophrenia ($n = 40$) into the group of participants who had a DIS/DSM-III disorder *but who did not have social phobia*. They reasoned, quite justifiably, that "the pervasive quality of schizophrenia and its associated social deficits could obscure the clinical relevance of comorbid social phobia and detract from reliability and validity of the social phobia diagnosis" (p. 283). This decision reduced the number of social phobic participants by about 10% but actually increased the similarity of the DIS social phobia diagnosis to that in DSM-III. In their analysis, which included the complete data from the four sites that examined social phobia, 361 of 13,537 individuals were determined to have had social phobia at some time in their lives, a lifetime prevalence rate of 2.4%.

Other Studies Using the DIS. Several other studies have examined the prevalence of social phobia and other psychiatric disorders using the DIS. Lifetime prevalence rates in Puerto Rico (1.6%; Canino et al., 1987), Edmonton, Canada (1.7%; Bland, Orn, & Newman, 1988), Christchurch, New Zealand (3.0%; J. Wells, Bushnell, Hornblow, Joyce, & Oakley-Browne, 1989), Iceland (3.5%; Stefánsson, Líndal, Björnsson, & Guðmundsdóttir, 1991), and a community outside of Paris, France (4.1%; Lépine & Lellouch, 1995) fell roughly in the range defined by the four ECA study sites (1.8%–3.2%; Schneier et al., 1992). However, prevalence rates reported for Seoul, Korea (0.5%; Lee et al., 1990a), for rural settings in Korea (0.7%; Lee et al., 1990b), and for Taipei and small town and rural settings in Taiwan (0.4%–0.6%; Hwu, Yeh, & Chang, 1989) were considerably lower. Walker and Stein (1995) and Chapman, Mannuzza, and Fyer (1995) both argue that the severe stigma associated with mental illness and the emphasis on privacy in these cultures may account for these low prevalence rates.

Studies Using Instruments Other Than the DIS. Faravelli, Guerrini Degl'Innocenti, and Giardinelli (1989) administered a structured interview based on the Schedule for Affective Disorders and Schizophrenia, Lifetime Version (Spitzer & Endicott, 1978), to more than 1,000 individuals registered with general practitioners in Florence, Italy. DSM-III hierarchical decision rules were strictly applied, and only one diagnosis was assigned per participant, making this study the most conservative examination of the prevalence of social phobia. Lifetime prevalence of social phobia was 1%.

Pollard and Henderson (1988) conducted a telephone survey of 500 residents of St. Louis. Their diagnostic interview was developed to address DSM-III criteria, but, as with the DIS, the match was less than perfect. Four situations relevant to social phobia were probed by Pollard and Henderson: (1) public speaking or performing, (2) writing in front of others, (3) eating in restaurants, and (4) using public rest rooms. A diagnosis of social phobia was assigned if the respondent reported becoming "very nervous" in one or more of the situations, attributed his or her discomfort to a fear of criticism or embarrassment, and stated that he or she avoided or would avoid the situation if at all possible. Respondents also had to agree that their fear caused them significant distress, as indicated in DSM-III. Accordingly, the authors reported that 2.0% of their sample met criteria for social phobia at the time of the interview (prevalence assessed at the time of the interview is referred to as "point prevalence"). If the significant-distress criterion was not applied, 22.6% of the sample endorsed significant social fears. Although the majority of these individuals did not meet DSM-III criteria for social phobia, it is noteworthy that fears of these situations (mostly of public speaking or performing) were so common in a community sample.

Summary of DSM-III Prevalence Studies. Fourteen studies of the prevalence of DSM-III social phobia have been reviewed. Lifetime prevalence was reported in 12 of these studies, with a range of 0.5% to 4.1% (summarized in Table 1.2). It is interesting to note that the five studies reporting the lowest lifetime prevalence were all conducted in non-English-speaking countries or territories and that the median prevalence in these five studies was only 0.7%. The median for studies conducted in English-speaking countries other than the United States was substantially higher (3.0%).

PREVALENCE OF DSM-III-R SOCIAL PHOBIA IN THE COMMUNITY

Much less work has been conducted on the prevalence of DSM-III-R social phobia. To date, only five studies have been reported (Kessler et al., 1994; Offord et al., 1996; Stein et al., 1994; Wacker, Müllejans, Klein, & Battegay, 1992; Weiller, Bisserbe, Boyer, Lépine, & Lecrubier, 1996).

Kessler et al. (1994), Offord et al. (1996), Wacker et al. (1992), and Weiller et al. (1996) employed the Composite International Diagnostic Interview (CIDI; Robins et al., 1988; World Health Organization, 1990) in their studies of the prevalence of psychiatric disorders. The CIDI, like its predecessor the DIS, is a highly structured diagnostic interview intended for use by lay interviewers. The CIDI social phobia section examines participants' responses to each of six social situations: (1) speaking in public, (2) using public rest rooms, (3) eating or drinking in public, (4) talking to people with concern that you might sound foolish or have nothing to say, (5) writing while being observed, and (6) participating in a meeting or class or going to a party.

Kessler et al.'s (1994) study, dubbed the National Comorbidity Survey, is the most ambitious undertaking of its kind since the ECA study (Walker & Stein,

TABLE 1.2. Lifetime Prevalence of DSM-III Social Phobia in Several Studies

Authors	Location	Diagnostic interview	Sample size	Prevalence rate (%)
Bland et al. (1988)	Edmonton, Canada	DIS	3,258	1.7
Bourdon et al. (1988)	4 ECA sites	DIS	13,537	3.0
Canino et al. (1987)	Puerto Rico	DIS	1,513	1.6
Davidson et al. (1993)	Durham ECA site	DIS	3,801	3.8
Faravelli et al. (1989)	Florence, Italy	SADS-L	1,110	1.0
Hwu et al. (1989)	Taipei, Taiwan	DIS	5,005	0.6
	Small towns	DIS	3,004	0.5
	Rural villages	DIS	2,995	0.4
Lee et al. (1990a)	Seoul, Korea	DIS	3,134	0.5
Lee et al. (1990b)	Rural Korea	DIS	1,966	0.7
Lépine & Lellouch (1995)	Paris, France	DIS	1,787	4.1
Schneier et al. (1992)	4 ECA sites	DIS	13,537	2.4
Stefánsson et al. (1991)	Iceland	DIS	862	3.5
J. Wells et al. (1989)	Christchurch, New Zealand	DIS	1,498	3.0

Note. DIS, Diagnostic Interview Schedule; ECA, National Institute of Mental Health Epidemiologic Catchment Area Study; SADS-L, Schedule for Affective Disorders and Schizophrenia, Lifetime Version. Bourdon et al. (1988) reported prevalence rates separately for men and women. Prevalence rate for these authors was calculated from data provided in their paper. Schneier et al. (1992) excluded individuals with both social phobia and schizophrenia from their social phobia sample, but other authors did not.

1995). These investigators conducted CIDI interviews with 8,098 persons spread across the United States, ages 15–54, who were part of a national probability sample. In Kessler et al.'s (1994) report, 12-month and lifetime prevalences of 14 psychiatric disorders are presented (see data for anxiety and affective disorders in Table 1.3). DSM-III-R social phobia was determined to be very common. In fact, whether 12-month or lifetime figures were consulted, social phobia was the third most prevalent psychiatric disorder assessed in this study. The 12-month prevalence rate was 7.9%, surpassed only by major depressive episode and simple phobia. The lifetime rate was 13.3%, surpassed only by major depressive episode and alcohol dependence. Wacker et al. (1992) reported an even greater lifetime prevalence of social phobia (16.0%) in their sample of 470 residents of Basel, Switzerland. Weiller et al. (1996) reported that 14.4% of patients in primary care settings in Paris, France, met criteria for a lifetime diagnosis of DSM-III-R social phobia. These figures are substantially higher than those reported for DSM-III social pho-

TABLE 1.3. Lifetime and 12-Month Prevalence Rates for Social Phobia and Other DSM-III-R Anxiety and Affective Disorders in the National Comorbidity Survey

Disorder	Men		Women		Total	
	Lifetime	12-month	Lifetime	12-month	Lifetime	12 month
Social phobia	11.1	6.6	15.5	9.1	13.3	7.9
Other anxiety disorders						
Panic disorder	2.0	1.3	5.0	3.2	3.5	2.3
Agoraphobia without panic	3.5	1.7	7.0	3.8	5.3	2.8
Simple phobia	6.7	4.4	15.7	13.2	11.3	8.8
Generalized anxiety disorder	3.6	2.0	6.6	4.3	5.1	3.1
Any anxiety disorder	19.2	11.8	30.5	22.6	24.9	17.2
Affective disorders						
Major depressive episode	12.7	7.7	21.3	12.9	17.1	10.3
Manic episode	1.6	1.4	1.7	1.3	1.6	1.3
Dysthymia	4.8	2.1	8.0	3.0	6.4	2.5
Any affective disorder	14.7	8.5	23.9	14.1	19.3	11.3

Note. Numbers represent percentage of National Comorbidity Survey sample who met criteria for selected disorders. Adapted from "Lifetime and 12-Month Prevalence of DSM-III-R Psychiatric Disorders in the United States," by R. C. Kessler et al., 1994, *Archives of General Psychiatry, 51*, p. 12. Copyright 1994 by the American Medical Association. Adapted by permission.

bia, probably a combined result of the increased breadth of social phobia in DSM-III-R and the increased depth of assessment of feared situations in the CIDI.

Stein et al. (1994), in a study that will be described in more detail subsequently, conducted a telephone survey of social anxiety among 526 residents of Winnepeg, Manitoba, Canada. Questions were designed to allow the estimation of the point prevalence of DSM-III-R social phobia, which was determined to be 7.1%, similar to the 12-month rate reported by Kessler et al. (1994). Offord et al. (1996) reported a 12-month prevalence rate of 6.7% among the 9,953 respondents interviewed with the CIDI as part of the Mental Health Supplement to the Ontario Health Survey. In this study, social phobia was the most prevalent of the 14 psychiatric disorders assessed.

PREVALENCE OF DSM-IV SOCIAL PHOBIA IN THE COMMUNITY

The prevalence of DSM-IV social phobia was examined in the Early Developmental Stages of Psychopathology (EDSP) study (Wittchen et al., 1999). As part of this study, a DSM-IV version of the CIDI was administered to a community sample of 3,021 adolescents and young adults (ages 14–24) in metropolitan Munich, Germany. The 12-month prevalence rate for social phobia was 5.2%; the lifetime prevalence rate was 7.3%. Although these rates are substantial, they are lower than those reported in the studies of DSM-III-R social phobia. The authors suggest that this may be the case because they employed stricter criteria for the assessment of impairment and distress and a more refined approach to the assessment of anxiety symptoms. It is also possible that these rates are somewhat lower because a smaller percentage of the total sample was old enough at the time to have survived the period of risk.

GENDER DIFFERENCES IN THE PREVALENCE OF SOCIAL PHOBIA

Most of the studies reviewed previously also examined differences in the prevalence of social phobia between men and women. In the initial report of the ECA study by Myers et al. (1984), 6-month prevalence rates for men were 0.9%–1.7%, whereas rates for women were 1.5%–2.6%. However, the significance of this difference was not reported. In the report of the ECA study by Schneier et al. (1992), lifetime prevalence of DSM-III social phobia was significantly higher for women (3.1%) than for men (2.0%). However, in an earlier analysis of these same data, but one that did not reclassify persons with both social phobia and schizophrenia as did Schneier et al. (1992), the difference in prevalence between men (2.3%) and women (3.2%) was not significant (Bourdon et al., 1988). Davidson et al. (1993) reported that lifetime social phobia was significantly more common among women but did not provide gender-specific prevalence rates. In the three ECA studies of lifetime prevalence of DSM-III social phobia, between 61% and 70% of individuals with social phobia were female. In other studies, the findings for gender differences in prevalence of DSM-III social phobia were mixed. In both urban and rural samples in Korea (Lee et al., 1990a) and in the French sample (Lépine & Lellouch, 1995), the prevalence rate for women was higher than for men. This was also the case in metropolitan Taipei, but not in the small towns and rural villages of Taiwan (Hwu et al., 1989). There were no significant gender differences in prevalence reported in either Puerto Rico (Canino et al., 1987), Iceland (Stefánsson et al., 1991), or Edmonton (Bland et al., 1988).

Gender differences in prevalence were also noted by Kessler et al. (1994) in their study of DSM-III-R social phobia. Twelve-month and lifetime rates for women (9.1% and 15.5%, respectively) were greater than the same rates for men (6.6% and 11.1%, respectively). In the Ontario Health Survey (Offord et al., 1996), the 12-month prevalence rates for women and men were 7.9% and 5.4%, respectively. However, Weiller et al. (1996) found no difference in lifetime prevalence for men (14.6%) and women (14.2%) in primary care settings. Gender differences in prevalence were also noted in the EDSP study of DSM-IV social phobia. Lifetime prevalence was 9.5% for women, compared with only 4.9% for men. Twelve-month rates were 7.2% for women and 3.2% for men.

Although not entirely uniform, these data suggest that social phobia in the community is more common among women than men. However, this does not appear to be the case in samples of individuals awaiting treatment for social phobia. For instance, Marks (1970) reported that 50% of treatment-seeking persons with social phobia were male, whereas only 25% of agoraphobics and 5% of persons with animal phobias were male. In another series of 199 patients referred for behavioral treatment (Solyom, Ledwidge, & Solyom, 1986), roughly half (47%) of the persons with social phobia were male, whereas the large majority of agoraphobics (86%) and simple phobics (78%) were female. Similarly, Heimberg (1989) reported that 47% of participants in studies of the cognitive-behavioral treatment of social phobia were male, although much variability existed from study to study. Reasons for the difference in gender distribution of social phobia in the community versus the clinic are not entirely clear. However, it has been speculated that social phobia may be more likely to interfere with instrumental role functioning in men than in women, thus leading men to seek treatment for social phobia with increased frequency (Turk et al., 1998).

COHORT DIFFERENCES IN THE PREVALENCE OF SOCIAL PHOBIA

Several reports have examined differences across birth cohorts in the prevalence of social phobia in the National Comorbidity Survey (Magee, Eaton, Wittchen, McGonagle, & Kessler, 1996), the Ontario Health Survey (Offord et al., 1996), the ECA study (Schneier et al., 1992), and the French study of Lépine and Lellouch (1995). Regardless of differences in diagnostic criteria, structured interviews, or cultures, the findings are quite robust. Prevalence rates were higher in the youngest cohorts. For example, in the Ontario Health Survey, the 12-month prevalence of DSM-III-R social phobia among women ages 15–24 was 12.7%, compared with 7.1% for women ages 25–44 and 5.9% for women ages 45–64. Among men, these figures were 8.2%, 6.1%, and 2.3%, respectively. In the National Comorbidity Survey, the lifetime prevalence of social phobia in the 15–24 age group was 14.9%, declining to 12.2% among respondents ages 45–54 (Magee et al., 1996). Curiously, cohort effects were evident only in the subgroup of social phobics with ages at onset of 16 or greater. As has been noted for major depressive disorder (Wickramaratne, Weissman, Leaf, & Holford, 1989), the prevalence of social phobia appears to be on the rise. In a recent reanalysis of data from the National Comorbidity Survey, we showed that this increase was entirely accounted for by persons with social phobia who feared social situations above and beyond those that require public speaking (Heimberg, Stein, Hiripi, & Kessler, 2000).

Feared Situations

SITUATIONS FEARED BY PERSONS IN THE COMMUNITY

Two studies have examined the prevalence of fears of specific social situations in the community at large (Pollard & Henderson, 1988; Stein et al., 1994). Pollard and Henderson reported that 22.6% of their telephone survey sample endorsed significant fear in at least one of the four situations assessed. Specifically, 20.6% reported fears of public speaking or performing, 2.8% fears of writing in public, 1.2% fears of eating in restaurants, and 0.2% fears of using public rest rooms.

Stein et al. (1994) examined the reactions of their 526 respondents to seven social situations. They selected situations so as to include all situations assessed by Pollard and Henderson (1988)—except for use of public rest rooms, which was deemed too rare—and all situations examined in the ECA studies. In addition, the situations "attending social gatherings" and "dealing with people in authority" were queried. Respondents were asked to indicate if they were "much more nervous than other people," "somewhat more nervous than other people," or "about the same as other people" in these situations. Sixty-one percent of respondents reported being either much more or somewhat more nervous than other people in at least one of the seven situations. Public speaking was, by far, the most feared situation, resulting in responses of "much more" or "somewhat more" nervousness than other people in 55% of respondents, and it was also most likely to be selected as the situation that made respondents most uncomfortable or nervous (80.5%). Excluding public speaking, however, 45.2% of respondents still reported that they were either much more or somewhat more nervous than other people in at least one social situation. Women were significantly more likely than men to report that they were either much more or somewhat more nervous than other people in at least one situation, but many respondents also reported fears in multiple situations. Of those individuals reporting social fears, 31.4% reported fear of a single situation, 28.9% reported fears of two situations, 21.4% fears of three situations, 9.6% fears of four situations, and 8.7% fears of five or more situations.

SITUATIONS FEARED BY PERSONS WITH SOCIAL PHOBIA

Several studies have examined the nature of the situations that cause anxiety among people with social phobia. The earliest of these studies (Amies, Gelder, & Shaw, 1983) compared the responses of 87 social phobics and 57 agoraphobics to a fear survey schedule. Interestingly, social phobics reported greater fear in the following situations: (1) being introduced, (2) meeting people in authority, (3) using the telephone, (4) having visitors come to one's home, (5) being watched doing something, (6) being teased, (7) eating at home with acquaintances, (8) eating at home with family, (9) writing in front of others, and (10) speaking in public.

Agoraphobics reported greater fear than social phobics in the following situations: (1) being alone, (2) being in unfamiliar places, (3) crossing streets, (4) using public transportation, (5) going into department stores, (6) being in crowds, (7) being in open spaces, and (8) being in small shops. Of course, it is these very types of differences that lead to the diagnosis of social phobia versus agoraphobia.

S. Turner et al. (1986a) also examined the types of situations feared by a sample of 21 DSM-III social phobics and reported that the overwhelming majority of individuals feared and/or avoided speaking in front of others, in both formal and informal circumstances. S. Turner et al. (1986a) also reported that their social phobic participants generally reported avoidance and/or distress in more than one situation. Only 9.5% of their participants reported distress in a single situation, whereas 42.9% reported distress in two situations, 38.9% reported distress in three situations, and 9.5% reported distress in four situations.

Schneier et al. (1992) examined the specific situations feared by DSM-III social phobics identified in the ECA study. Keep in mind that the DIS addressed only three social situations. Fear of speaking in front of a small group of familiar people was endorsed by 57.1% of participants with social phobia, whereas speaking to strangers or meeting new people was endorsed by 42.1%, and eating in front of other people was endorsed by 24.7%. In contrast to the findings of S. Turner et al. (1986a), presented previously, the large majority of social phobics (79.5%) reported fear in only one of the three situations, 17.2% of the sample reported fear in two of the situations, and 3.3% reported fear in all three DIS situations. It is interesting to speculate whether the difference in the findings of S. Turner et al. (1986a) and Schneier et al. (1992) represents variation in the number of situations assessed or whether it might be a function of differences between persons with social phobia in the community (most of whom have not sought out treatment) and clients with social phobia in the treatment clinic. In fact, it may be this very issue, the larger number of situations feared and the potentially larger interference as a result, that separates the person with social phobia who seeks treatment from the one who does not.

Holt et al. (1992b) examined responses of 91 DSM-III social phobics to the 24-item Liebowitz Social Anxiety Scale (Liebowitz, 1987). However, rather than examining clients' fears in specific situations, as is typical of this type of research, Holt et al. (1992b) assessed clients' fears in classes of related situations that they labeled "situational domains." Each domain was represented by four to five situations from the clinician-administered Liebowitz Social Anxiety Scale, and the client had to endorse at least moderate fear in all or all but one situation in a domain to be judged as anxious in that domain. Four situational domains were identified: (1) formal speaking and interaction (e.g., giving a report to a group or speaking up at a meeting), (2) informal speaking and interaction (e.g., meeting strangers or going to a party), (3) assertive interaction (e.g., expressing disagreement or disapproval to people one does not know very well or talking to people in authority), and (4) observation of behavior by others (working, writing, eating, drinking in public or while being observed). Formal speaking and interaction produced the most frequent anxiety, with 70.3% of clients classified as anxious in that domain. Significant anxiety was also reported in the informal speaking and interaction domain by 46.2% of clients, in the assertive interaction domain by 30%, and in the observation of behavior by others domain by 22%. When anxiety was reported in only a single domain, it was most likely to be formal speaking and interaction (73.6% of the time), and when anxiety was present in multiple domains, formal speaking and interaction was highly likely to be one of them (94.3% of the time). Fifty-eight percent of clients were anxious in more than one domain.

SITUATIONS FEARED BY MEN VERSUS WOMEN WITH SOCIAL PHOBIA

As discussed previously, there may be differences in the frequency with which men and women experience social phobia and in the likelihood that they will seek out treatment. However, it is also important to know whether or not men and women with social phobia differ in other ways. Turk et al. (1998) assessed 108 men and 104 women who sought treatment for social phobia. The gender groups were similar on duration of social fear, previous treatment history, and the presence or absence of comorbid anxiety or affective disorders. Women did score higher on one questionnaire measure of social phobia and anxiety reported during a behavioral test, but the genders did not differ on four other questionnaire measures. Thus it seems fair to say that the difference between the men and the women in the severity of their social phobia was not large. However, there were differences between men and women in their reports of anxiety in specific situations. In response to the Liebowitz Social Anxiety Scale, women reported greater anxiety than men in the following situations: talking to authority; acting, performing, or giving a talk in front of an audience; working while being observed; being the center of attention; speaking up at a meeting; giving a report to a group; giving a party; entering a room after others were seated; and expressing disagreement or disapproval to people they do not know very well. Men reported greater anxiety than women urinating in public rest rooms and returning goods to a store.

The Etiology of Social Phobia

What are the causes of social phobia? This question has been addressed by researchers from two perspectives: First, is social phobia inherited? Second, does the environment in which a child is brought up contribute to the development of social phobia, and, if so, what is the nature of this contribution?

Genetic Contributions

In the first published study of the heritability of social phobia, Reich and Yates (1988) interviewed 17 clients with DSM-III social phobia, 88 clients with panic disorder, and 10 normal controls about the occurrence of various psychiatric disorders in their relatives. Although the percentages were small, individuals with social phobia identified significantly more relatives with social phobia (6.6%) than did the clients with panic disorder (0.4%). There was also a trend for individuals with social phobia to report more relatives with social phobia than did individuals in the normal group. The failure to find a significant difference between participants with social phobia and normal controls may have been an artifact of the small size of the normal sample, as only one relative of a normal participant was reported to have social phobia.

Fyer, Mannuzza, Chapman, Liebowitz, and Klein (1993) examined the occurrence of social phobia in first-degree relatives of clients and nonclinical controls by administering a structured diagnostic interview to the relatives themselves. This procedure is much superior to that of Reich and Yates (1988), who administered a structured interview to clients that inquired about their relatives. Eighty-three relatives of thirty clients who met criteria for DSM-III-R social phobia but no other anxiety disorder and 231 relatives of 77 not-ill controls were interviewed. In fact, there was a threefold increased risk of social phobia among clients' relatives (16%) compared with those of control participants (5%). However, there was no increased risk for any of the other anxiety disorders among relatives of clients with social phobia. Thus there appears to be a familial contribution to the development of at least some cases of social phobia. Furthermore, this contribution appears to be specific to social phobia and not a general propensity to development of anxiety. Fyer, Mannuzza, Chapman, Martin, and Klein (1995) examined the rates of social phobia, simple phobia, and panic disorder with agoraphobia in first-degree relatives of probands with each of these disorders and normal controls. Whereas the rate of social phobia was elevated in the relatives of social phobia probands, this was not the case for relatives of probands with simple phobia or panic disorder with agoraphobia (see also Fyer et al., 1996).

Mannuzza et al. (1995) conducted a further family study in which they focused on differential risk for social phobia among first-degree relatives of clients with generalized versus nongeneralized social phobia, compared with the relatives of the same group of not-ill controls employed by Fyer et al. (1993). Whether their analyses focused on the number of relatives with social phobia or the number of families in which at least one relative had social phobia, the results were the same. The relatives of clients with generalized social phobia (16% of relatives; 36% of families) were significantly more likely to have social phobia than either the relatives of clients with nongeneralized social phobia (6% of relatives; 13% of families) or not-ill controls (6% of relatives; 19% of families).

These data suggest that the earlier report by Fyer et al. (1993) might be accounted for by the probable high percentage of individuals with generalized social phobia in their sample.

Stein et al. (1998) conducted a direct-interview family study of 106 first-degree relatives of 23 probands with generalized social phobia and 74 first-degree relatives of 24 comparison participants without social phobia. There were no differences in the frequency of discrete or nongeneralized forms of social phobia. However, relatives of probands with generalized social phobia were 10 times more likely (26.4%) to meet criteria for generalized social phobia than were the relatives of control probands (2.7%). Similarly, 19.8% of relatives of generalized social phobics, but no relatives of control probands, met criteria for APD. These data are summarized in Figure 1.1.

These studies certainly suggest that social phobia has a familial component. However, they cannot determine whether this component has genetic or environmental roots. Studies comparing identical (monozygotic) and fraternal (dizygotic) twins are necessary for that purpose. Three studies (K. Phillips, Fulker, & Rose, 1987; Rose & Ditto, 1983; Torgersen, 1979) have examined the responses of monozygotic and dizygotic twins to fear survey schedules, and each has found some support for a genetic component in the self-report of social fears. However, only three studies of social phobia in twins have thus far been conducted (Andrews, Stewart, Allen, & Henderson, 1990; Kendler, Neale, Kessler, Heath, & Eaves, 1992; Torgersen, 1983). Neither Torgersen (1983) nor Andrews et al. (1990) found evidence of direct inheritance of social phobia or other anxiety disorders, although both studies did find some support for genetic transmission of a predisposition toward trait anxiousness. The Torgersen (1983) study was limited by the inclusion of only four social phobic probands, and although the total sample in Andrews et al. (1990) was a respectable 446, the number of probands with social phobia was still modest ($n = 33$). In the large-scale and carefully controlled study by Kendler et al. (1992), more than 2,000 female twins from the Virginia Twin Registry received structured diagnostic interviews, administered by clinicians uninformed regarding the diagnosis of the other twin. DSM-III social phobia was diagnosed in 11.5% of twins (a very high percentage for DSM-III social phobia). In fact, the concordance rate for social phobia was higher among monozygotic (24%) than dizogotic (15%) twins, suggesting that there is a degree of genetic transmission of social phobia. Further analyses suggested that 21% of the variance in liability to social phobia was due to genetic factors that are specific to social phobia and that an additional 10% of the variance was attributable to genetic factors common to all phobias. To put these numbers in perspective, 39% of the variance in liability to agoraphobia was accounted for by genetic factors. However, these figures are substantially lower than those reported in studies of bipolar disorder or schizophrenia, which have usually ranged from 60% to 90% (Kendler et al., 1992). Environmental factors were found to account for the remaining variance in liability to social phobia.

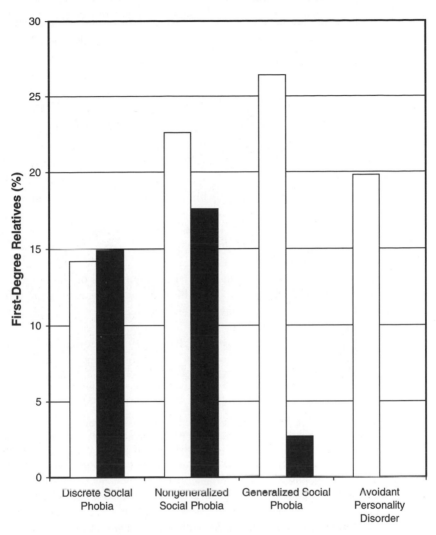

FIGURE 1.1. First-degree relatives of probands with and without social phobia or avoidant personality disorder who had social phobia or avoidant personality disorder. From "A Direct-Interview Family Study of Generalized Social Phobia," by M. B. Stein et al., 1998, *American Journal of Psychiatry, 155,* p. 93. Copyright 1998 by the American Psychiatric Association. Reprinted by permission.

Environmental Contributions

What might these environmental factors be? One area of considerable attention has been the child-rearing practices of parents of persons with social phobia. Do parents act in a way that may predispose the child to develop social phobia? Several studies (Arrindell, Emmelkamp, Monsma, & Brilman, 1983; Arrindell et al., 1989; Bruch & Heimberg, 1994; Bruch, Heimberg, Berger, & Collins, 1989; Leung, Heimberg, Holt, & Bruch, 1994; Lieb et al., 2000; Parker, 1979; Stravynski, Elie, & Franche, 1989; also see the review by Hudson & Rapee, 2000) suggest that this might, in fact, be the case. Keep in mind, however, that these studies almost universally suffer from the same flaw. They ask adult clients, many of whom have suffered with their emotional problems for several years and some of whom have received treatment in the interim, to recall their parents' behavior while they were growing up. Although some studies suggest that this type of material may be recalled with accuracy (Brewin, Andrews, & Gotlib, 1993; Gerlsma, Kramer, Scholing, & Emmelkamp, 1994) and others (Rapee & Melville, 1997) have reported substantial agreement between adults with social phobia and their mothers in terms of retrospective recall, the alternative explanations that clients' current state somehow influenced their recall of childhood experiences or that clients' childhood difficulties influenced (rather than were caused by) parents' child-rearing behavior cannot be ruled out without appropriately conducted longitudinal studies.

In the first of these retrospective studies, Parker (1979) theorized that a lack of parental affection combined with parents' tendency to be overly controlling or overprotective might predispose the child toward the development of social phobia:

> It would appear reasonable to suggest that a child exposed to parental characteristics of low care and overprotection, which inhibit the development of a satisfying parent-child bond, might subsequently experience greater difficulty in interpersonal situations and experience anxiety in social situations. Parental overprotection, by restricting the usual developmental process of independence, autonomy, and social competence, might further promote any diathesis to a social phobia. (Parker, 1979, p. 559)

In fact, Parker found some support for this hypothesis, as individuals with social phobia described their parents as less affectionate and more controlling in comparison with the parents of normal controls. Arrindell et al. (1983) similarly reported that individuals with social phobia described their parents as less emotionally warm, more rejecting, and more overprotective than did normal controls. In both these studies, clients with agoraphobia were included and differed less from controls than did the clients with social phobia. However, there was no direct comparison between clients with social phobia and those with agoraphobia. In a follow-up study by Arrindell et al. (1989), individuals with social phobia described their parents' behavior as significantly less affectionate and more rejecting when compared with descriptions of parents' behavior provided by individuals with agoraphobia.

In our laboratory, we have conducted a series of studies designed to test theoretical propositions (derived from the work of social psychologist Arnold Buss) about the child-rearing behavior of the parents of individuals with social phobia. Buss (1980, 1986) argued that sensitivity to social evaluation during childhood may be fostered by parental child-rearing attitudes and behavior that serve to isolate the child, that emphasize the importance of others' opinions regarding appropriate behavior, and that deemphasize family sociability (the involvement of the family unit in shared social activities with other families). Isolation from other children may prevent the child from engaging in situations through which peer social skills may be acquired and social fears extinguished, whereas low family sociability may have a similar impact on interactions with both adults and children. Excessive parental admonitions about the importance of others' opinions may sensitize the child to the negative aspects of attention from and scrutiny by others. Buss also hypothesized that socially anxious parents may contribute to the development of children's concerns about social evaluation both by modeling and by limiting interactions with other families in order to keep their own anxiety in check.

In our first study, Bruch et al. (1989) examined the responses of 21 clients with generalized social phobia and 22 clients with agoraphobia to a questionnaire designed to assess these concerns. Clients with social phobia described their mothers as more fearful and avoidant of social situations than did clients with agoraphobia. Furthermore, clients with social phobia described their parents as more likely to isolate them from normal social experiences, as more concerned about the opinions of others, and as placing less emphasis on socializing as a family unit in comparison with the parents of clients with agoraphobia.

Bruch and Heimberg (1994) extended this line of research in a comparison of 34 clients with generalized social phobia, 36 clients with nongeneralized social phobia, and 39 nonanxious controls. They also examined another parental behavior that might potentially be related to social-evaluative fears—the use of shame as a mode of discipline. Both groups of clients with social phobia described their parents as placing more emphasis on the opinions of others and as more likely to use shame tactics than did the nonanxious participants, but on these two dimensions, the generalized and nongeneralized groups did not differ from each other. Both groups of clients with social phobia also described their parents as less likely to emphasize family social activities than did nonanxious participants. However, clients with generalized social phobia described their parents as significantly more extreme on this dimension than did clients with nongeneralized social phobia. Individuals with generalized social phobia also described their parents as more likely to isolate them from other children than either those with nongeneralized social phobia or nonanxious controls. As in the study by Bruch et al. (1989), the mothers of individuals with social phobia were rated as more fearful and avoidant of social situations, but this was the case only for the mothers of clients with generalized social phobia. The mothers of clients with nongeneralized social phobia were no more fearful or avoidant than the mothers of nonanxious controls. Few participants reported anxiety in their fathers, suggesting that other aspects of paternal behavior should be further investigated.

Thus the study by Bruch and Heimberg (1994) revealed some interesting areas of similarity and difference between clients with generalized and nongeneralized social phobia. In areas representing the psychological influence of parents on children (emphasis on others' opinions, shame), there were no differences between subtypes. However, clients with generalized social phobia described their parents as less likely to place them in the company of other children or other families. They also described their mothers as more socially anxious and avoidant, suggesting that the mothers might have acted in this fashion as a means of controlling their own anxiety. It is tempting to speculate that what parents say to children may predispose them to social phobia and that what they prevent children from doing may contribute to the spread of fear across the range of social interaction.

We must qualify this speculation because of the results of the last study in this series. Our first two studies and all studies by other investigators employed either American or western European participants. Is it possible that the specific types of parental behavior associated with social anxiety might be more or less culture specific? Leung et al. (1994) addressed this question by administering Bruch and Heimberg's questionnaire to three groups of participants—people with social phobia who were of American descent, comparison participants of American descent, and comparison participants of Chinese American descent. People with social phobia who were of American descent and American comparison participants differed as expected, that is, those with social phobia described their parents as more isolating, more shaming, more concerned with others' opinions, and less likely to emphasize family social activities. However, we expected different responses from the Chinese American participants, whose culture emphasizes respect for age and authority, a strong social orientation, and the need for the maintenance of social harmony more than do Western cultures (see Leung et al., 1994, for a more thorough discussion). Chinese Americans described their parents as emphasizing others' opinions, using shame tactics, and isolating them from other children in a manner similar to that reported by the American group that had been diagnosed with social phobia. However, unlike the social phobia group, they described their parents as strongly emphasizing family sociability. Overall, the magnitude of the correlation between these parenting variables and participants' social anxiety was a great deal smaller for the Chinese American group. This study was a humbling lesson in our own ethnocentricity, and it suggests that the behavior of parents that may contribute to social anxiety in their children is the behavior that makes them aware of their differences from other children and of how well (or poorly) they fit in. Certainly, these behaviors may vary from culture to culture. Another caveat to these studies is that parenting behavior is complex and may itself have genetic components (Kendler, 1996) and that it may be at least partially responsive to, rather than a determinant of, the behavior of the child.

Various studies have also reported a link between the presence of psychopathology in parents and the development of social phobia in offspring (Davidson et al., 1993; Wittchen et al., 1999). Lieb et al. (2000) explored this issue in greater detail, using data that were collected from more than 1,000 community adolescents. As suggested by research reviewed earlier, children of parents with social phobia were significantly more likely to also have social phobia than were children whose parents did not have the disorder. Although the presence of social phobia in the parent was the best predictor of social phobia in the adolescent, other anxiety disorders, depressive disorders, and alcohol use disorders in parents were also associated with social phobia in their children.

Lieb et al. (2000) also reported that respondents with social phobia were more likely than those without to describe their parents as overprotective and rejecting. That these judgments were made by respondents who were still under the influence of their parents is significant, given the retrospective nature of all other studies on this topic. It is also interesting to note that the association between parental rejection and adolescents' social phobia was significantly greater when parents were affected by psychopathology of any kind.

Behavioral Inhibition

Social phobia appears to run in families. Genetics and environmental factors both appear to make meaningful contributions. In all probability, however, social phobia is not itself directly transmitted. More likely, the child inherits, learns, or otherwise develops a predisposition to experience social anxiety in the "right" set of circumstances; but what might this predisposition be? A likely candidate is known as "behavioral inhibition to the unfamiliar" (Rosenbaum, Biederman, Pollock, & Hirshfeld, 1994).

Behavioral inhibition is a temperament, "a response disposition characterized by early manifested traits enduring over time, having impact on later personality, and most likely having important heritable components" (Rosenbaum et al., 1994, p. 12). Jerome Kagan and his colleagues at the Harvard Infant Study Laboratory have studied two cohorts of children, identified at either 21 or 31 months of age, over the course of several years (Kagan, Resnick, & Snidman, 1988). These children were classified at entry into the study as either "behaviorally inhibited" (i.e., characterized by a tendency toward withdrawal when confronted with novel or unfamiliar settings, people, or objects) or "uninhibited" (i.e., characterized by approach toward novel stimuli or persons). Followed for more than a decade thus far, the majority of these children have retained their original classifications. By the time they were ready for school, behaviorally inhibited children were described as cautious, quiet, and introverted. They also showed more reactivity of the sympathetic nervous system and muscle tension in response to psychological stress than uninhibited children. Rosenbaum and his group pursued the notion that behavioral inhibition might present a potential diathesis for the development of anxiety disorders (Rosenbaum, Biederman, Hirshfeld, Bolduc, & Chaloff, 1991a).

Of the many studies conducted by this group, two seem most relevant to the current context. First, the rates of various forms of psychopathology among behaviorally inhibited and uninhibited children, as well as among nonpsychiatric pediatric clients who served as a normal control group, were examined (Biederman et al., 1990). Behaviorally inhibited children drawn from either clinical or nonclinical samples exhibited increased risk for the presence of overanxious disorder of childhood, phobic disorders, and multiple anxiety disorders, despite the fact that a number of these children had been classified as behaviorally inhibited several years earlier. Specific fears reported by the behaviorally inhibited children who met criteria for phobia included standing up and speaking in front of the class (55.5%), meeting strangers (44%), and being called on in class (33.3%), situations clearly of concern to persons with social phobia. This general pattern was still evident when the children were reassessed after another 3 years (Biederman et al., 1993).

Second, Rosenbaum et al. (1991b) hypothesized that, if behavioral inhibition is an anxiety diathesis, the parents of behaviorally inhibited children should show an increased rate of anxiety disorders compared with the parents of uninhibited or control-group children. In fact, the parents of inhibited children demonstrated increased risk for the diagnosis of multiple anxiety disorders, childhood anxiety disorder, and anxiety disorder continuing from childhood into adulthood. As adults, the parents had a significantly higher rate of social phobia, but not of simple phobia or panic disorder with agoraphobia, as demonstrated in Figure 1.2.

More recent research suggests a potentially strong relationship between behavioral inhibition and the later development of social phobia. C. Schwartz, Snidman, and Kagan (1999) administered a structured diagnostic interview to seventy-four 13-year-olds who had been classified as behaviorally inhibited or uninhibited 11 years earlier as part of Kagan's original studies. Sixty-one percent of the children previously classified as behaviorally inhibited met criteria for generalized social phobia, compared with only 27% of the children previously classified as uninhibited. In another study by these investigators (C. Schwartz, Snidman, & Kagan, 1996), the children previously classified as inhibited showed information processing biases similar to those demonstrated by adults with social phobia (see Chapter 4). Another recent study suggests that a history of behavioral inhibition may be specifically related to social anxiety in young adulthood (Mick & Telch, 1998). In that study, undergraduate students were classified into one of four groups on the basis of their responses to the Social Phobia and Anxiety Inventory (S. Turner, Beidel, Dancu, & Stanley, 1989a) and the Penn State Worry

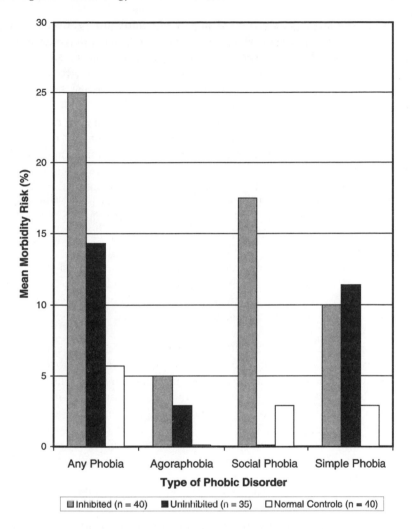

FIGURE 1.2. Morbidity risk of phobic disorders in parents of inhibited, uninhibited, and normal control children. Adapted from "The Etiology of Social Phobia," by J. F. Rosenbaum, J. Biederman, R. A. Pollock, and D. R. Hirshfeld, 1994, *Journal of Clinical Psychiatry, 55*(6, Suppl.), p. 14. Copyright 1994 by Physicians Postgraduate Press. Adapted by permission.

Questionnaire (Meyer, Miller, Metzger, & Borkovec, 1990). These four groups were characterized by high social anxiety, high generalized anxiety and worry, both, or neither. Participants also completed the Retrospective Self-Report of Inhibition (RSRI; Reznick, Hegeman, Kaufman, Woods, & Jacobs, 1992), a 30-item questionnaire assessing a broad range of childhood behaviors associated with behavioral inhibition. The two groups with high social anxiety reported greater inhibition than the generalized anxiety or control groups. Because the so-cial-anxiety group and the social-anxiety-plus-generalized-anxiety group did not differ from each other, it appears that these indices of behavioral inhibition in childhood were specifically related to current social, but not general, anxiety. In the EDSP study (Wittchen et al., 1999), high scores on the RSRI were most pre-dictive of a diagnosis of generalized social phobia. Clearly, further research is needed.

Note

1. Strictly speaking, the "continuum concept" is viable only when considering the simi-larities between shy persons and persons whose social phobias are characterized by generalized fears of social interaction. It is difficult to apply this notion to the person with social phobia who fears formal public speaking or working while being observed but who does not fear interactions in dyads or small groups.

2

Subtypes of Social Phobia, Comorbidity, and Impairment

Subtypes of Social Phobia

DSM-III-R expanded the breadth of social phobia as a diagnostic category by allowing persons with broadly based interpersonal anxiety to be classified as having the disorder. These individuals, who would have been assigned to the Axis II category of avoidant personality disorder in DSM-III, were further described as having the generalized subtype of social phobia. Since that time, a great deal of research has been devoted to the study of the possible differences between persons with generalized social phobia and other social phobias in terms of clinical course, presentation, and treatment response.

DSM III R defined generalized social phobia as the fear of most social situations. This definition was little more than a general guideline, as no further elaboration of the meaning of "most" or of "situations" was provided. DSM-IV goes only a bit further:

> **Generalized.** This specifier can be used when the fears are related to most social situations (e.g., initiating or maintaining conversations, participating in small groups, dating, speaking to authority figures, attending parties). Individuals with Social Phobia, Generalized, usually fear both public performance situations and social interactional situations. Because individuals with Social Phobia often do not spontaneously report the full range of their social fears, it is useful for the clinician to review a list of social and performance situations with the individual. . . . Individuals with Social Phobia, Generalized, may be more likely to manifest deficits in social skills and to have severe social and work impairment. (APA, 1994, pp. 412–413)

Individuals with social phobia who do not meet the criteria for the generalized subtype have been labeled "discrete," "limited," "circumscribed," and "specific" by different investigators. These labels suggest that this group of persons with social phobia fears a small number of very specific situations, such as public speaking or eating or drinking in public, but may otherwise function quite normally. This concept is, in fact, quite similar to the narrow definition of social phobia presented in DSM-III. It also implies that persons with social phobia can be completely and totally subdivided into two groups, one fearing only a limited number of situations and the other fearing most social situations. However, this dichotomy contradicts our clinical and research experience, in which we often see individuals with social phobia who fear a significant number of situations but who also report that there are important situations in which they are not fearful. These people seem to fall between the two groups and are exemplified by the man who is anxious in any interaction involving women but who is "OK" in social interactions in the work setting or involving only other men. As a result, Heimberg and Holt prepared a report for the group working on the diagnostic criteria for social phobia in DSM-IV in which they defined a third subtype, *nongeneralized social phobia* (see Heimberg et al., 1993). Individuals in this group (1) may or may not have fears in discrete performance situations, (2) experience clinically significant interpersonal anxiety, but (3) demonstrate at least one broad domain of social functioning in which they do not experience clinically meaningful anxiety. Several studies have shown important differences between persons with generalized and nongeneralized social phobia defined in this manner. However, the DSM-IV work group elected not to adopt a three-group subtyping for social phobia for lack of empirical data differentiating nongeneralized and more specific types of social phobia (Schneier et al., 1996, 1998). DSM-IV (APA, p. 413) states that "individuals whose clinical manifestations do not meet the definition of Generalized compose a heterogeneous group that includes persons who fear a single performance situation as well as those who fear several, but not most, social situations."

These controversies notwithstanding, several studies demonstrate differences between persons with generalized and nongeneralized/specific social phobia (E. Brown, Heimberg, & Juster, 1995; Gelernter, Stein, Tancer, & Uhde, 1992; Heimberg, Hope, Dodge, & Becker, 1990c; Herbert, Hope, & Bellack, 1992b; Holt, Heimberg, & Hope, 1992a; Levin et al., 1993; Mannuzza et al., 1995; Schneier, Spitzer, Gibbon, Fyer, & Liebowitz, 1991; Tran & Chambless, 1995; S. Turner, Beidel, & Townsley, 1992). See Heimberg et al. (1993) and Heimberg (1996) for detailed summaries of these studies. Here we review only a few studies that we believe to be representative of the larger group.

Heimberg et al. (1990c) reported a comparison of 35 clients with generalized social phobia and 22 clients with public-speaking phobias. Clients with generalized social phobia were younger, less educated, and less likely to be employed than public-speaking phobics. Clinical assessors rated their anxiety as more severe and as resulting in greater functional impairment. They appeared more anxious, more depressed and more concerned about negative social evaluation, and they endorsed more negative and fewer positive self-statements regarding social interaction.

In response to a behavioral test in which clients were asked to enact a situation that was highly anxiety-evoking for them, both clients with generalized social phobia and public-speaking phobics rated themselves as highly anxious and their performance as inadequate. However, observers rated clients with generalized social phobia as more anxious and as performing more poorly than public-speaking phobics. If the ratings of observers are compared with clients' own self-evaluations, an interesting pattern emerges. Observers appeared to agree with the negative judgments made by clients with generalized social phobia about their own performance. However, they disagreed with public-speaking phobics' extremely negative self-evaluations. If we think of the observers as representing consensual "reality," it appears that the public-speaking phobics were characterized by a greater tendency toward a negatively biased view of their performance, whereas the clients with generalized social phobia were characterized by more objectively poor performance.

Physiological responses during the behavioral test were also examined. Physiological arousal was defined as the degree of change in heart rate from baseline assessment during the behavioral test (i.e., heart rate reactivity). Although clients with generalized social phobia appeared more impaired on the other measures described previously, they showed less heart rate reactivity (4–5 beats per minute) in the first minute of the behavioral test than the public-speaking phobics (19–20 beats per minute). As can be seen in Figure 2.1, public-speaking phobics' surge of arousal decreased over time, but they did not return to baseline levels during the behavioral test.

Because the specifics of our behavioral test were individually determined for each client, differences in heart rate response could have been the result of differential task demands during the behavioral test (e.g., different amounts of physical effort required by different test situations). However, our finding for heart rate was substantially replicated by Levin et al. (1993), who examined heart rate responses of clients with generalized social phobia, public-speaking phobics, and normal controls when they were giving speeches. Although clients with generalized social phobia reported greater subjective anxiety, public-speaking phobics showed greater heart rate than either clients with generalized social phobia or normal controls during the speech. However, in this study, they also differed in resting heart rate measured before the speech task, suggesting that a key difference between subtypes may lie in the degree of anticipatory arousal.

One of the larger studies of subtypes of social phobia was conducted by E. Brown et al. (1995), who compared 38 clients with nongeneralized social phobia and 64 clients with generalized social phobia (28 of whom also received a diagnosis of APD; see the next section) on a broad range of questionnaire, interview,

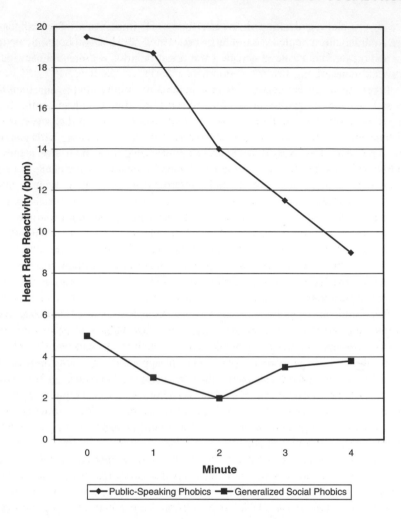

FIGURE 2.1. Heart rate reactivity of generalized social phobics and public-speaking phobics in response to the individualized behavioral test. From "DSM-III-R Subtypes of Social Phobia: Comparison of Generalized Social Phobics and Public Speaking Phobics," by R. G. Heimberg, D. A. Hope, C. S. Dodge, and R. E. Becker, 1990, *Journal of Nervous and Mental Disease, 178*, p. 176. Copyright 1990 by Lippincott Williams & Wilkins. Reprinted by permission.

and behavior test measures. Clients with generalized social phobia were rated as more anxious by clinical assessors on several measures, including the Hamilton (1959) Anxiety Scale, the Clinician's Severity Rating from the Anxiety Disorders Interview Schedule—Revised (DiNardo & Barlow, 1988), and several subscales of the Liebowitz Social Anxiety Scale (Liebowitz, 1987). They also achieved more extreme scores on several questionnaire measures of social anxiety and avoidance, including the Social Avoidance and Distress Scale and the Fear of Negative Evaluation Scale (Watson & Friend, 1969), the Social Phobia Scale and the Social Interaction Anxiety Scale (Mattick & Clarke, 1998), and the Social Phobia subscale of the Fear Questionnaire (Marks & Mathews, 1979). Clients with generalized social phobia were also judged to be more depressed than clients with nongeneralized social phobia, both in their own responses to the Beck Depression Inventory (A. T. Beck, Ward, Mendelson, Mock, & Erbaugh, 1961) and when they were rated by clinical assessors on the Hamilton (1960) Rating Scale for Depression. Although the other studies cited previously may agree or disagree with the findings of E. Brown et al. (1995) on specific measures, all support the pattern of greater severity and impairment among clients with generalized social phobia.

The available data do not yet answer the question of whether these subtypes represent truly different subcategories of social phobia or whether they simply represent differences in severity that might be viewed dimensionally rather than categorically (but consider the results of the studies of heart rate during behavior tests and see the family studies by Mannuzza et al., 1995, and Stein et al., 1998, reviewed in Chapter 1). However, the distinction between generalized and nongeneralized social phobia may have implications for treatment outcome. This question was addressed by E. Brown et al. (1995) and Hope, Herbert, and White (1995b), with both studies drawing similar conclusions. E. Brown et al. (1995) treated 40 clients with generalized social phobia and 23 clients with nongeneralized social phobia using cognitive-behavioral group therapy, or CBGT, the protocol we describe in Part II of this book. Across self-report, interview, and behavior test measures, the pattern was the same. Clients with generalized social phobia were more impaired before treatment began. Despite the fact that several of them made substantial gains, they remained more impaired as a group after treatment ended. Seventy-nine percent of clients with nongeneralized social phobia, compared with only 44% of clients with generalized social phobia, were determined to have improved to a clinically significant degree by the end of the 12-week treatment. Hope et al. (1995b) also reported this pattern. Clients with generalized social phobia were more impaired prior to treatment. Although they improved to a similar degree, they remained more impaired after treatment than clients with nongeneralized social phobia.[1]

Most studies of subtypes of social phobia have examined clinical samples, but a few studies have examined subtypes of social phobia in the community. Stein, Walker, and Forde (1996) conducted a telephone survey similar to their previous one (Stein et al., 1994). This time they focused on persons who endorsed public-speaking anxiety as their primary concern and reported that these individuals experienced substantial distress and impaired functioning despite the specific nature of their fears. Kessler et al. (1998) examined subtypes of social phobia in the National Comorbidity Survey. Latent class analysis identified two groups of persons with social phobia: those with public speaking fears only and those with at least one additional social fear. Approximately two-thirds of persons with lifetime social phobia fell into the latter category. Although the two groups did not differ in age at onset, the group with other social fears reported a longer time to offset (i.e., their social phobias either were still ongoing at interview or had lasted longer than those of the public-speaking phobic group before diminishing). This group also reported greater interference in functioning as a result of their fears, and their fears were strongly associated with lower income and education. It is among this more impaired group that the prevalence of social phobia appears to be increasing in younger cohorts (Heimberg et al., 2000). Finally, Wittchen et al. (1999) examined generalized and nongeneralized social phobia in the EDSP study. Persons with generalized social phobia reported an earlier age of onset, greater persistence of symptoms, more comorbid diagnoses, greater impairment, and more frequent seeking of mental health treatment. They were also more likely to report early separation from either parent and parental history of mental disorder.

Generalized Social Phobia and Avoidant Personality Disorder

No discussion of social phobia and its subtypes is complete without reference to the issue of the relationship between social phobia and avoidant personality disorder (APD), a theme reviewed by us (Heimberg, 1996; Heimberg et al., 1993) and by other authors as well (Johnson, Turner, Beidel, & Lydiard, 1995; Mattick & Newman, 1991). Recall that DSM-III limited social phobia to fears of specific social situations and assigned more diffuse interpersonal anxiety to APD. In DSM-III, APD was characterized (p. 323) by "hypersensitivity to potential rejection, humiliation, or shame; an unwillingness to enter into relationships unless given unusually strong guarantees of uncritical acceptance; social withdrawal in spite of a desire for affection and acceptance, and low self-esteem." Thus the focus of APD in DSM-III was on fear of personal relationships rather than fear of humiliation or embarrassment in specific social situations.

DSM-III-R added the generalized subtype to social phobia and removed the rule that social phobia could not be diagnosed in the presence of APD. Several changes were also made to the criteria for APD. The number of criteria for APD was increased from five to seven, but the number of criteria that had to be met in order to receive the diagnosis decreased from five to four. Thus it became easier (percentagewise) for the diagnosis of APD to be assigned. Furthermore, as the criteria for social phobia broadened to include fears of social interaction, the criteria for APD were redirected away from personal relationships and low self-esteem and toward discomfort and fear of negative evaluation in social interaction. It should be expected that DSM-III-R diagnoses of social phobia and APD should be assigned to the same person with some frequency, simply because the criteria for the two disorders are quite similar. This situation remains basically unchanged in DSM-IV. In fact, Hazen and Stein (1995) suggest that minor changes to the criteria for APD in DSM-IV may actually increase the overlap between the two disorders. DSM-IV criteria for APD are presented in Table 2.1.

Overlap between Generalized Social Phobia and Avoidant Personality Disorder

Several investigators have noted a high degree of overlap between social phobia and APD (Alnaes & Torgersen, 1988; Brooks, Baltazar, & Munjack, 1989; Sanderson, Wetzler, Beck, & Betz, 1994; S. Turner, Beidel, Borden, Stanley, & Jacob, 1991). However, this comparison seems most sensible when subtypes of social phobia are taken into account. Because generalized social phobia is defined as the fear of most social situations and APD is described as "a pervasive pattern of social discomfort, fear of negative evaluation, and timidity" (APA, 1987, p. 352), most of the overlap between social phobia and APD should involve the generalized subtype.

Six studies have examined the rate of diagnosis of APD in samples of clients with generalized and nongeneralized or specific social phobia and support the prediction of a greater association between APD and the generalized type (E. Brown et al., 1995; Herbert et al., 1992b; Holt et al., 1992a; Schneier et al., 1991; Tran & Chambless, 1995; S. Turner et al., 1992). Despite differences in sample characteristics, assessment methods, and definitions of subtypes of so-

TABLE 2.1. DSM-IV Diagnostic Criteria for Avoidant Personality Disorder (301.82)

A pervasive pattern of social inhibition, feelings of inadequacy, and hypersensitivity to negative evaluation, beginning by early adulthood and present in a variety of contexts, as indicated by four (or more) of the following:

1. avoids occupational activities that involve significant interpersonal contact, because of fears of criticism, disapproval, or rejection
2. is unwilling to get involved with people unless certain of being liked
3. shows restraint within intimate relationships because of the fear of being shamed or ridiculed
4. is preoccupied with being criticized or rejected in social settings
5. is inhibited in new interpersonal situations because of feelings of inadequacy
6. views self as socially inept, personally unappealing, or inferior to others
7. is unusually reluctant to take personal risks or to engage in any new activities because they might prove embarrassing.

Note. From the *Diagnostic and Statistical Manual of Mental Disorders* (4th ed., pp. 664–665), by the American Psychiatric Association, 1994, Washington, DC: Author. Copyright 1994 by the American Psychiatric Association. Reprinted by permission.

cial phobia (see Heimberg et al., 1993), all studies found a preponderance of APD among clients with generalized compared with nongeneralized social phobia (see Table 2.2). The frequency of APD among clients with generalized social phobia ranged from 25% to 89% (median = 52.5%), whereas the frequency of APD clients with nongeneralized social phobia ranged from 0% to 44% (median = 17.5%).

A study by Jansen, Arntz, Merckelbach, and Mersch (1994) examined the frequency of APD in 32 clients with social phobia (30 with the generalized type). This study also included another anxiety disorder group—85 clients with panic disorder—for purposes of comparison. Thirty-one percent of the clients with social phobia received a diagnosis of APD compared with 23.5% of the clients with panic disorder, a nonsignificant difference. Those with social phobia did, however, receive higher scores on avoidant personality features than did clients with panic disorder. This finding is difficult to interpret because the rate of APD in the social phobia sample was substantially below the median figure previously cited and because a higher-than-expected percentage of clients with social phobia were married. Nevertheless, APD was diagnosed with some frequency in anxious clients without social phobia, a phenomenon that has been reported by other investigators as well (Alnaes & Torgersen, 1988; Renneberg, Chambless, & Gracely, 1992).[2]

TABLE 2.2. Overview of Studies Examining the Overlap between Social Phobia and Avoidant Personality Disorder

Authors	Diagnosis of APD	N	Generalized APD	Generalized No APD	Nongeneralized[a] APD	Nongeneralized[a] No APD
Brown et al. (1995)	PDE	108	28(44)	36(56)	6(14)	38(86)
Herbert et al. (1992b)	SCID-II	23	10(71)	4(29)	4(44)	5(56)
Holt et al. (1992a)	PDE	33	10(50)	10(50)	3(23)	10(77)
Schneier et al. (1991)	SCID-II	50	32(89)	4(11)	3(21)	11(79)
Tran & Chambless (1995)	MCMI	46	16(55)	13(45)	1(6)	16(94)
Turner et al. (1992)	SCID-II	89	15(25)	46(75)	0(0)	28(100)

Note. APD, avoidant personality disorder; MCMI, Millon Clinical Multiaxial Inventory; PDE, Personality Disorders Examination; SCID-II, Structured Clinical Interview for DSM-III-R Personality Disorders. Numbers in parentheses are percentages of patients with generalized or nongeneralized social phobia with or without APD. Updated from "The Issue of Subtypes in the Diagnosis of Social Phobia," by R. G. Heimberg, C. S. Holt, F. R. Schneier, R. L. Spitzer, and M. R. Liebowitz, 1993, *Journal of Anxiety Disorders, 7*, p. 259. Copyright 1993 by Elsevier Science. Adapted by permission.

[a]The group to which generalized social phobics were compared varied from study to study. Examination of each study suggests that comparison-group participants experienced anxiety in social interactional situations (i.e., nongeneralized social phobia) with the exception of participants examined by Turner et al. (1992) and Tran and Chambless (1995) (i.e., circumscribed social phobia).

Diagnostic Criteria for Avoidant Personality Disorder

Three studies have examined the endorsement of the diagnostic criteria for APD among clients with generalized and nongeneralized social phobia. Schneier et al. (1991) reported that clients with generalized social phobia endorsed four of the seven APD criteria significantly more frequently than did clients with nongeneralized social phobia. However, the high rate of overlap between generalized social phobia and APD in that study (89%) makes this finding difficult to interpret. Holt et al. (1992a) and E. Brown et al. (1995) examined the endorsement of these criteria during structured interviews in samples of clients with nongeneralized social phobia and clients with generalized social phobia with and without APD. The findings of these two studies were very similar, so only the data from the larger E. Brown et al. (1995) study are reported here (see Table 2.3). Those with generalized social phobia and APD endorsed only three criteria significantly more frequently than did those with generalized social phobia without APD: Criterion 3 (unwilling to get involved with others unless certain of being liked), Criterion 4 (avoids social or occupational activities that involve significant interpersonal contact), and Criterion 6 (fears being embarrassed by blushing, crying, or showing signs of anxiety in front of others). Individuals with generalized social phobia and APD also endorsed Criterion 1 (easily hurt by criticism or disapproval), Criterion 5 (reticent in social situations), and Criterion 7 (exaggerates risks of activities outside usual routine) more frequently than individuals with nongeneralized social phobia, but they did not differ from individuals with generalized social phobia without APD.

Criteria 1, 2 (no close friends or confidants other than first-degree relatives), and 7 were endorsed by less than 11% of participants and thus have little relevance to the diagnosis of APD among clients with generalized social phobia. Criterion 5 was the most frequently endorsed, but it did not separate those with generalized social phobia with APD from those without APD. The remaining criteria (3, 4, and 6), although they did distinguish between these groups, were endorsed with decreasing frequency by clients with generalized social phobia with APD, clients with generalized social phobia without APD, and clients with nongeneralized social phobia. This pattern leaves open the possibility that differences in endorsement frequency are related to the severity of social phobia, with greater severity associated with a greater likelihood of endorsing the criteria for APD.

Clinical Presentation

Several of the studies cited herein also administered large assessment batteries to individuals with generalized social phobia both with and without APD. As discussed in the section on subtypes of social phobia, both generalized groups routinely exhibited greater anxiety and impairment than did a nongeneralized social

TABLE 2.3. DSM-III-R Criteria for APD Endorsed by Patients Grouped According to the Presence of APD and Subtype of Social Phobia

APD criteria	GSP/APD ($n = 28$)	GSP only ($n = 36$)	NSP ($n = 38$)
1. Is easily hurt by criticism or disapproval	6_a (21)	2_{ab} (6)	0_b (0)
2. Has no close friends or confidants (or only one) other than first-degree relatives	2 (7)	0 (0)	0 (0)
3. Is unwilling to get involved with people unless certain of being liked	18_a (64)	6_b (17)	5_b (13)
4. Avoids social or occupational activities that involve significant interpersonal contact	14_a (50)	6_b (17)	4_b (11)
5. Is reticent in social situations because of a fear of saying something inappropriate or foolish or of being unable to answer a question	22_a (79)	20_a (56)	10_b (26)
6. Fears being embarrassed by blushing, crying, or showing signs of anxiety in front of other people	14_a (50)	9_b (25)	8_b (21)
7. Exaggerates the potential difficulties, physical dangers, or risks involved in doing something ordinary but outside his or her usual routine	7_a (25)	3_{ab} (8)	1_b (3)

Note. APD, avoidant personality disorder; GSP, generalized social phobia; NSP, nongeneralized social phobia. Frequencies with different subscripts are significantly different ($p < .05$) according to Fisher's exact test. Numbers in parentheses are percentages of participants in each group. From "Social Phobia Subtype and Avoidant Personality Disorder: Effect on Severity of Social Phobia, Impairment, and Outcome of Cognitive-Behavioral Treatment," by E. J. Brown, R. G. Heimberg, and H. R. Juster, 1995, *Behavior Therapy, 26,* p. 479. Copyright 1995 by the Association for Advancement of Behavior Therapy. Reprinted by permission.

phobia group. However, the differences between clients with generalized social phobia with and without APD have been considerably less notable than the similarities, and inconsistent findings across studies have been the rule.

Scores on questionnaire measures of social anxiety and avoidance among individuals with generalized social phobia have been higher for those with APD than for those without APD (Herbert et al., 1992b), higher on only one of several measures (Holt et al., 1992a; S. Turner et al., 1992), or not at all different (E. Brown et al., 1995; Tran & Chambless, 1995). Similarly, three studies (Herbert et al., 1992b; Feske, Perry, Chambless, Renneberg, & Goldstein, 1996; Tran & Chambless, 1995) reported greater self-rated depression among those with both generalized social phobia and APD, but this finding was not replicated by three others (E. Brown et al., 1995; Holt et al., 1992a; S. Turner et al., 1992). Individuals with both generalized social phobia and APD have scored higher on measures of interpersonal sensitivity and lower on measures of social adjustment than those with social phobia but without APD (Feske et al., 1996; Herbert et al., 1992b; S. Turner et al., 1992).

Several measures completed by clinical assessors have suggested greater severity of symptoms and impairment among individuals with both generalized social phobia and APD. Although neither S. Turner et al. (1992) or E. Brown et al. (1995) reported differences between those with generalized social phobia with and without APD on the Hamilton (1959) Anxiety Scale, several other differences have been reported. These include differences on measures of global functioning (Herbert et al., 1992b; Tran & Chambless, 1995) and severity of social phobia (E. Brown et al., 1995; Holt et al., 1992a; S. Turner et al., 1992), as well as on subscales of the Liebowitz Social Anxiety Scale (E. Brown et al., 1995; Holt et al., 1992a). Although a number of differences occurred between clients with generalized social phobia with and without APD, these findings must be interpreted with caution because the clinical assessor also determined the diagnosis of APD in several of these studies.

Most of these studies also examined the anxiety and performance of participants during behavioral tests. Although Herbert et al. (1992b) reported that individuals having generalized social phobia with APD demonstrated greater anxiety during their behavioral test situations than those with generalized social phobia without APD, this finding was not replicated in four of the other studies. No study employing DSM-III-R criteria reported differences in the quality of behavior test performance. Cognitive assessment measures administered after behavioral tests have failed to distinguish between individuals who had generalized social phobia with or without APD (see also McNeil et al., 1995a).

Avoidant Personality Disorder and Response to Cognitive-Behavioral Treatment among Clients with Social Phobia

In a preliminary study, R. Turner (1987) reported that personality disorders (diagnosed on the basis of DSM-III criteria and responses to the Minnesota Multiphasic Personality Inventory) had a negative impact on the outcome of cognitive-behavioral treatment of social phobia. In more recent studies, Hope et al. (1995b), E. Brown et al. (1995), Lucas and Telch (1993), and Feske et al. (1996) examined the impact of APD on the outcome of cognitive-behavioral treatment of social phobia. With the exception of Feske et al. (1996), these studies used CBGT.

Although Lucas and Telch (1993) reported that APD was significantly and negatively associated with outcome in their study of CBGT, individually administered cognitive-behavioral treatment, and an educational-supportive control treatment, they did not include social phobia subtype in their prediction equation. Because clients with generalized social phobia are more likely to have APD than clients with nongeneralized social phobia, subtype differences in response to treatment may have accounted, at least in part, for their results. Feske et al. (1996) did report that individuals who had generalized social phobia with APD began treatment more impaired than individuals who had generalized social phobia without APD and remained that way, despite significant improvement, at posttest and 3-month follow-up assessments. Treatment in this study consisted of 32–42 hours of group exposure, relaxation training, systematic desensitization, and social skills training. Neither E. Brown et al. (1995) nor Hope et al. (1995b) found an effect for APD on CBGT outcome. However, in the study by E. Brown et al. (1995), 8 of 17 clients with generalized social phobia who met criteria for APD before treatment no longer did so after completing treatment. Thus the four studies examining the impact of APD on the outcome of cognitive-behavioral treatments for social phobia have produced equivocal and conflicting results.

Comments

The authors of the studies of APD and generalized social phobia, as well as Widiger (1992) and Heimberg (1996), have wrestled with the question of whether or not generalized social phobia and APD are truly different. Because the two diagnoses do not co-occur 100% of the time, they do not appear to be exactly the same thing. APD can co-occur with nongeneralized social phobia, and APD occurs in the context of Axis I disorders other than social phobia. However, the two diagnoses refer to the same general domain of symptoms. S. Turner et al. (1992) assert that the diagnostic criteria are just too similar, and they are correct. Herbert et al. (1992b) suggest that the two diagnostic categories are not sufficiently conceptually distinct to be validly separated. The problem is simple enough: The client who currently receives both diagnoses does not suffer from two distinct and comorbid mental disorders but instead exhibits a set of symptoms that meets the criteria for two diagnoses. It seems that the data are best accounted for if we consider generalized social phobia with APD to be a more severe instance of generalized social phobia, quantitatively but not qualitatively different. However, as noted by Heimberg (1996), it is time for researchers and clinicians who work with these two disorders to closely examine the implications of placing severe social anxiety simultaneously on both Axes I and II and to make the difficult decision about where it fits best.

Comorbidity of Social Phobia with Other Psychiatric Disorders

Axis I Disorders

OTHER ANXIETY DISORDERS

Several investigators have examined the rates of co-occurrence of social phobia and other anxiety disorders in clinical samples (Barlow, 1994; T. Brown &

Barlow, 1992; de Ruiter, Rijken, Garsssen, van Schaik, & Kraaimaat, 1989; Sanderson, DiNardo, Rapee, & Barlow, 1990; S. Turner et al., 1991), and this question has been addressed in the ECA study (Schneier et al., 1992), the National
Comorbidity Survey (Magee et al., 1996), and the EDSP study (Wittchen et al.,
1999).

In the ECA study, social phobia increased the relative risk of each of the
other anxiety disorders that were examined, and, in the case of agoraphobia, the
increase was more than elevenfold (odds ratio = 11.81). Among individuals with
social phobia, 59% received an additional diagnosis of simple phobia, 49.6% a
diagnosis of panic disorder or agoraphobia, and 11.1% a diagnosis of obsessive–
compulsive disorder. In the National Comorbidity Survey, 56.7% of persons with
social phobia met criteria for another anxiety disorder (Magee et al., 1996).
Thirty-eight percent received an additional diagnosis of simple phobia, 23.3%
agoraphobia, 15.8% posttraumatic stress disorder, 13.3% generalized anxiety disorder, and 10.9% panic disorder. In the EDSP study, 49.9% of respondents with
social phobia met criteria for another anxiety disorder, most commonly specific
phobia (43.6%).

The largest of the clinical studies was reported by T. Brown and Barlow
(1992). Their sample of 468 DSM-III-R anxiety disorder clients included 76 clients with social phobia. Seventeen percent of the clients with social phobia received an additional diagnosis of generalized anxiety disorder, 9% a diagnosis of
simple phobia, and 9% a diagnosis of panic disorder (with or without agoraphobia). S. Turner et al. (1991) also reported that generalized anxiety disorder was
the most frequent secondary diagnosis assigned to a sample of 71 individuals
with DSM-III-R social phobia, although they reported a somewhat higher percentage (33.3%).

The rates of comorbid diagnoses in these clinical samples seem low, especially given the higher rates in the epidemiological samples. At least for panic
disorder, other investigators have reported higher rates of occurrence in samples
of persons with social phobia. Van Ameringen, Mancini, Styan, and Donison
(1991) reported that 49.1% of their sample of clients with social phobia also had
a lifetime diagnosis of panic disorder with or without agoraphobia. Interestingly,
Stein, Shea, and Uhde (1989) reported a similar percentage (46%) of social phobia diagnoses in their sample of clients with panic disorder.

Mannuzza and colleagues (1995) have examined comorbid anxiety disorders in clinical samples of individuals with either generalized or nongeneralized
social phobia. The two groups differed in the frequency of lifetime diagnoses of
panic disorder. Thirty-four percent of individuals with nongeneralized social
phobia had panic disorder, compared with only 15% of individuals with generalized social phobia. This finding is consistent with the earlier reports by Heimberg
et al. (1990c) and Levin et al. (1993) that public-speaking phobics experienced
greater cardiac arousal in anticipation of and during behavioral tests than did individuals with generalized social phobia.

Differential diagnosis of social phobia and panic disorder has been discussed by several authors. Mannuzza, Fyer, Liebowitz, and Klein (1990) suggest that clients with social phobia and those with panic disorder who present for treatment differ in age of onset (those with social phobia are younger) and gender ratio (more clients with panic disorder are female). They also note differences in the phenomenology of the two disorders. First, clients with social phobia and clients with panic disorder differ in the focus of their fears even when they are frightened of the same situations; those with social phobia fear embarrassment and humiliation, whereas those with panic disorder are mostly concerned with the implications of the situation for the occurrence of panic attacks or for their physical well-being. Second, individuals with social phobia and individuals with panic disorder differ in their responses to the presence of others. Those with social phobia often report feeling more comfortable alone and may experience a respite from embarrassment or humiliation. Clients with panic disorder, in contrast, may feel comforted in the presence of others, who may be able to provide assistance to them in times of need. Finally, the typical somatic symptoms reported by individuals with social phobia and by those with panic disorder or agoraphobia may differ (Amies et al., 1983; Reich, Noyes, & Yates, 1988). Blushing, muscle twitching, and dry mouth occur more frequently in social phobia. Difficulty breathing, dizziness, palpitations, chest pains, tinnitus, blurred vision, headaches, and fears of dying, going crazy, or losing control are more common in panic disorder and agoraphobia. Reich et al. (1988) also reported on symptoms that differentiated clients with social phobia from clients with generalized anxiety disorder. Sweating and dyspnea were more frequently reported by clients with social phobia, whereas headaches and fear of dying were more common among the clients with generalized anxiety disorder.

Hazen and Stein (1995) note that clients with either social phobia or panic disorder may experience panic attacks, but the nature of these attacks differs. In social phobia, panic attacks are situationally bound or situationally predisposed; that is, they occur only during or in anticipation of feared situations. In panic disorder, attacks of this sort may occur, especially later in the course of the disorder; but there must be a history of at least one episode of panic that is spontaneous (i.e., unexpected and apparently out of the blue). Furthermore, individuals with social phobia are unlikely to be awakened from sleep by nocturnal panic attacks (Heckelman & Schneier, 1995).

It should come as no surprise that the situationally bound panic attacks experienced by persons with social phobia have a great impact on their lives. Because these panic attacks are elicited by specific feared situations, they seem very predictable to the person. That is, the person with social phobia who is confronted with the need to speak in front of a group "knows" with great certainty that a panic attack will occur and is very likely to believe that he or she will be both overwhelmed and embarrassed by it. This "certainty" is less likely to be experienced by persons who experience the spontaneous panic attacks that define panic disorder or by persons who become highly anxious in their feared social situations but do not experience panic attacks. Based on this reasoning, we recently studied 133 clients with social phobia (Jack, Heimberg, & Mennin, 1999). Fifty-seven experienced panic attacks, but only in feared social situations, 61 did not experience panic attacks, and 15 had spontaneous panic attacks (that is, they had secondary panic disorder). Clients with social phobia who experienced situational panic attacks reported greater fear and avoidance of social situations, were more distressed and impaired by their social anxiety, and reported greater fear of the symptoms of anxiety than clients with social phobia who did not experience panic attacks. Because we had found in an earlier study (E. Brown, Juster, Heimberg, & Winning, 1998) that people with social phobia reported greater hopelessness than persons with no mental disorder, we also wanted to know whether situational panic attacks would affect hopelessness. The clients who experienced panic attacks in their feared social situations reported greater hopelessness than either the clients without panic attacks or the clients with secondary panic disorder. The certainty that a panic attack will occur in feared situations may lead the person with social phobia to believe that he or she will always experience pain, never be able to rise above it, and never be able to achieve the gratification from which he or she is blocked by the imminent panic attack.

DEPRESSION AND SUICIDALITY

Estimates of the rates of depression among persons with social phobia vary widely from study to study. In the ECA study (Schneier et al., 1992), 16.6% of individuals with social phobia received a comorbid diagnosis of major depressive disorder, compared with 4.0% of individuals without social phobia. In the National Comorbidity Survey (Kessler, Stang, Wittchen, Stein, & Walters, 1999; Magee et al., 1996), a stunning 41.4% of persons with social phobia met criteria for any affective disorder (37.2% major depressive disorder). In the EDSP study (Wittchen et al., 1999), 31.1% of adolescents and young adults with social phobia met criteria for any affective disorder (25.5% major depressive disorder). In clinical samples, rates of comorbid major depression vary from 3% (S. Turner et al., 1991) to 11% (T. Brown & Barlow, 1992) to 35% (Stein, Tancer, Gelernter, Vittone, & Uhde, 1990) to 70% (Van Ameringen et al., 1991), but the reasons for this variability are unclear. According to Mannuzza et al. (1995), clients with generalized social phobia are more likely to have had a major depressive episode during their lifetimes (57%) than are clients with nongeneralized social phobia (37%), and the majority of these episodes may be of the atypical type (i.e., characterized by symptoms of rejection sensitivity, leaden paralysis, hypersomnia, or increased appetite). Holt et al. (1992a) and E. Brown et al. (1995) both reported that clients with generalized social phobia and APD were more likely than clients who had generalized social phobia without APD and clients with nongeneralized social phobia to have a comorbid mood disorder (major depression or dysthymia). Social phobia had an earlier onset than depression in 70.9% of persons with both disorders in the ECA study (Schneier et al., 1992), 68.9% of persons with both disorders in the National Comorbidity Survey (Kessler et al., 1999), and 81.6% of persons with both disorders in the EDSP study (Wittchen et al., 1999), suggesting that many individuals with social phobia develop major depression (and/or dysthymia) as a consequence of their social phobias. Stein et al. (2001) examined the notion that preexisting social phobia may increase the odds of later development of a depressive disorder (either major depression or dysthymia) using data from 2,548 respondents to the EDSP study who were reinterviewed after 34–50 months. In fact, the presence of social phobia at the initial interview greatly increased the odds that the respondent would meet criteria for a depressive disorder at reinterview in the 18–24 age group. Dilsaver, Qamar, and Del Medico (1992) have demonstrated that the reverse pattern is also possible. In that study, 45% of clients with major depression exhibited clinically significant fears of humiliation and embarrassment during their episodes.

In the ECA study, dysthymia occurred in 12.5% of individuals with social phobia, compared with 3.1% of individuals without social phobia. In the National Comorbidity Survey, the corresponding figure was 14.6% (Magee et al., 1996); in the EDSP study, it was 10.9% (Wittchen et al., 1999). In clinical samples, rates of 6% (S. Turner et al., 1991), 13% (T. Brown & Barlow, 1992), and 21% (Sanderson et al., 1990) have been reported. Dysthymia may be a result of the failures to attain interpersonal and occupational goals that are common among people with social phobia.

The ECA study also examined respondents' thoughts about suicide and their history of previous suicide attempts. When asked whether they thought a lot about death, felt like they wanted to die, or felt so low they wanted to commit suicide, individuals with social phobia were more likely to say yes than individuals without social phobia. Rates of actual suicide attempts were not elevated in individuals with social phobia relative to persons without social phobia unless the person with social phobia also had at least one other diagnosis of mental disorder. However, the suicide attempt rate for these "comorbid social phobics" was more than five times higher than the rate for individuals without social phobia (Schneier et al., 1992). Amies et al. (1983) reported that "parasuicidal acts" were more common among clients with DSM-III social phobia (14%) than among clients with agoraphobia (2%), but Cox, Direnfeld, Swinson, and Norton (1994) painted a somewhat different picture in their study of clients with DSM-III-R social phobia and panic disorder. Thirty-four percent of their clients with social phobia, compared with 31% of their clients with panic disorder, reported suicidal ideation within the past year. Although actual suicide attempts were rare within the past year, 12% of those with social phobia (18% of those with panic disorder) reported that they had attempted suicide at some other point in their lives. Clients who had made past suicide attempts were also more likely to report past psychiatric hospitalizations and treatment for depression than those who did not attempt suicide.

Social phobia may also contribute to the likelihood of suicide attempts among persons with other psychiatric disorders. In an analysis of epidemiological data from the United States, Canada, Puerto Rico, and Korea, Weissman and colleagues (1996) reported that persons with any psychiatric disorder were between 1.9 and 4.1 times as likely to attempt suicide if social phobia was present as a comorbid diagnosis. Furthermore, in the EDSP study, comorbid social phobia and depression at initial interview was associated with greater likelihood of the persistence or reoccurrence of depressive symptoms and of suicide attempts during the follow-up interval than was baseline depression alone (Stein et al., 2001).

ALCOHOLISM

The co-occurrence of alcoholism and social phobia has been well documented, although reported rates of alcoholism in social phobia have varied widely (Kushner, Sher, & Beitman, 1990). Amies et al. (1983, p. 177) reported that alcohol was "taken in excess" by 20% of their sample of individuals with social phobia. Schneier, Martin, Liebowitz, Gorman, and Fyer (1989) examined the past history of alcoholism in 98 outpatients who met DSM-III-R criteria for social phobia and found 16 of them to meet Research Diagnostic Criteria (Spitzer, Endicott, & Robins, 1978) for a lifetime diagnosis of alcoholism. Schneier et al. (1992) reported that 18% of individuals with DSM-III social phobia in the ECA study were comorbid for alcohol abuse. Additionally, the relative risk of alcoholism was 2.2 times greater for individuals with social phobia than for persons with no mental disorder. In the National Comorbidity Survey (Magee et al., 1996), 34.8% of persons with social phobia met criteria for either alcohol abuse (10.9%) or dependence (23.9%). Thyer et al. (1986) administered the Michigan Alcoholism Screening Test (MAST; Selzer, 1971) to a variety of anxiety clients, including clients with DSM-III social phobia. Four of 11 (36%) clients with social phobia achieved a score of 5 or higher on the MAST, considered to be indicative of alcoholism. In the study by Mannuzza et al. (1995), the lifetime rate of alcoholism among individuals with generalized social phobia (25%) was four times the rate among individuals with non-generalized social phobia (6%).

The occurrence of social phobia among individuals with alcohol problems has also been reported in several studies. Chambless, Cherney, Caputo, and Rheinstein (1987) reported that 19% of inpatient alcoholics met DSM-III criteria for social phobia, whereas Mullaney and Trippett (1979) and Smail, Stockwell, Canter, and Hodgson (1984) reported figures of 24% and 41%, respectively. In contrast, Stravynski, Lamontagne, and Lavallee (1986) reported that only 7.8% of their sample of 173 abstinent outpatient alcoholics met DSM-III criteria for social phobia. In several of these studies, the mean age of onset of social phobia was significantly earlier than the mean age of onset of alcohol problems.

Research on alcohol use among individuals with social phobia has largely ignored the impact of social context on alcohol consumption. S. Turner et al. (1986a) reported that a significant percentage of people with social phobia used alcohol to relieve anxiety in social situations. Forty-six percent used alcohol to feel more sociable at a party, and 50% reported alcohol consumption to relieve anticipatory anxiety before attending a social event. Smail et al. (1984) reported that 57% of individuals with social phobia deliberately used alcohol before talking to people in authority, 42% used alcohol while eating with other people, and 43% used alcohol when speaking or acting in front of an audience. Holle, Heimberg, Sweet, and Holt (1995) examined the intent to use alcohol by clients with social phobia and community controls across a number of social and nonsocial situations. Compared with controls, people with social phobia reported greater intent to drink alcohol while attending social events involving the presence of strangers.

Axis II Disorders Other Than Avoidant Personality Disorder

Research on personality disorders other than APD that may be comorbid with social phobia is relatively sparse, but the few studies that have been conducted agree that personality disorders are a frequent occurrence among individuals with social phobia.

S. Turner et al. (1991) administered the *Structured Clinical Interview for DSM-III-R Personality Disorders* (SCID-II; Spitzer, Williams, Gibbon, & First, 1990) to 71 individuals with social phobia. Thirty-seven percent met criteria for at least one Axis II diagnosis, and an additional 51% met several criteria, although not in sufficient numbers to qualify for a formal diagnosis. Although APD (22.1%) was the most common Axis II diagnosis, obsessive–compulsive personality disorder was also common (13.2%).

Sanderson et al. (1994) examined the frequency of SCID-II personality disorders in 355 clients with a variety of anxiety disorders. Personality disorders were diagnosed significantly more frequently (61%) among clients with social phobia than among any other anxiety disorder group except clients with generalized anxiety disorder (49%). The majority of these diagnoses were from Cluster C (avoidant, dependent, obsessive–compulsive). Again, APD was most common (37%), but dependent personality disorder was also frequent (18%), a finding also reported by Jansen et al. (1994) and Tran and Chambless (1995).

One word of caution is worthwhile when we attempt to understand the frequency of comorbid personality disorders in social phobia. Overall rates of personality disorders as reported herein include clients who met criteria for APD. Because it is unclear whether or not APD is truly different from generalized social phobia (see the earlier discussion), it might be best to subtract APD rates from the overall rates. However, data have not been reported in these studies in a manner that facilitates such recalculations, as many clients meet criteria for more than one personality disorder.

Personal Characteristics and Functional Impairment

In this section, we describe the personal characteristics of individuals with social phobia (other than gender, which was previously discussed) and the impact that social phobia has on their lives. Several authors (Hazen & Stein, 1995; Liebowitz et al., 1985; Schneier et al., 1992, 1994; S. Turner et al., 1986a; Wittchen & Beloch, 1996) have described the impaired functioning of individuals with social phobia. Schneier et al. (1994) noted that the majority of a sample of persons with social phobia seeking treatment at an anxiety disorders specialty clinic reported at least moderate impairment at some time in their lives in the areas of education, employment, family relationships, marriage and romantic relationships, and friendships. Degree of impairment was significantly related to the severity of social anxiety symptoms.

Age at Onset

Hazen and Stein (1995) reviewed 15 studies exploring age at onset of social phobia. The mean age at onset reported in those studies ranged from 13 to 24 years, with the majority of studies reporting onset before age 20. In the ECA study, mean age at onset was 15.5 years (Schneier et al., 1992); the median was 12.0 years (Bourdon et al., 1988). However, closer examination of the ECA data reveals two peaks in the age-at-onset distribution—one during the interval between 0 and 5 years of age and the other between ages 11 and 15 (see Figure 2.2). The peak at ages 0–5 represents the typically high percentage of individuals who cannot remember a specific onset or who report that their social phobia has been present for their entire lives.

The previous findings notwithstanding, the onset of social phobia typically occurs later than the onset of small animal phobias but earlier than the onset of panic disorder or agoraphobia (Gelernter et al., 1992; Lelliott, McNamee, & Marks, 1991; Marks & Gelder, 1966; Öst, 1987; Thyer, Parrish, Curtis, Nesse, & Cameron, 1985). In several studies, individuals with generalized social phobia have also reported an earlier age at onset than individuals with nongeneralized social phobia, although the presence of APD appears to make little difference in the age at onset of generalized social phobia (E. Brown et al., 1995; Holt et al., 1992a; Mannuzza et al., 1995; Wittchen et al., 1999). For instance, in the study by E. Brown et al. (1995), the age at onset for generalized social phobia (with or without APD) was 14.9 years, whereas the age at onset for nongeneralized social phobia was 21.6 years. This difference was not apparent in the epidemiological study of social phobia disorder subtypes by Kessler et al. (1998) reviewed previously.

Duration of Disorder

S. Turner et al. (1986a) report that their sample of 21 clients with DSM-III social phobia had experienced social distress for a mean of 20.9 years and had avoided

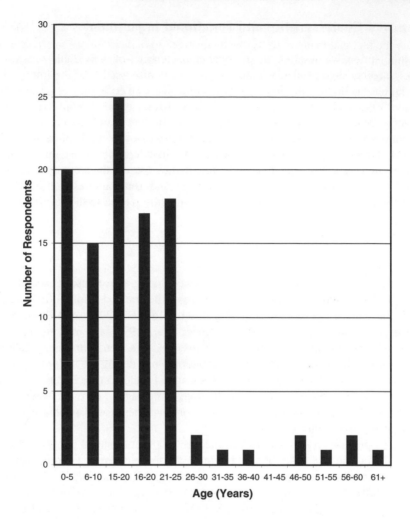

FIGURE 2.2. Epidemiologic Catchment Area study: Age of onset of social phobia in participants without agoraphobia or simple phobia (*n* = 97). Adapted from "Social Phobia: Comorbidity and Morbidity in an Epidemiologic Sample," by F. R. Schneier, J. Johnson, C. D. Hornig, M. R. Liebowitz, and M. M. Weissman, 1992, *Archives of General Psychiatry, 49*, p. 284. Copyright 1992 by the American Medical Association. Adapted by permission.

difficult situations for a mean of 15.3 years. In the ECA study, respondents with social phobia had experienced symptoms for a mean of 19.4 years (Davidson et al., 1993). Hazen and Stein (1995) report several other studies of the duration of social phobia, with a range from 10 to 21.4 years. Social phobia appears to run a chronic, unremitting course (Liebowitz et al., 1985), with evidence of considerable long-term morbidity (Reich, Goldenberg, Vasile, Goisman, & Keller, 1994).

Reich et al. (1994) followed 140 clients with social phobia for 65 weeks, and despite the fact that many of these clients received psychiatric or psychotherapeutic treatment in the community, only 11% were judged to have achieved complete remission by the end of the study.

From a slightly different perspective, Rapee (1995) reports that the mean age of presentation for treatment of social phobia appears to be around 30 years of age. Thus clients with social phobia seek treatment 15 to 25 years after the onset of their disorder, considerably later than do clients with panic disorder. Rapee (1995) suggests that this difference may be explained by the relative distress caused by social phobia and by panic disorder, by less public awareness of social phobia as a treatable disorder, or by the fact that persons with social phobia are more likely to view their disorder as an immutable part of their personality.

Marital Status and Other Interpersonal Relationships

Social phobia might reasonably be expected to interfere in the development of romantic relationships. In fact, 50% of the unmarried participants in the study by S. Turner et al. (1986a) believed that their social phobias limited their functioning in this area, as they felt hesitant to engage in social activities and unable to establish the degree of intimacy necessary for the development of long-term relationships. Shy university students have been found to interact less with students of the opposite sex than nonshy students (Dodge, Heimberg, Nyman, & O'Brien, 1987), and in a 30-year longitudinal study of shy individuals (Caspi, Elder, & Bem, 1988), shy men (but not shy women) married about 3 years later than nonshy men (see also Kerr, Lambert, & Bem, 1996). In epidemiological studies (Davidson et al., 1993; Schneier et al., 1992), individuals with social phobia have been less likely to be married than individuals without social phobia. In clincial samples (Amies et al., 1983; Lelliott et al., 1991; Solyom et al., 1986), clients with social phobia have been less likely to marry than clients with other anxiety disorders, although in the study by Gelernter et al. (1992), those with social phobia only tended ($p < .07$) to be less likely to have ever married than clients with panic disorder. In one study (Lelliott et al., 1991), individuals with social phobia also had fewer children than individuals with agoraphobia. Individuals with comorbid generalized social phobia and APD are less likely to be married than individuals with social phobia who do not meet criteria for APD (E. Brown et al., 1995; Tran & Chambless, 1995), and individuals with generalized social phobia were less likely to be married than individuals with nongeneralized social phobia in one study (Mannuzza et al., 1995). Seventy percent of individuals with social phobia also report impairment in nonromantic social relationships (S. Turner et al., 1986a).

Education

In the study by S. Turner et al. (1986a), 84.6% of clients with social phobia reported significant impairment in academic functioning. They stated that their fear prevented them from getting better grades by inhibiting their participation in class discussion. They felt unable to speak up in class, to join clubs or organizations, or to seek positions of leadership within these organizations. In our clinical practice and research, we have frequently seen university students with social phobia who avoid speaking with professors when they need guidance or tutorial assistance or who have foregone further education when they learned that they would be required to speak in front of the class. Schneier et al. (1992) reported that individuals with social phobia obtained less education than other individuals assessed in the ECA study. Davidson et al. (1993) also reported that persons with social phobia were more likely than persons without social phobia to have experienced a broad range of academic and behavioral difficulties during their school years. In the study by Stein et al. (1994), persons who reported being much more nervous than other people in at least one situation were less likely than nonanxious persons to have attended a university (15% vs. 43%), even when controlling for age and gender. This was also the case for public-speaking-fearful persons in the follow-up telephone survey by Stein et al. (1996). Individuals with generalized social phobia were less educated than individuals with circumscribed public-speaking phobias (Heimberg et al., 1990c).

Employment and Career Functioning

In the study by S. Turner et al. (1986a), 92% of individuals with social phobia reported significant impairment in occupational functioning. Inability to engage in group discussion or make presentations was believed to result in lack of career advancement or in being passed over for promotions. Shy college students have also been shown to be less likely to express interest in careers with an interpersonal orientation than nonshy students (S. Phillips & Bruch, 1988). In the longitudinal study by Caspi and colleagues (1988), shy men entered a steady career 3 years later than nonshy men and were more likely to change careers and to achieve less in their careers. Shy women were less likely to enter the workforce or to reenter it after childbirth than nonshy women. In a series of 11 clients with DSM-III social phobia, Liebowitz et al. (1985) reported that 2 were unable to work and 6 were blocked from career advancement by their social fears. Davidson et al. (1993) reported that persons with social phobia were more likely than persons without social phobia to be repeatedly fired from jobs and to be repeatedly late or absent from work, and Schneier et al. (1992) reported that those with the disorder were more likely to be of lower socioeconomic status and to receive welfare or disability payments than persons without the disorder. In the study by Stein et al. (1994), persons who reported being much more nervous than other people in at least one situation were less likely than nonanxious persons to earn $20,000 or more a year (35% vs. 70%). Individuals with generalized social phobia were less likely to be employed than individuals with circumscribed public-speaking phobias (Heimberg et al., 1990c). Individuals with comorbid generalized social phobia and APD also earned less money per year than individuals with social phobia alone (E. Brown et al., 1995), although social phobia was not associated with lower income in the National Comorbidity Survey (Magee et al., 1996). Furthermore, persons with social phobia report more days missed from work and more days of reduced productivity at work than persons without mental disorder (Stein, McQuaid, Laffaye, & McCahill, 1999), suggesting that the economic burden of social phobia is not limited to the client himself or herself but is shared by his or her employer and society at large (Greenberg et al., 1999).

Treatment Utilization

Despite the distress and impairment attendant to social phobia, individuals with this disorder are unlikely to seek treatment. In their community survey of individuals with anxiety disorders, Pollard, Henderson, Frank, and Margolis (1989) reported that only 8% of individuals with social phobia or fears of social situations sought out professional help. At the Durham, North Carolina, site of the ECA study (Davidson et al., 1993), people with social phobia were more likely to seek help from a variety of sources (friend or relative, nonpsychiatric physician, psychiatrist or therapist, clergyman, mental health clinic, emergency room, social service agency) than people without social phobia. However, help was rarely sought for social anxiety specifically. Of the 32 individuals with social phobia who reported seeing their doctors for psychological problems, only 3 admitted seeking help for social anxiety. Only 19% of persons with social phobia in the National Comorbidity Survey (Magee et al., 1996) and 21.5% of persons with social phobia in the EDSP study (Wittchen et al., 1999) had sought professional help for their anxiety at some time in their lives.

Notes

1. We have often speculated about the nature of differences between persons with generalized versus nongeneralized social phobia and what about these differences may be important from a cognitive-behavioral clinical perspective. Clearly, persons with generalized social phobia have more severe symptoms and are more functionally impaired. However, we also wonder whether the meaningful difference between them will someday be shown to be in the realm of cognitive structure. Is it possible that the difference between them is that the person with nongeneralized social phobia understands that not all situations in life involve negative evaluation by others and may thus more easily entertain alternative beliefs about feared situations than persons with generalized social phobia who reject this belief? Informally, we have remarked more than once that it is sometimes quite difficult to engage persons with generalized social phobia in the treatment process. The pervasiveness of their pessimism about social situations may provide few opportunities to "pry" their schemata open with our "cognitive

crowbars." The more pervasive negative belief might not only contribute to severity and impairment but also might suggest that there is a need for more intense and prolonged treatment for persons with generalized social phobia.

2. Although it is technically possible to obtain a diagnosis of APD without meeting criteria for social phobia, we have yet to meet the person for whom this description seems correct. Given the large degree of overlap between the criteria sets, we can only wonder about the nature of the participants in these studies.

3

Cognitive Function in Social Phobia

Cognitive-behavioral group therapy for social phobia is based, in part, on the notion that there are difficulties in the individual's view of self and others that require modification. A model of the role of cognition in social phobia will be described in Chapter 5, but it is first necessary to show that these difficulties exist. And exist they do! In this chapter and the next, we review many of the problematic aspects of cognitive functioning among individuals with social phobia. For the purposes of discussion, these may be subdivided into three categories: (1) negative cognitive content, (2) errors of judgment or interpretation, and (3) dysfunctions of cognitive process. The first two areas are discussed in this chapter, the third in Chapter 4. In our review of these areas, we demonstrate the nature of these difficulties and how they may affect the functioning of individuals with social phobia.

Negative Cognitive Content

Thought Frequency

Assessments of the content of the thoughts of socially anxious individuals show that it is decidedly tilted toward the negative. That is, socially anxious persons report a much higher frequency of negative thoughts than positive thoughts. This was first demonstrated among socially anxious college students who were asked to write down the thoughts that occurred to them in anticipation of role-played social interactions (Cacioppo, Glass, & Merluzzi, 1979; Heimberg, Acerra, & Holstein, 1985). Similar results were obtained when socially anxious participants completed the Social Interaction Self-Statement Test (SISST; Glass, Merluzzi,

Biever, & Larsen, 1982), a questionnaire assessing the frequency of positive and negative thoughts experienced during a role-played social interaction. Importantly, this pattern of cognition has been repeatedly demonstrated in samples of clients with social phobia (Dodge, Hope, Heimberg, & Becker, 1988; Glass & Furlong, 1990; S. Turner et al., 1986b). Figure 3.1 presents the SISST scores from a sample of 28 clients with social phobia who sought treatment at our clinic (Dodge et al., 1988) and compares them with the scores of 50 normal participants

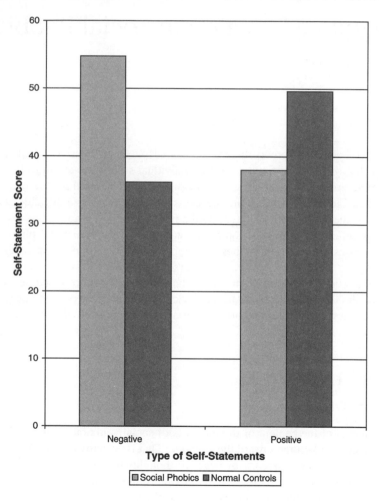

FIGURE 3.1. Social Interaction Self-Statement Test positive and negative self-statement scores of social phobics and normal control participants. Adapted from "Evaluation of the Social Interaction Self-Statement Test with a Social Phobic Population," by C. S. Dodge, D. A. Hope, R. G. Heimberg, and R. E. Becker, 1988, *Cognitive Therapy and Research, 12,* p. 216. Copyright 1988 by Kluwer Academic/Plenum Publishers. Adapted by permission.

who completed the SISST as part of another study. Several points are evident from inspection of these data: (1) clients with social phobia report that negative self-statements occur to them more frequently than positive self-statements, (2) negative self-statements occur more frequently to clients with social phobia than to normal participants, (3) positive self-statements occur less frequently to clients with social phobia than similar statements occur to normal participants, and (4) normal participants report that positive self-statements occur to them more frequently than negative self-statements. Clearly, the thought content of persons with social phobia and of normal individuals is different.

Thought Balance

Another way of evaluating the content of the internal dialogue of people with social phobia is to examine the relative proportion of positive and negative thoughts. R. Schwartz (1986; R. Schwartz & Garamoni, 1989) has put forward a theory of States of Mind (SOM) suggesting that a preponderance of positive thoughts is a marker of good adjustment. A ratio of positive thoughts to the sum of positive and negative thoughts (P/[P + N]; the "SOM ratio") approximating 0.62 is described as ideal because it serves to make threat (as indexed by negative thoughts) salient but puts them in the context of a positive and optimistic approach to life. Increasing proportions of negative thoughts (or decreasing SOM ratios) are related to more and more severe psychopathology. The mean SOM ratio of people with social phobia, based on thoughts listed after completing a role play of a personally relevant anxiety-evoking situation, was only 0.28, a very negative score (Heimberg, Bruch, Hope, & Dombeck, 1990a). The SOM ratio was also significantly related to several measures of the severity of social phobia. Interestingly, when scores on the SISST were utilized to calculate the SOM ratio, the ratio was less negative. Bruch, Heimberg, and Hope (1991) demonstrated that treatment of social phobia with CBGT results in significant and sustained improvement in SOM ratios.

Thought Content

Stopa and Clark (1993), in a study that is discussed at several points in this chapter, examined the specific content of thoughts experienced by clients with social phobia after they had participated in an interaction with a female research assistant. Clients were also asked to imagine themselves in three hypothetical social situations and report on their thoughts associated with each. The thoughts of clients with social phobia were compared with those of normal participants, as well as with those of a control group of clients with anxiety disorders other than social phobia, making it possible to determine if the pattern of thinking experienced by clients with social phobia is specific to the disorder or related to a more generic aspect of anxiety.

Participants' thought content during the interaction was coded into a number of categories, including positive, negative, and neutral thoughts about the self, about the conversation partner, and about the conversation partner's evaluation of the participant. Thoughts related to coping and avoidance were also coded. Participants with social phobia differed from both anxious and normal control participants in the number of negative self-evaluative thoughts recorded (see Figure 3.2). It should not be surprising that participants with social phobia would record more negative self-evaluative thoughts, and, in fact, they recorded more than four times as many of these thoughts than either anxious or normal controls. Negative thoughts about what the conversation partner thought about the participant were recorded very infrequently and did not differ among groups. Because social phobia is defined as a marked fear of situations in which the person may be exposed to unfamiliar people or scrutiny by others, this was an unexpected outcome. Similar results were noted in response to the hypothetical situations, and individuals with social phobia also recorded more thoughts about avoidance and fewer thoughts about coping. This pattern of findings led Stopa and Clark (1993, p. 264) to speculate that

> social phobics' thoughts are not data driven but function rather like an automatic programme which is activated in a social situation. That is, once in a social situation social phobics tend to run through a repertoire of negative thoughts without really paying attention to what is happening in the situation.

They go on to suggest (p. 265) that

> the prospect of meeting a stranger triggers anticipatory thoughts which focus on negative evaluation of the self. These thoughts produce anxiety which, in turn, leads to thoughts about avoidance. This focus on negative thoughts interferes with adaptive behaviour because it prevents the social phobic from formulating a plan of how to deal with the encounter, and thus further increases anxiety and stimulates more negative judgments about the self.

Although participants recorded few negative thoughts about how they were being evaluated by the other person in the conversation or hypothetical situations, we maintain a strong belief in the notion that people with social phobia are very concerned about others' evaluation. The most striking conclusion we reach from Stopa and Clark's data is that people with social phobia may substitute their own negative self-perceptions for the thoughts they believe others are having about them. Of course, this pattern would create a closed system that neither utilizes nor is modified by disconfirmatory information!

Although negative thoughts about being evaluated by the conversation partner did not play a big role in the Stopa and Clark (1993) study, thoughts about the other person in an interaction may still be important. For instance, Leary, Kowalski, and Campbell (1988) found that socially anxious persons maintain a

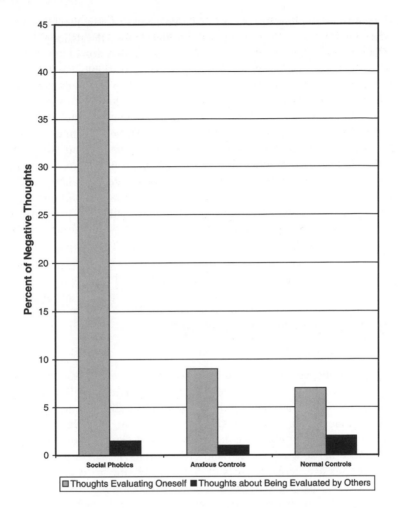

FIGURE 3.2. Negative self-evaluative thoughts and negative thoughts about being evaluated by the conversation partner recorded by social phobics, anxious controls, and normal controls. Adapted from "Cognitive Processes in Social Phobia," by L. Stopa and D. M. Clark, 1993, *Behaviour Research and Therapy, 31*, p. 260. Copyright 1993 by Elsevier Science. Adapted by permission.

generalized belief that people tend to evaluate others unfavorably. In their study, socially anxious undergraduates thought they would be evaluated more negatively than nonanxious participants, regardless of the extent of their initial contact with a potential interactant. They also believed that potential interactants would evaluate other people just as unfavorably. The difference may be that individuals with social phobia believe that other people have "what it takes" to overcome these negative evaluations but are equally convinced that they themselves do not (see the later section on "Perfectionism and Standards of Evaluation").

Concern about others' evaluations may also be a function of the characteristics of the other person or of the situation. Russell, Cutrona, and Jones (1986) evaluated the types of situations that were most likely to elicit symptoms of shyness in susceptible persons. Their results suggest that two dimensions best characterize difficult and anxiety-evoking situations: novelty and perception of the other person as highly attractive or successful. Mahone, Bruch, and Heimberg (1993) further evaluated this notion and examined how both negative thoughts about the self and positive thoughts about the attributes of the other person could contribute to social anxiety experienced by undergraduate men during an interaction with an undergraduate woman. Negative self-referent thoughts accounted for significant variance in participants' ratings of anxiety and self-efficacy. However, positive thoughts about the woman accounted for significant variance in behavioral signs of anxiety displayed during the interaction. The more positive attributes of the woman that participants recorded during a thought listing task, the more anxious they were during the subsequent interaction.

Errors of Judgment and Interpretation

Attributions of Causality and Control

Attributions for the causes of events have occupied a central position in research on depression for the past two decades (Abramson, Seligman, & Teasdale, 1978). However, maladaptive attributions do not seem to be the exclusive province of depressed persons. For instance, Girodo, Dotzenroth, and Stein (1981) and Teglasi and Hoffman (1982) have demonstrated that shy persons attribute social failures to internal sources (i.e., to themselves or some aspect of themselves) and social successes to external sources (e.g., to chance, the good graces of others, etc.). Of course, this is a very good way of demonstrating to yourself that the world is beyond your control. Perceptions of control (or the lack of it) are central to several theories of anxiety (e.g., Barlow, 2002).

Several years ago, we decided to examine the attributional style of clients with social phobia and other anxiety disorders (Heimberg et al., 1989). We administered a slightly modified version of the Attributional Style Questionnaire (ASQ; Peterson et al., 1982) to clients with DSM-III social phobia, clients with panic disorder, clients with agoraphobia, depressed clients, and normal controls. There were many between-group differences in this complicated study, and we highlight only the ones comparing clients with social phobia and normal controls. Individuals with social phobia attributed the causes of negative events to sources that were more internal, more global (having to do with more aspects of life), and more stable (permanent) than did normal controls. They also saw themselves as more responsible for these negative outcomes and viewed the negative outcomes as more important than did the normal group. Differences were smaller in the analysis of attributions for positive outcomes, but individuals with social phobia were less likely to attribute these events to internal sources than normal controls and saw themselves as less likely to be able to control the occurrence of these positive events in the future.

We have since conducted two further studies of attributions of control in social phobia (Cloitre, Heimberg, Liebowitz, & Gitow, 1992b; Leung & Heimberg, 1996). Cloitre et al. (1992b) administered Levenson's (1973) Locus of Control Scale (LOCS) to groups of clients with social phobia and panic disorder, as well as to a group of normal control participants. The LOCS measures attributions to internal versus external sources for a broad range of both positive and negative events. It also features additional subscales that measure two different aspects of the external control of events: (1) *Chance*, or the belief that events are essentially randomly determined, and (2) *Powerful Others*, or the belief that events are essentially controllable but only by persons other than the participant. Not surprisingly, the normal control group achieved higher Internality scores than either group of anxious clients. However, clients with social phobia and clients with panic disorder differed from each other and from normal participants in their pattern of external attributions. Clients with panic disorder differed from clients with social phobia and from normal controls by making the most extreme attributions to Chance, an attribution entirely consistent with their experience of panic attacks that strike them "out of the blue." Clients with social phobia, on the other hand, differed from clients with panic disorder and from normal controls by making the strongest endorsement of attributions to Powerful Others. Thus individuals with social phobia appear to believe in orderly and controllable events; they just do not believe that they, personally, have the ability to exert this control. Leung and Heimberg (1996) reported essentially the same findings in additional groups of individuals with social phobia and normal controls.

Subjective Probability and Cost of Events

Lucock and Salkovskis (1988) asked individuals with social phobia to estimate the likelihood of the occurrence of social and nonsocial events that were either positive or negative in nature. An example of a negative social event was, "You will have a serious disagreement with a friend in the next six months" (p. 299). Of course, if a person believes that negative events are more likely to occur, then it is reasonable to speculate that he or she would be more anxious and more hypervigilant about when and where these events might happen. In fact, participants with social phobia rated the probability of negative social events as greater than did a matched group of control participants and also rated the probability of positive events as lower. Cognitive-behavioral treatment resulted in reduced ratings of the probabilities of negative social events.

Foa, Franklin, Perry, and Herbert (1996) carried the study of subjective probability of negative social and nonsocial events a step further and also examined participants' evaluations of the subjective cost of these events. Subjective cost refers to the question of how bad an event would be if it were to actually happen to the person; it may be considered an index of catastrophic thinking about the consequences of events. Fifteen clients with generalized social phobia and 15 gender-matched control participants completed the Probability/Cost Questionnaire (PCQ), a measure adapted from similar previous work by Butler and Mathews (1983) and McNally and Foa (1987). The PCQ contains 40 items, 20 concerning negative social events (e.g., "Someone you know won't say hello to you," "During a job interview, you will freeze") and 20 negative nonsocial events. Subjective probability and cost are rated on 0–8 Likert-type scales.

Like Lucock and Salkovskis (1988), Foa et al. (1996) found that individuals with social phobia differed from normal controls in their assessment of the probability of negative social and nonsocial events (see Figure 3.3). Specifically, individuals with social phobia rated negative social events as more likely than did control participants. They also rated negative social events as significantly more likely than negative nonsocial events, a pattern that was not evident in the control group.

Figure 3.4 displays participants' ratings of the subjective cost of the negative social and nonsocial events. Again, individuals with generalized social phobia rated the negative social events as more costly than the control group did. They also tended to see nonsocial events as more costly, but this difference was small. Interestingly, participants with social phobia viewed negative social events as more costly than negative nonsocial events, whereas control participants had the opposite view. Negative nonsocial events were viewed as more costly.

In summary, individuals with social phobia saw negative social events as both more probable and more costly than normal controls. In Foa et al.'s (1996) study, individuals with social phobia then received a treatment very similar to CBGT. Control participants were retested after a similar interval. After treatment, the probability and cost estimates made by people with social phobia were reduced, but they remained elevated above the level of control participants' ratings. Further analyses by Foa et al. (1996) suggested that change in cost estimates was the greater predictor of change in the severity of social phobia, but this finding was not replicated in a study by McManus, Clark, and Hackmann (2000).

Poulton and Andrews (1994) examined ratings of probability and cost of an upcoming negative event among individuals with social phobia. Forty-six clients with social phobia and a control group of 27 non–social phobic stutterers were asked to complete probability and cost ratings of five possible outcomes 15 minutes before giving a speech to a small audience. Ratings were also completed after the speech (with instructions that they be completed on the basis of how participants felt halfway through their speeches) and again the next day. Thus, participants provided ratings for the time periods before, during, and after the speech for the following items: (1) "People will find fault with you," (2) "People

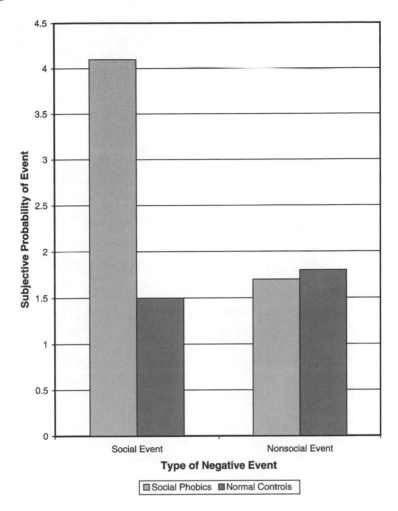

FIGURE 3.3. Ratings of the subjective probability of negative social and nonsocial events by social phobics and normal control participants. Adapted from "Cognitive Biases in Generalized Social Phobia," by E. B. Foa, M. E. Franklin, K. J. Perry, and J. D. Herbert, 1996, *Journal of Abnormal Psychology, 105,* p. 436. Copyright 1996 by the American Psychological Association. Adapted by permission.

will see you as incompetent or foolish," (3) "People will see that you are anxious and not like you," (4) "People will laugh at you," and (5) "You will make a scene in front of others." The cross-product of cost and probability ratings was taken as an index of "danger appraisal."

As expected, clients with social phobia made greater appraisals of danger at each point than did the participants who stuttered. Participants who stuttered saw

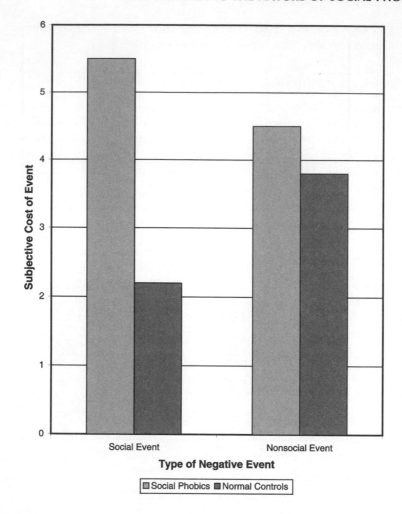

FIGURE 3.4. Ratings of the subjective cost of negative social and nonsocial events by social phobics and normal control participants. Adapted from "Cognitive Biases in Generalized Social Phobia," by E. B. Foa, M. E. Franklin, K. J. Perry, and J. D. Herbert, 1996, *Journal of Abnormal Psychology, 105,* p. 436. Copyright 1996 by the American Psychological
Association. Adapted by permission.

their greatest danger during the actual speech. Participants with social phobia, on
the other hand, saw the greatest danger before the speech and became progressively less anxious. Poulton and Andrews (1994) correctly point out that the
cognitions experienced by people with social phobia prior to feared events may
motivate avoidance and should be very significant points of intervention in cognitive-behavioral treatment. Andrews, Freed, and Teesson (1994) substantially rep-

licated these patterns in a different sample of clients with social phobia, clients with other anxiety disorders, and nonanxious controls.

Biased Interpretation of Ambiguous Events

Several years ago, Butler and Mathews (1983) demonstrated that generally anxious clients showed a negative bias in the interpretation of ambiguous events. That is, when asked to choose between various interpretations of situations that were inherently unclear, they would routinely select the negative interpretation. Stopa and Clark (2000) and Amir, Foa, and Coles (1998b) have examined this phenomenon in samples of people with social phobia. In the study by Stopa and Clark, clients with social phobia were more likely to choose negative interpretations of ambiguous social events ("You have visitors round for a meal and they leave sooner than expected") than were other anxious clients or nonanxious controls, but there were no group differences for ambiguous nonsocial events ("A letter marked 'urgent' arrives at your home"). Amir and colleagues (1998b) reported similar findings in their comparison of clients with generalized social phobia, clients with obsessive–compulsive disorder, and nonanxious controls. Furthermore, clients with social phobia showed no preference for negative interpretations when asked to view the events as happening to "the typical person" rather than happening to themselves.

Using a far different methodology, Hirsch and Mathews (1997, 2000) also examined judgment biases in social situations and have come up with some unique conclusions. In their 1997 investigation (Study 1), socially anxious individuals were presented with sentences describing job interviews, including critical ambiguous sentences. These ambiguous sentences ended with a word that could result in either a positive or negative meaning of the sentence. Participants were asked to decide as quickly as possible if this final word could grammatically complete the sentence. The socially anxious participants responded to both negative and positive words at the same rate, whereas a nonanxious comparison group responded to positive words more quickly than negative words. This pattern of findings was replicated in a sample of individuals with social phobia by Hirsch and Mathews (2000). In a second study using a lexical decision task, Hirsch and Mathews (1997) again found evidence for a positive inferential bias in their nonanxious group, but there was no evidence of negative bias in the socially anxious group.

Hirsch and Mathews draw on the literature on text comprehension to explain their findings. They suggest that their nonanxious participants made positively biased inferences "on-line," that is, at the time the information was encountered. They propose that this positive bias serves as a protective factor, maintaining a "positive and confident mood state" (1997, p. 1131). In contrast, socially anxious individuals may not make on-line inferences at all. Rather, their interpretations may be based on other information, such as preexisting negative beliefs about themselves. The failure to make positively biased on-line inferences may further contribute to difficulties with social anxiety.

Biased Interpretation of Others' Emotions and Judgments

If socially anxious persons are indeed concerned about the evaluations they receive from others, then it becomes important for them to be able to accurately read the nonverbal communications of others, especially negative ones. The ability to accurately judge how others are feeling should give the person an important means to minimize negative evaluations or other unpleasant social consequences. This notion was investigated in a creative study by Winton, Clark, and Edelmann (1995). These investigators presented slides of persons portraying negative emotions (anger, sadness, disgust, contempt, and fear) and neutral emotions to high and low socially anxious students, grouped according to their scores on the Fear of Negative Evaluation (FNE) Scale. Participants were asked simply to indicate if each slide's emotion was negative or neutral in a forced-choice format. Interestingly, there was no overall difference between groups in accuracy of emotion identification. This failure to find a group difference was accounted for by the fact that socially anxious individuals were significantly better than less anxious participants at identifying negative emotions, but at the same time, they were significantly worse at identifying neutral emotions. Winton et al. (1995) then conducted further analyses that revealed that this pattern was not the result of socially anxious participants' more finely tuned ability to identify negative emotions. Instead, it appeared to be the result of a bias toward identifying emotions as negative regardless of the actual emotion expressed. That is, when in doubt, they chose "negative." One way to always be aware of social threat is to assume it is always present. Recall that Leary et al. (1988) reported that socially anxious persons expected others to evaluate everyone negatively. However, this strategy is another example of how the person with social phobia may construct a world that is highly threatening but that may bear little resemblance to the world as it is (Stopa & Clark, 1993).

In another recent study, Roth, Antony, and Swinson (2001) asked clients with social phobia to judge how their anxiety symptoms are interpreted by others. Predictably, they were more likely than control participants to think that others interpreted their anxiety symptoms as indicative of intense anxiety or mental illness. When asked how they interpret the anxiety they observe in others, however, they interpreted it as being indicative of a normal physical state.

Self-Evaluation of Performance

Several studies have now examined the evaluations that people make of their public performances and how these evaluations compare with those given by observers (Alden & Wallace, 1995; J. V. Clark & Arkowitz, 1975; Glasgow &

Arkowitz, 1975; Heimberg et al., 1990c; Hope, Heimberg, & Bruch, 1995a; Rapee & Lim, 1992; Stopa & Clark, 1993). We look closely at only a couple of the studies that included people with social phobia.

Rapee and Lim (1992) asked 28 individuals with social phobia and 33 nonanxious controls to give a speech in front of small groups of other participants. Speakers and audience members provided two sorts of evaluations of each speaker's performance: (1) ratings of specific public-speaking behaviors (e.g., kept eye contact with audience, had a clear speaking voice), and (2) global ratings (e.g., kept audience interested, generally spoke well). On specific items, speakers with social phobia were judged more poorly than nonanxious control speakers, both when they rated themselves and when the audience members provided the ratings. Ratings of global items produced a different result. Although speakers with social phobia were again rated more poorly than control participants, the magnitude of this difference was much larger for self-ratings than for ratings by audience members. That is, people with social phobia were much harder on themselves than the audience members were.

In the study by Stopa and Clark (1993), clients with social phobia, anxious control participants, and nonanxious controls had a conversation with a female research assistant. After the conversation, participants completed rating scales of both positive (e.g., friendly, confident, relaxed, attractive, warm) and negative (e.g., nervous, awkward, uncomfortable) aspects of their interpersonal behavior. An independent observer later completed the same ratings from videotape. Individuals with social phobia rated their own behavior more negatively and less positively than did anxious and nonanxious control participants when asked to rate their own behavior. The observer also rated the behavior of participants with social phobia as more negative than that of both control groups and as less positive than that of the nonanxious controls. However, when social phobics' ratings of their own behavior were compared with the ratings of their behavior provided by the observer, their self-ratings were again significantly more negative and less positive. In contrast, neither anxious nor nonanxious control participants differed from the observer in the evaluation of their negative behavior, and both rated their positive behavior more positively than did the observer. The findings for negative behaviors are summarized in Figure 3.5.

The studies by Rapee and Lim (1992) and Stopa and Clark (1993) converge to suggest that, in both public speaking and social interactional contexts, two different processes are at work. First, to a degree, the social behavior of people with social phobia may be less competent than that of nonanxious persons (or, in the Stopa & Clark study, of anxious controls). However, it remains unclear whether this is an actual deficit in the capacity to perform or the result of negative cognitions, physiological arousal, or other inhibitory or disruptive factors. We have previously (Heimberg & Juster, 1995; Turk, Fresco, & Heimberg, 1999) raised the concern that *performance* deficits, as demonstrated in studies such as those of Rapee and Lim (1992) and Stopa and Clark (1993),

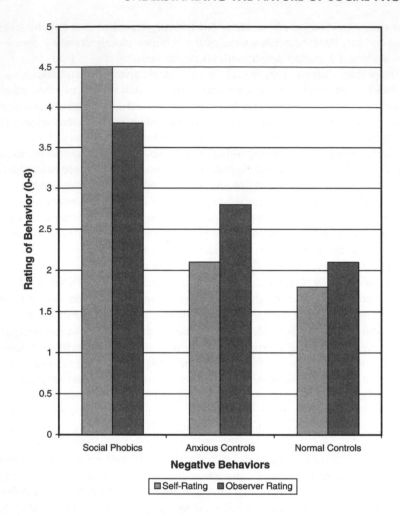

FIGURE 3.5. Ratings of the negative social behavior of social phobics, participants with other anxiety disorders, and normal controls as evaluated by participants and observers. Adapted from "Cognitive Processes in Social Phobia," by L. Stopa and D. M. Clark, 1993, *Behaviour Research and Therapy, 31,* p. 263. Copyright 1993 by Elsevier Science. Adapted by permission.

may be confused with *social skills* deficits, a judgment of performance capacity that is inferred from inadequate social behavior. At present, the data for performance deficits are strong, the data for deficient capacity weak and open to multiple interpretations.

Second, individuals with social phobia appear to expand on this difference when making global judgments about themselves, rating themselves more extremely negatively than they are rated by other persons. According to Stopa and

Clark (1993, p. 265), they have "distorted self-perceptions of their own behaviour which can only serve to increase the probability of further negative self-evaluations, more anxiety, and further deterioration in social performance." Clearly, these two processes, performance deficits and distorted self-perception, can only serve to potentiate each other. Of interest, Heimberg et al. (1990c) have noted that negatively biased self-evaluation is more pronounced in nongeneralized social phobics, whereas performance deficits may be more likely to characterize generalized social phobics.

Rapee and Hayman (1996) conducted a series of studies suggesting that the tendency of people with social phobia to rate themselves more harshly than others rate them may be influenced by the source of information on which their ratings are based. In one study, socially anxious and nonanxious students rated their own public-speaking performances both from memory and after viewing their efforts on videotape. Socially anxious participants showed the expected negative bias when rating from memory. However, the self-evaluations of both groups of participants were more positive and more in line with the ratings of observers after they had viewed their videotapes. In another study, socially anxious students gave a speech, rated the speech either from memory or from video, and then gave a second speech. As in the earlier study, ratings of the first speech from video were more positive and more similar to observer ratings than evaluations made from memory. Importantly, students who rated their first speech from videotape evaluated themselves more positively (from memory) after the second speech. Hope et al. (1995a) have also demonstrated that the discrepancy between self- and observer ratings of performance disappears after cognitive-behavioral treatment for social phobia.

Reactions to Feedback

R. Smith and Sarason (1975) examined the reactions of socially anxious college students to negative interpersonal feedback. Social anxiety was determined on the basis of responses to the FNE Scale. Participants were presented with feedback that they might have received in a hypothetical experiment about the amount of insight they had about the way they might behave in a novel social situation. The feedback included 10 rating scales—7 of which were rated toward the negative end of the scale—and this feedback was then itself rated by the participants. Socially anxious individuals rated the feedback as less favorable and indicated that they would feel worse about it than nonanxious participants did. They also rated themselves as significantly more likely to receive such an evaluation than did nonanxious participants. Rapee, McCallum, Melville, Ravenscroft, and Rodney (1994, Experiment 3) recently failed to replicate these findings in a sample of clients with social phobia compared with normal controls. However, as noted by Rapee et al. (1994), the two studies employed different mixes of positive and negative feedback—70% for R. Smith and Sarason (1975), 50% for Rapee et al. (1994).

Perfectionism and Standards of Evaluation

Perfectionistic thinking has been implicated in several accounts of social phobia (D. M. Clark & Wells, 1995; Juster, Brown, & Heimberg, 1996a), and several empirical demonstrations have appeared in the literature. Juster et al. (1996b) and Lundh and Öst (1996b) each compared the responses of clients with social phobia and control participants on a measure of perfectionism devised by Frost, Marten, Lahart, and Rosenblate (1990), who define perfectionism as the tendency to set excessively high standards and to be overly self-critical of failure to meet those standards. In both studies, individuals with social phobia scored higher than controls on scales measuring catastrophic concern about the consequences of making mistakes, doubts about the correct course of action to take in a situation, and parental criticism. Persons with social phobia also achieved higher scores on these scales than clients with panic disorder, obsessive–compulsive disorder, or specific phobia in another study (Antony, Purdon, Huta, & Swinson, 1998). Juster et al. (1996b) also reported that high scores on the scales measuring concern over mistakes and doubt about actions were correlated with high scores on several measures of social anxiety.

Alden, Bieling, and Wallace (1994) administered a different measure of perfectionism to a sample of undergraduates. The scale developed by Hewitt and Flett (1991) assesses perfectionistic expectations that one holds for oneself (self-oriented perfectionism), that one holds for others (other-oriented perfectionism), and that the person believes are held for him or her by others (socially prescribed perfectionism). Socially anxious students earned higher perfectionism scores than nonanxious students, but only in the area of socially prescribed perfectionism. This finding was later replicated in samples of clients with social phobia and normal controls (Antony et al., 1998; Bieling & Alden, 1997). It may be that the standards that one believes are held by others are more central to social anxiety than the standards one holds for oneself. Several studies by Alden's research group address this important issue.

In one of the first studies by this group, Alden and Wallace (1991) presented participants with a standard-setting manipulation. That is, they showed participants a videotape of same-sex dyads conversing and getting to know each other. Dyads differed in the degree of conversational skills they displayed. Participants were led to expect that they would soon engage in a similar interaction and were either told that they should attempt to match the performance of either a highly skilled person (high standard) or a less skilled person (low standard), or they were told nothing at all (no standard). Participants were allowed to stop the conversation whenever they wished, and duration of the conversation served as an index of persistence versus withdrawal. Nonanxious participants persisted longer in the low-standard and no-standard conditions than in the high-standard condition, suggesting that they persisted longest when they perceived the greatest probability of positive outcomes. They also persisted longer than the anxious participants in the low-standard and no-standard conditions. Anxious participants showed no differences in persistence in response to the various standards, being generally quick to withdraw.

Important differences arose on participants' self-ratings of their performance in the interaction. Anxious participants rated their success in the interaction no differently than did nonanxious participants. Nevertheless, they reported less comfort and a lesser sense of control over the interaction than their nonanxious peers did. Although they were quicker to terminate the interaction than nonanxious participants, they actually reported a greater sense of pressure to continue beyond the point at which they would have liked to have stopped. Alden and Wallace (1991) reconcile these complex results by suggesting that the anxious participants were more likely to believe that the experimenter held unarticulated expectations for them that they were unable to meet. The perception of these unarticulated expectations appeared to motivate withdrawal from the situation despite the fact that anxious participants viewed their performance as successful.

This study examined the impact of externally imposed standards, but it is the person's own internally generated standards or thoughts about others' standards for them that may be most related to social anxiety. Therefore, Wallace and Alden (1991) examined the discrepancy between self-standards and self-efficacy in social situations. Male participants were told that they would soon have a get-acquainted interaction with a female participant. First, however, they were to interact with a female research assistant as a way to practice for the upcoming experimental interaction. After the "practice" interaction, participants rated their sense of self-efficacy for the upcoming interaction. Using a video-anchored rating scale similar to the one used by Alden and Wallace (1991), participants rated their own (personal) standard for their performance and their perception of the experimenter's standards for them. They also rated the performance that they thought most people would succeed in achieving in the upcoming interaction (social comparison standard).

Nonanxious participants in this study rated themselves quite highly and expected their performance to surpass the standard, whether it was their own, the experimenter's, or the social comparison standard. Socially anxious participants were not so positive. However, they believed that their performance would equal that of most other people (social comparison standard) and that they would be able to match their own personal standard. Consistent with the previous study, socially anxious participants rated their performances as falling short of what the experimenter expected of them. According to Wallace and Alden (1991, p. 250), "social comparative processes and concerns about meeting one's own standards may be of less concern to socially anxious men than concerns about falling short of others' expectations." This finding was essentially replicated by Alden et al. (1994; see also Doerfler & Aron, 1995).

Wallace and Alden (1995, 1997) extended this line of research in a very im-

portant and creative direction. Most nonanxious persons might be expected to increase their expectation of meeting standards of evaluation as a result of prior
success. However, this was not the case among socially anxious students
(Wallace & Alden, 1995) or people with social phobia (Wallace & Alden, 1997).
In the clinical study, clients with generalized social phobia and control participants interacted with an experimental assistant of the opposite sex, and the success of the interaction was manipulated by the behavior of the assistant (e.g.,
warm and receptive vs. cold and aloof) and by the feedback given to the participant by the experimenter. The key finding was the following: Clients with generalized social phobia rated others' standards for them as higher after the successful
interaction than before, but they did not show a similar increase in ratings of their
ability. Control participants did not show this pattern, and clients with social phobia did not show it after failed interactions. Thus, whereas for most of us "nothing succeeds like success," for people with social phobia, success seems only to
up the ante for future interactions. They expect others to expect more from them,
but because success does not lead to improved self-appraisal, they do not believe
they have more to give. In a most paradoxical way, success becomes the basis for
the prediction of future failure.

Safety Behaviors

A. Wells and colleagues (1995) have noted that individuals with social phobia
may be exposed to feared situations repeatedly in everyday life but that this naturally occurring exposure does not usually lead to the reduction of social fears.
These authors suggest several potential reasons for this outcome (attentional bias
for fear-congruent information, self-focused attention, discounting of positive experiences) but they highlight the role of in-situation safety behaviors. In-situation
safety behaviors are those behaviors engaged in by the person while in the feared
situation that have the misleading appearance of helping him or her to better
manage anxiety or better cope with the situation. Examples include gripping a
glass very tightly while drinking in order to keep one's hands from shaking, tens-
ing one's leg muscles and leaning against the nearest solid object when feeling
dizzy and worried about the possibility of fainting, and speaking little in social
situations for fear of saying the wrong thing and evoking others' evaluative wrath
(D. M. Clark & Wells, 1995; A. Wells et al., 1995). If the feared consequence
does not occur, the person tends to attribute this happy outcome to the safety
behavior. However, this may be a serious error of judgment, as safety behaviors
may actually have a number of harmful effects (A. Wells et al., 1995). First, they
may serve to maintain anxiety because they prevent the person from engaging in
a straightforward analysis of the situation and learning that the feared consequence may not have occurred even though the safety behaviors were not performed. Second, the safety behaviors may actually increase the probability that
the feared consequence might happen. The person who grips the glass tightly

might actually experience heightened muscle tension and an increased tremor. The person who speaks little in social encounters may be viewed by others as aloof, uncaring, or above it all.

Alden and Beiling (1998) recently conducted an experimental evaluation of safety behaviors. If these behaviors are strategically implemented, as suggested by A. Wells et al. (1995), we should observe that socially anxious persons implement them more in negative situations than in positive situations. If safety behaviors are counterproductive, their use should be related to less favorable ratings of the socially anxious person by others. In their study, socially anxious and nonanxious persons engaged in a get-to-know-you interaction with an experimental confederate. Through the use of an instructional manipulation, the situation was set up to focus on either the critical nature of the other person or the positive atmosphere that is generated when two similar people share with each other. Several items of importance arose from the analyses. Socially anxious participants were more likely to endorse self-protective motivational goals than nonanxious persons, as has been demonstrated in previous social psychological (Arkin, Appelman, & Burger, 1980) and clinical (Meleshko & Alden, 1993) research. In the negative appraisal condition, but not in the positive appraisal condition, socially anxious participants disclosed information about less intimate topics than did nonanxious individuals, and this pattern of disclosure was associated with less liking of the participant by the confederate.

In the clinical arena, A. Wells et al. (1995) treated eight clients with social phobia via exposure to their feared situations. Two sessions of exposure were administered in a crossover design, one with standard instructions to remain in the feared situation for a planned period of time and the other also including specific instructions to prevent clients from engaging in their habitual in-situation safety behaviors. Regardless of which type of exposure instructions were given first, instructions to reduce safety behaviors led to greater reductions in anxiety and in the strength of clients' beliefs that their feared outcomes would occur. More recently, these findings were essentially replicated in a study of an intensive group treatment (10 full days within 3 weeks) for social phobia (Morgan & Raffle, 1999). The group receiving specific education about the importance of dropping safety behaviors demonstrated more improvement than the group without such instructions.

Partner Similarity and Interpersonal Attraction

One of the most robust findings in the social psychology literature is that people are most attracted to others whom they believe to be similar to themselves (Byrne, 1961; Byrne & Nelson, 1965). Using Byrne's (1961) interpersonal attraction paradigm, we tested the hypothesis that socially anxious persons would be less likely to show this strong effect than nonanxious persons because their preoccupation with themselves and whether they would be evaluated by the other person would interfere with their ability to make interpersonal judgments (Heimberg et al., 1985). Socially anxious and nonanxious students were told that they would soon meet a person of the opposite sex and that the two of them would be expected to interact. The study was described as concerned with "interpersonal perception" and with testing the notion that, given certain information about another person, one could make rather accurate predictions about that person's intelligence, morality, likeability, and so forth. Each participant then completed a questionnaire about age, background, interests, social relationships, and self-perceived attractiveness to the opposite gender. This questionnaire was to be exchanged for the one completed by the other person. However, that person was fictitious, and the participant was provided with a questionnaire completed so that the responses provided by the "other person" would be highly similar or dissimilar to his or her own. Participants were then asked to complete a measure of their attraction to this person whom they believed they were soon to meet.

In fact, our prediction was strongly supported. Nonanxious individuals showed a large difference in attraction to similar and dissimilar partners, replicating the expected similarity-attraction effect. However, socially anxious participants showed absolutely no preference for one type of partner over the other. Furthermore, their ratings were in the middle of the range defined by nonanxious participants' ratings of similar and dissimilar partners, suggesting that they established little sense of either attraction or lack of attraction to either partner. The design of this study did not permit us to completely determine whether socially anxious individuals could not perceive the range of differences between similar and dissimilar partners (although anxious males rated similar partners as more anxious than they rated dissimilar ones), did not attend to them, could not recall them, or could not utilize them effectively when it came to making judgments of attraction. However, it is clear that they did not make the discrimination that nonanxious participants made. Whatever one may think about a preference for similar versus dissimilar others, this inability to make consensual social decisions would predict that socially anxious persons might be vulnerable to making poor relationship choices, choices that might act to increase the aversiveness of interactions with others.

4

Dysfunctional Cognitive Processes in Social Phobia

Most cognitive theories of anxiety focus not only on the content of conscious thought or the judgments that people make about events in their lives but also on more fundamental aspects of our cognitive "equipment" and how it works. Detailed discussion of these theories is beyond the scope of this book, and interested readers are referred to an excellent book on the topic by Williams, Watts, MacLeod, and Mathews (1997). Briefly, the theories of anxiety and emotion put forth by A. T. Beck, Emery, and Greenberg (1985) and Bower (1981, 1987) suggest that anxious individuals should be hypervigilant to threatening information in the environment and should selectively devote attentional capacity to the processing of this information. A. T. Beck et al. (1985) assert that cognitive structures called schemata filter stimulus input such that attention is preferentially directed toward schema-congruent information, that is, toward information that suggests that the world is a dangerous place. For persons with social phobia, this dangerous place is filled with the prospect of social failure, negative evaluation, or rejection. Furthermore, schema-congruent interpretation of ambiguous information and recall of schema-congruent memories should be facilitated. Bower's theory of spreading activation suggests that emotional material is organized into a network of interconnected "nodes." Stimulation of a node by environmental input or emotional state should stimulate other nodes connected to it. Thus any emotional state should facilitate the perception of, attention to, and processing of emotion-related semantic material. A large and expanding body of research in the anxiety disorders has examined these phenomena. Here we review attentional bias toward socially threatening material and whether or not biased memory for social events is shown among persons with social phobia. A third, and relatively new, area of inquiry concerns the perspective taken by persons with social phobia when they recall events in their lives. Do they visualize events as if through their own eyes or through the eyes of an observer?

Attentional Bias toward Social Threat

One of the most frequently utilized tasks for the examination of attentional bias in anxiety-disordered clients has been a modified version of the Stroop color-naming task (Stroop, 1935). In the original task, participants are asked to name the ink color in which words, which are also the names of colors, are printed. When the word *red* is printed in the color *green*, interference is produced between the required color-naming response and the overlearned, but task-irrelevant, reading response, and the result is increased processing and prolonged response times. Otherwise stated, interference is produced to the extent that the meaning of the word attracts attention. Mathews and McLeod (1985) first demonstrated that anxious participants show a similar, although smaller, degree of interference when asked to name the colors in which anxiety-evoking words are presented. These theorists have explained the phenomenon of slowed color naming of threatening words by anxious persons by suggesting that the meaning of these very personally important words captures their attention and interferes with task-relevant responding (i.e., color naming). Since that time, a number of investigators have employed the modified Stroop task to examine attentional bias toward disorder-relevant threat cues among clients with a variety of anxiety disorders (see Williams, Mathews, & MacLeod, 1996, for a review). Only a handful of Stroop studies have been conducted with persons with social phobia.

Mattia, Heimberg, and Hope (1993) examined the color-naming responses of 29 individuals with social phobia and 50 community residents who were age- and gender-matched to the participants with social phobia and screened to assure that they were not themselves socially anxious. Socially threatening words ("boring," "foolish," "inferior," "stupid," "failure"), threatening words related to personal physical and mental health ("insane," "doctor," "illness," "fatal," "hospital"), and neutral words selected to match the social and health threat words on length and frequency of usage served as stimuli. Over the course of the task, a total of 99 words of each type was presented. Words of each type were presented simultaneously on a computer monitor. A "threat index" was calculated for each type of threat word by subtracting the total time required to color-name matched neutral words from the total time required to color-name threat words, such that a higher threat index represents greater interference with color naming.

Compared with the normal controls, the participants with social phobia showed slowed color-naming responses for social-threat, health-threat, and neutral words, suggesting either that they were less efficient at information processing in general or that they may have experienced anxiety over being evaluated in multiple aspects of the task. However, the slowing effect was magnified when they were color-naming social-threat words. Participants with social phobia displayed substantially greater interference (i.e., higher threat index) in the processing of social-threat words than normal participants but about the same amount when processing disorder-irrelevant health-threat words. These results have since been replicated with other samples of clients and matched controls (Amir et al., 1996; Lundh & Öst, 1996b). Interestingly, Amir et al. (1996) demonstrated that slowed color naming of social-threat words is suppressed when individuals with social phobia are made anxious by the prospect of giving a speech. Presumably, the bigger threat of having to give a speech captured their attention to a greater extent than did the Stroop words!

Hope, Rapee, Heimberg, and Dombeck (1990b) examined whether social-threat interference was specific to individuals with social phobia. Sixteen clients with social phobia and 15 clients with panic disorder completed a very similar version of the Stroop task described previously (with the exception that stimulus words were presented on printed cards rather than via computer screen). Both client groups showed substantial interference when color-naming color words. However, they showed very different patterns of interference when color-naming social-threat and health-threat words (see Figure 4.1). Clients with social phobia showed the greatest interference when color-naming social-threat words and virtually none when color-naming health-threat words. Clients with panic disorder demonstrated the reverse pattern, exhibiting the greatest interference in response to health-threat words, although they did show a statistically nonsignificant degree of interference with social-threat words, as well. Interestingly, interference when color-naming social-threat words was significantly correlated with the degree of self-reported avoidance behavior among clients with social phobia.

McNeil et al. (1995a) conducted another study of Stroop response among individuals with social phobia. In this study, several different types of social-threat words were employed. First, McNeil et al. administered the social-threat words employed by Mattia et al. (1993), listed previously, which were taken to represent negative social evaluation. They also presented threat words that were specific to public speaking (e.g., "speech," "audience"), words that referred to general social interactional settings (e.g., "party," "conversation"), and neutral words matched to the words in each of the social-threat categories. These Stroop stimuli were presented to 12 clients whose social phobias were specific to fears of speaking in public ("circumscribed speech phobics") and 25 clients with generalized social phobia (8 of whom also met criteria for avoidant personality disorder). Two findings are of interest. First, there were no differences between clients with generalized social phobia with and without avoidant personality disorder for any of these tests, suggesting that these two subgroups of clients are not different in terms of attentional bias. Second, both groups of individuals with generalized social phobia showed significantly more interference than the clients with cir-

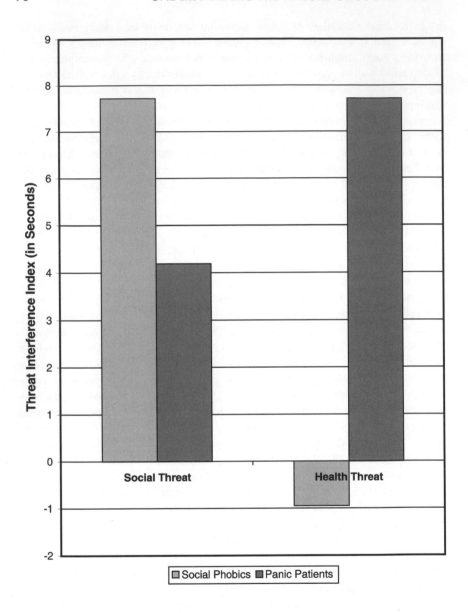

FIGURE 4.1. Color-naming latencies of social phobics and patients with panic disorder for social-threat and health-threat words. Threat index is equal to the total time required to color-name control words subtracted from the total time required to color-name threat words. Adapted from data presented in "Representations of the Self in Social Phobia: Vulnerability to Social Threat," by D. A. Hope, R. M. Rapee, R. G. Heimberg, and M. Dombeck, 1990, *Cognitive Therapy and Research, 14*, p. 184. Copyright 1990 by Kluwer Academic/Plenum Publishers. Adapted by permission.

cumscribed speech phobias when color-naming general social interactional words, a finding that further supports those of Hope et al. (1990b) and Mattia et al. (1993), suggesting that attentional bias may be specific to the stimuli feared by the individual. No differences in degree of interference were noted among clients with social phobia in color-naming the speech words or negative evaluative words.

In each of the preceding studies, words of a specific stimulus type were presented as a block, either on printed cards or computer monitors. However, there is no necessity that the stimulus words be presented in that way, especially since the advent of personal computers. Most investigators now present word stimuli to the computer screen one at a time and randomly intermix words of different stimulus types. Cassiday, McNally, and Zeitlin (1992) examined the impact of blocked versus randomized presentation orders on the color-naming latencies of rape victims with and without posttraumatic stress disorder, and we have recently done the same with individuals with social phobia (Holle, Neely, & Heimberg, 1997). We also examined whether part of the difference in color-naming social-threat versus neutral words that had been demonstrated in previous studies might have been due to the fact that social-threat words are inherently more closely related to each other than randomly selected neutral words. Social-threat words, related neutral words (all words were members of the class of animal names), and unrelated neutral words were presented to 24 participants with social phobia in either randomized or blocked format. Several findings emerged from this study. First, there were no differences in color-naming latencies for the different word types when words were presented in the random format. However, there were large differences in color-naming latencies between word types in the blocked presentation format. Social-threat words led to the slowest color-naming times, slower than animal names and unrelated neutral words. Animal names also resulted in slower color-naming times than unrelated neutral words. Thus words that have some relatedness to each other may "prime" each other (that is, they may stimulate each other in semantic memory), and this phenomenon may account for some, but not all, of the interference produced by color-naming social-threat words.

Participants with social phobia were also slower to color-name social-threat words in the blocked format than in the random format, and this finding led us to further examine the process of color-naming in the blocked format. The blocked condition involved the presentation of words from the same category for 48 consecutive trials. Figure 4.2 displays the color-naming latencies for each word type in blocks of six trials, and the pattern is quite interesting. Although the relative speed of color-naming the different word stimuli remained the same across trials (social-threat words slower than animal names slower than unrelated neutral words), the absolute time it took to complete the color-naming task increased over time. The average time it took to color-name a social-threat word increased from 633 milliseconds to 698 milliseconds, a large difference in studies of this

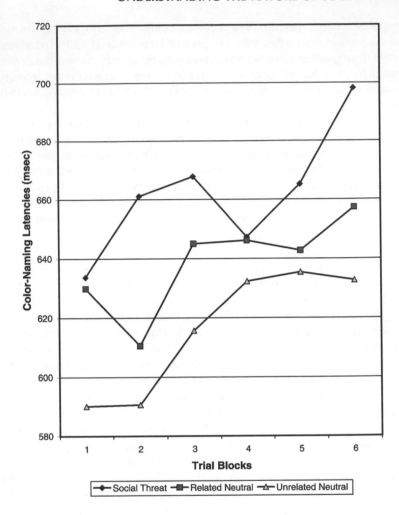

FIGURE 4.2. Color-naming latencies for social threat, related neutral, and unrelated neutral words across blocks of six trials. From "The Effects of Blocked versus Random Presentation and Semantic Relatedness of Stimulus Words on Response to a Modified Stroop Task among Social Phobics," by C. Holle, J. H. Neely, and R. G. Heimberg, 1997, *Cognitive Therapy and Research, 21*, p. 691. Copyright 1997 by Kluwer Academic/Plenum Publishers. Reprinted by permission.

type, and similar increases were noted for both categories of neutral words. The reasons for this slowing are not entirely clear, but it may simply be that the task becomes fatiguing over time. Nevertheless, it is tempting to speculate that the individuals with social phobia, when called on to take part in a social situation that lasts for an extended period, might experience ever-increasing interference from perceived social threat. It may be that the person might find it increasingly difficult not to pay attention to the threatening aspect of the ongoing situation, a tendency that creates the perception of increasing danger or at least works against the possibility that the person might calm down on continued exposure to the situation. Although the behavioral and emotional implications of this finding remained to be explored in future research, this is an intriguing explanation of why people with social phobia often tell us that they have tried exposure to feared situations over and over again with little success.

None of the aforementioned studies included positively valenced words as a comparison condition. It has been suggested that attentional bias, as assessed by the modified Stroop task, may be a function of the "emotionality" of the words, rather than the threatening meaning of the words alone (Martin, Williams, & Clark, 1991). Maidenberg, Chen, Craske, Bohn, and Bystritsky (1996) used a modified Stroop task to examine the response latencies of clients with social phobia to seven categories of stimulus words: social threat, social positive, panic threat, panic positive, general threat, general positive, and neutral. Participants with social phobia rated the positive words as more emotional than the threatening words, stacking the odds in favor of finding longer response latencies for positive words than threatening words if the "emotionality" hypothesis were true. As demonstrated in previous research, individuals with social phobia showed longer response times to social-threat words than to neutral words. In contrast to what would be expected from the emotionality hypothesis, they did not demonstrate longer response times to social-positive words than to neutral words, and their response times to the social-positive words were similar to their response times to the panic-positive and general-positive words. This study, in combination with previous research, suggests that individuals with social phobia do not simply attend to all emotional information. Rather, they exhibit an attentional bias that favors the processing of threatening social information.

An interesting question to consider is whether interference with the color-naming of social-threat words is reduced as a result of successful treatment of social phobia. Mattia et al. (1993), in a second experiment, addressed this question. Participants in a treatment study received either CBGT, the monoamine oxidase inhibitor phenelzine, or a pill placebo. Small *n*s limited our ability to make statements about response to specific treatments. Clients were classified as responders or nonresponders to treatment on the basis of their responses to the Anxiety Disorders Interview Schedule—Revised (DiNardo & Barlow, 1988). Responders and nonresponders did not differ in the magnitude of their social-threat indices before treatment. However, responders showed a significant decrease in social-threat index scores by posttreatment, at which time their scores were also significantly lower than the scores of nonresponders.

In interpreting the results of studies utilizing the modified Stroop task, it is important to note that some authors (Cloitre, Heimberg, Holt, & Liebowitz, 1992a; de Ruiter & Brosschot, 1994) have questioned whether or not the Stroop task is a pure measure of attentional bias toward threatening stimuli. Cloitre et al. (1992a) suggest that slowed color-naming of threatening words not only may be the result of impaired attentional processes but also may be attributable to impairment or inhibition of the response system. De Ruiter and Brosschot (1994) assert that the Stroop task may tap both bias toward threat and anxiety-motivated avoidance of further elaboration of the same threatening material. Arguments such as these have led other investigators to employ other paradigms in their attempts to study attentional processes in social phobia and other anxiety disorders. One such example is the dot-probe paradigm, an experimental setup that has been employed in several studies of clients with generalized anxiety disorder (MacLeod, Mathews, & Tata, 1986), those with panic disorder (Asmundson, Sandler, Wilson, & Walker, 1992; J. G. Beck, Stanley, Averill, Baldwin, & Deagle, 1992), and high-anxious normals (MacLeod & Mathews, 1988). In the dot-probe paradigm, attentional allocation is separated from response inhibition because participants are required to make a neutral response (key press) to a neutral stimulus (visual dot probe; Elting & Hope, 1995; Heimberg, 1994). Typically the participant is instructed that word pairs will be briefly presented (e.g., 500 milliseconds) on the computer screen, separated vertically by a few centimeters. On seeing the words, the participant is to read the word in the upper position, thereby focusing attention in that area. On some trials, a small dot (the "dot probe") appears immediately following the offset of the word pair in the position of either the top or bottom word. The participant's task is to press a designated key as quickly as possible on detecting the probe. Selective attention to threat is measured by the difference in reaction time to the dot probe when it appears in the location formerly occupied by threat versus neutral words.

Asmundson and Stein (1994) presented social-threat words, health-threat words, and neutral words to participants with generalized social phobia and to normal control participants utilizing the dot-probe paradigm. Participants with social phobia responded more quickly to dot probes following social-threat words than to dot probes following health-threat or neutral words. Control participants did not demonstrate preferential allocation of attention to threatening stimuli of either type, as their reaction times to social-threat, health-threat, and neutral words did not differ (see Figure 4.3). Interestingly, these differences were noted only for word stimuli presented to the upper position, that is, the location of the words that the participants were asked to read. No differences occurred for words in the lower position, suggesting that attentional bias toward social threat in this study was related to active processing of the stimulus words.

The several studies reviewed here provide support for the notion that socially anxious individuals exhibit an attentional bias for threatening social cues. These experiments could be criticized, however, as lacking external validity. A recent study examined attentional bias among socially anxious individuals using a more naturalistic experimental situation. Similar to the dot-probe task, the experimental paradigm employed by Veljaca and Rapee (1998) was constructed so that attentional bias facilitated task performance. College undergraduates high and low in social anxiety were asked to give a 5-minute presentation to a three-

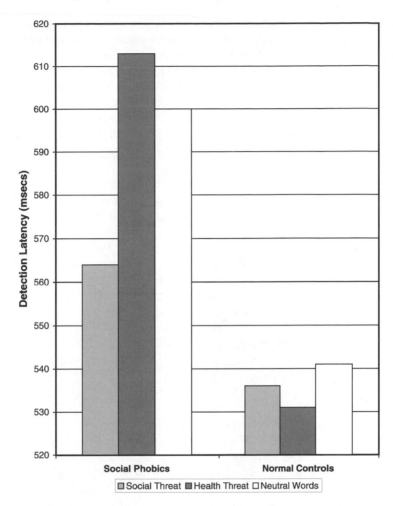

FIGURE 4.3. Probe detection latencies as a function of word type in social phobics and normal controls. Adapted from data presented in "Selective Processing of Social Threat in Patients with Generalized Social Phobia: Evaluation Using a Dot-Probe Paradigm," by G. J. G. Asmundson and M. B. Stein, 1994, *Journal of Anxiety Disorders, 8,* pp. 113–114. Copyright 1994 by Elsevier Science. Adapted by permission.

person audience. Members of the audience engaged in a total of seven behaviors suggesting a positive reaction (e.g., smiling, nodding) and seven behaviors suggesting a negative reaction (e.g., yawning, looking at their watches) to the speech. Participants indicated observation of these audience behaviors by pressing one button when a positive reaction was detected and another button when a negative reaction was detected. Participants high in social anxiety detected significantly more negative than positive audience reactions. Conversely, participants low in social anxiety detected significantly more positive than negative reactions (see Figure 4.4). Additional analyses revealed that socially anxious participants were more accurate at detecting negative reactions than positive reactions, whereas low-anxious participants were more accurate at the identification of positive behaviors. Socially anxious individuals also exhibited a response bias in that

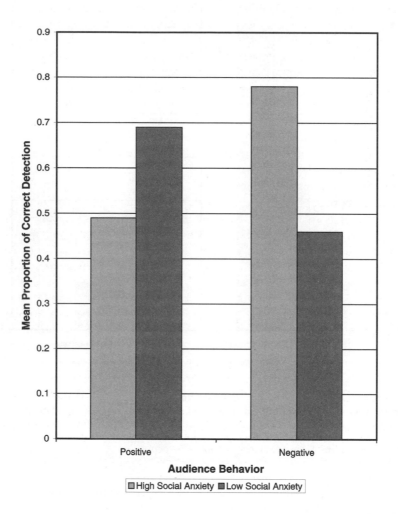

FIGURE 4.4. Mean proportion of correct detection as a function of audience behavior (negative vs. positive) and social anxiety level (high vs. low). From "Detection of Negative and Positive Audience Behaviors by Socially Anxious Subjects," by K. A. Veljaca and R. M. Rapee, 1998, *Behaviour Research and Therapy, 36,* p. 316. Copyright 1998 by Elsevier Science. Reprinted by permission.

they used more liberal criteria to report a reaction as negative than as positive, whereas low-anxious participants did not.

Veljaca and Rapee (1998) found evidence for greater accuracy for detecting social-threat cues, but Winton et al. (1995), in their study of the interpretation of others' emotions, did not. Differences in task demands may account for these disparate outcomes. In the Winton et al. (1995) study, participants examined one slide at a time, but very briefly (60 milliseconds). Such brief presentations should maximize uncertainty and minimize detection accuracy (Veljaca & Rapee, 1998). Furthermore, detection accuracy should be facilitated to the extent that attention is devoted to the stimulus. Veljaca and Rapee (1998) required participants to divide their attention among a variety of tasks (giving a speech, scanning for positive and negative reactions among three people, pressing buttons), demanding that they strategically determine to what their attention should be directed. Other studies of attentional allocation in anxious persons (MacLeod & Mathews, 1991; Mogg, Mathews, Eysenck, & May, 1991) suggest that it is in this type of task, in which participants must determine their own processing priorities, that attentional bias is most evident. Thus the heightened detection accuracy for negative information among socially anxious participants may reflect their biased attention toward those cues.

It has been suggested that, although anxious individuals may initially shift their attention toward fear-relevant stimuli, they may then strategically avoid elaborative processing of the threatening stimuli in order to reduce anxiety (Cloitre et al., 1992a; D. M. Clark & Wells, 1995; de Ruiter & Brosschot, 1994; Mogg, Bradley, Bono, & Painter, 1997). Amir, Foa, and Coles (1998a) examined this "vigilance-avoidance" hypothesis using a homograph paradigm (Gernsbacher, Varner, & Faust, 1990). Homographs are words that have multiple meanings (e.g., the word "chicken" can refer to a bird or a cowardly person). Participants were presented with a series of sentences, and each sentence was followed by a single word. The participants' task was to decide whether or not the stimulus word fit the meaning of the sentence. For half of the critical trials, the last word in the sentence was a nonhomograph, and the stimulus word following the sentence was a social-threat word (e.g., "She cut off the string." ABANDON). For the other half of the critical trials, the last word in the sentence was a homograph, and the stimulus word following the sentence implied the socially threatening meaning of the homograph but did not fit the meaning of the sentence (e.g., "She wrote down the mean." UNFRIENDLY). Longer response latencies to social-threat words following sentences ending in homographs than in nonhomographs are thought to represent automatic activation of the threatening meaning of the homograph. That is, automatic activation of the threatening meaning of the homograph interferes with decision making and increases response latency. Each stimulus word was presented at either a short (100-millisecond) or a long (850-millisecond) stimulus-onset asynchrony (SOA) in order to examine whether inhibition or avoidance of the threatening meaning of homographs occurs when enough time has elapsed for controlled processing. In fact, at the short SOA, clients with social phobia exhibited longer response latencies to social-threat words for sentences ending in socially relevant homographs than in nonhomographs. However, at the long SOA, clients with social phobia actually showed shorter response latencies to social-threat words for sentences ending in socially relevant homographs than in nonhomographs. These results suggest that, during early stages of processing, clients with social phobia have a bias toward the detection of threat-relevant information but, during later stages of processing, they are characterized by enhanced strategic avoidance of such information. In contrast, normal control participants responded to social-threat words following homograph and non-homograph sentences with similar response latencies at both short and long SOAs, suggesting that the threatening meaning of these words may never have been activated for them. These complex data are presented in Figure 4.5.

Yuen (1994) conducted a study that puts a twist on the standard investigation of attentional bias. High and low socially anxious students (classified according to scores on the FNE Scale) were presented with a dot-probe task in which negative and neutral facial expressions served as stimuli rather than threat and neutral words. To ensure that all participants were in a state of social anxiety during the experiment, they were led to believe that they would soon have to give a speech to a small audience. In contrast to Asmundson and Stein (1994) and all other dot-probe studies with anxious students and clients, the high socially anxious participants were *slower* at locating the dot probe if it appeared in the location previously occupied by the negative facial expression than if it appeared in the location at which the neutral face had been. Low-anxious participants showed no difference in reaction times between the two locations.

D. M. Clark and Wells (1995) attempt to resolve the discrepancy between the results of Yuen (1994) and other studies of attentional bias in anxiety with the following arguments. Word stimuli and faces are fundamentally different. Yuen's study of "face processing" may model attention to actual social cues, whereas the "word processing" studies may be more closely related to mental preoccupation with frightening ideas. Social phobics may show an attentional bias toward social-threat words not because they are hypervigilant for negative social cues but because they are ruminatively preoccupied with thoughts of negative self-evaluation. D. M. Clark and Wells (1995) also offer the alternative notion that Yuen's participants may have shown a vigilance-avoidance response to the negative facial expressions. Because the stimulus presentation time used in Yuen's study was 1 second (compared with 500 millisecond in Asmundson & Stein, 1994, and other studies using the dot-probe paradigm), it is possible that the avoidance portion of this response could have manifested itself in their study but not in others. It is also interesting to speculate that the slowed response to threatening faces might have occurred because the anxious participant acted as if he or she were trying to minimize "eye contact" with the negative face.

To further examine this issue, Mansell, Clark, Ehlers, and Chen (1999) further modified the dot-probe task. They presented negative, neutral, or positive

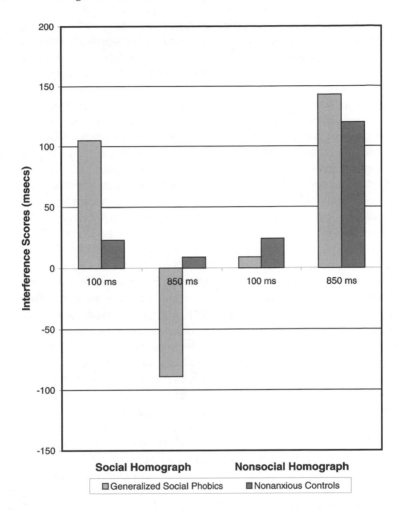

FIGURE 4.5. Mean interference scores of generalized social phobics (GSPs) and non-anxious controls (NACs) in response to social and nonsocial homographs at short (100 millisecond) and long (850 millisecond) stimulus onset asynchrony. From "Automatic Activation and Strategic Avoidance of Threat-Relevant Information in Social Phobia," by N. Amir, E. B. Foa, and M. E. Coles, 1998, *Journal of Abnormal Psychology, 107,* p. 288. Copyright 1998 by the American Psychological Association. Reprinted by permission.

faces in one screen location and pictures of household objects at another. Stimuli were presented for 500 milliseconds rather than 1 second. To examine whether the pattern reported by Yuen (1994) may have been the result of the induction of social threat, half of the participants were led to expect that they would soon give a speech, whereas the other half were not. High socially anxious students (classified according to scores on the FNE Scale), compared with low-anxious students, again showed a bias to direct their attention away from negative facial expressions. However, there were two additional findings of interest. First, this pattern was evident only when participants expected to give a speech and was absent otherwise. Second, they showed a similar pattern of slowed responding to positive facial expressions. Regarding the latter finding, the authors speculate that positive facial expressions, just like negative ones, mean that the other person is reacting to the participant in some way. Averting one's gaze may be a means to avoid that engagement. They also speculate that a positive facial expression may not be automatically interpreted as positive by socially anxious persons. A positive facial expression may signal that the other person is laughing at you!

Gilboa-Schechtman, Foa, and Amir (1999) have conducted the only study so far that examined attention to facial expressions in a clinical sample of persons with social phobia. They employed the "face-in-the-crowd" paradigm developed by Hansen and Hansen (1988). This paradigm involves the simultaneous presentation of 12 faces (all of the same person). On some trials, all 12 faces are identical. On target trials, one face differs from all the others; that is, it is a picture of the same person, but the person has a different facial expression. As a test of the hypothesis that persons with social phobia would show an attentional bias *toward* threatening faces, angry, disgusted, happy, and neutral facial expressions were presented in "crowds" that were otherwise composed of happy, angry, or neutral faces. Of greatest interest here is that individuals with social phobia, compared with nonanxious control participants, were faster to detect an angry face in a neutral crowd. They were also slower to detect a neutral face in an angry crowd. Both of these outcomes are consistent with an attentional bias toward threatening faces and at odds with the findings of Yuen (1994) and Mansell et al. (1999).

In summary, a growing but complex body of research suggests that socially anxious individuals demonstrate an attentional bias toward the detection of threatening social information. Some preliminary evidence suggests that they may exhibit a "vigilance-avoidance" pattern of information processing, characterized by automatic detection of threat followed by strategic avoidance of elaborative processing of such information (Amir et al., 1998a). Mogg and colleagues (1997) suggest that this pattern of processing might maintain anxiety by increasing the likelihood that threatening information will be detected but decreasing the likelihood that habituation to and objective evaluation of threatening information will occur.

Memory Bias for Threatening Social Information

If anxious persons demonstrate an attentional bias toward threat information, they may also show enhanced recall of threat information. However, empirical support for memory bias in the anxiety disorders is less consistent than it is for attentional bias. At present, there is support for enhanced recall of disorder-relevant threat information in panic disorder (Cloitre & Liebowitz, 1991; McNally, Foa, & Donnell, 1989) and posttraumatic stress disorder (Vrana, Roodman, & Beckham, 1995), but not in generalized anxiety disorder (Mogg & Mathews, 1990; Mogg, Mathews, & Weinman, 1987). The data for a memory bias in social anxiety and social phobia is confused at best.

Several studies have demonstrated preferential recall of negative information about the self in socially anxious undergraduates (Breck & Smith, 1983; O'Banion & Arkowitz, 1977; T. Smith, Ingram, & Brehm, 1983). Breck and Smith (1983), for instance, exposed socially anxious and nonanxious female students to a depth-of-processing task (Craik & Tulving, 1975). That is, several positive and negative trait adjectives were presented to participants, who were asked to judge whether or not a word was long, meaningful, or descriptive of themselves. Social-evaluative threat was also manipulated by informing some participants that they would later be asked to interact with a male stranger and might also be evaluated by him. The most theoretically interesting data concern the performance of participants on an unannounced free recall test, especially in regard to recall of adjectives judged to be self-descriptive. Socially anxious women recalled significantly more negative self-descriptive traits and significantly fewer positive self-descriptive traits than nonanxious women. The pattern for negative trait adjectives was most evident when participants were led to believe that they would soon interact with the male stranger.

T. Smith and colleagues (1983) also conducted a depth-of-processing study in which they asked socially anxious students, "Was the word read by a man or a woman?" "Does the word mean the same thing as _____?" "Does the word describe you?" and "Would your friends say the word describes you?" The first two questions were presumed to facilitate superficial processing. The third question should facilitate self-referent processing, similar to the question utilized by Breck and Smith (1983). The fourth question was intended to facilitate the processing of the word as related to evaluation by others, an important aspect of social anxiety ("public self-referent"). As in the previous study, Smith et al. (1983) manipulated social stress, this time by telling participants that they would each have to stand before an audience and talk about themselves while being evaluated by the audience members. In contrast to the findings of Breck and Smith (1983), socially anxious participants in the high-stress condition recalled more words processed with the public self-referent question but did not differ from nonanxious participants in the number of self-referent words recalled.

Studies in samples of clients with social phobia have been less likely to find support for a memory bias. Hope, Sigler, Penn, and Meier (1998) found enhanced recall of self-referent (but not public self-referent) social threat words. Although the design of their study was very similar to that of Smith et al. (1983), their results were more consistent with those of Breck and Smith (1983). However, other studies of memory bias in social phobia have come up empty. Cloitre, Cancienne, Heimberg, Holt, and Liebowitz (1995) found no evidence of biased recall of social-threat words in either a high-speed recognition task or a free-recall test, although the paradigm they employed was used successfully to examine recall biases in clients with panic disorder (Cloitre & Liebowitz, 1991). Rapee et al. (1994), in a comprehensive series of studies, found no evidence at all for memory bias in social phobia in recognition or recall tasks, on tests of implicit versus explicit memory, in recall of positive versus negative feedback after imagined public speaking, or on an autobiographical memory task.

Rapee et al. (1994), in their second experiment, failed to demonstrate enhanced memory for social-threat words on tests of explicit memory (or controlled/intentional memory processes) or implicit memory (or automatic memory processes). However, in a similar study, Lundh and Öst (1997) demonstrated an implicit memory bias among clients with nongeneralized social phobia. In these two studies, cued stem-completion tasks, in which participants are instructed to complete word stems from their memory of the words on a previously presented list, were employed to tap explicit memory, whereas uncued stem-completion tasks, in which participants are instructed to complete each word stem with the first appropriate word that comes to mind, were employed to tap implicit memory. Although the research provides little evidence that socially anxious and nonanxious persons differ in terms of explicit memory for social threat, it is harder to draw conclusions with regard to implicit memory. Tasks such as the uncued stem-completion task have been criticized because they may tap into multiple processes that affect memory. They may actually assess a combination of intentional and automatic processes (Jacoby, Toth, & Yonelinas, 1993), making the results of the "implicit" portion of these studies difficult to interpret.

Amir, Foa, and Coles (2001) conducted a study using a noise judgment paradigm (Jacoby, Allan, Collins, & Larwill, 1988), which is an implicit memory task less likely to be contaminated by explicit memory processes than the uncued word-stem-completion task. Clients with generalized social phobia and normal controls listened to and repeated neutral sentences (e.g., "The manual tells you how to set up the tent") and socially threatening sentences (e.g., "The classmate asks you to go for drinks"). In the test phase, participants were presented with sentences masked by white noise at different volumes and were asked to rate the volume of the white noise. Both neutral and social-threat sentences were presented in the test phase; half of these sentences were novel ("new"), and half had been previously presented ("old"). In this paradigm, lower noise ratings for old sentences than for new sentences are interpreted to indicate implicit memory for the old sentences. In fact, individuals with generalized social phobia gave lower noise ratings to old social-threat sentences than to old neutral sentences. Normal controls did not rate old threat and neutral sentences differently. These results suggest that individuals with generalized social phobia may demonstrate an implicit memory bias for disorder-specific threatening information.

Recent attention has been devoted to memory for facial expressions. As noted earlier, faces may be more meaningful stimuli than the words used in most studies of information processing, and it may therefore be easier to demonstrate memory biases for faces, if they do exist. In one study, clients with generalized social phobia, unlike nonanxious controls, demonstrated better recognition memory for angry or disgusted facial expressions than for neutral or happy facial expressions (Foa, Gilboa-Schechtman, Amir, & Freshman, 2000). In a similar study, Lundh and Öst (1996a) found that clients with social phobia and normal controls made similar judgments regarding how "critical" or "accepting" a face appeared to be. However, in a later recognition memory task, clients with social phobia recognized a higher proportion of faces they had previously rated as "critical" than faces they had previously rated as "accepting." In contrast, normal controls tended to recognize a higher proportion of faces they had previously rated as "accepting." This study is particularly interesting because, together with another study by this research group, it suggests that the way a person encodes a stimulus is very important in determining whether it will be recalled. Lundh, Thulin, Czyzykow, and Öst (1998) administered the same task to clients who had panic disorder with agoraphobia. In contrast to the performance of clients with social phobia, clients with agoraphobia showed no difference in recall of faces they had previously rated as "critical" versus "accepting." However, they recalled more faces that they had previously rated as "safe" than faces that they had rated as "unsafe" (the concept of "safe" persons is very important to persons with agoraphobia, whereas the concept of "critical" vs. "accepting" is not).

The literature on memory bias in social phobia and the other anxiety disorders is more completely reviewed by Coles and Heimberg (2002). The best studies converge to suggest that persons with social phobia do tend to recall faces or words that are initially encoded as being relevant to the self (e.g., negative self-referent words) or that may be relevant to their safety or lack of it (e.g., critical faces) in biased fashion. However, much more study is needed.

Disrupted Memory for Information about the Social Environment

Whether or not a memory bias for social threat exists, other aspects of memory are also worthy of our research attention. One such aspect concerns whether memory for everyday information is disrupted among people with social phobia. One might hypothesize that socially anxious persons would be so self-focused during social interactions that they would have difficulty recalling information from these interactions. (Note that this hypothesis implies that poor recall may be a function of poor encoding and not a problem of memory per se). In fact, several studies have examined this very phenomenon. Stopa and Clark (1993) examined the recall of people with social phobia after the conversation with the research assistant, described earlier. Neither a recognition test of items the assistant wore during the conversation and of items and sounds present in the laboratory or a recall test of the content of the conversation yielded significant findings. However, several other studies have provided more supportive evidence. Kimble and Zehr (1982) reported that socially anxious persons were less able to recall the names of persons to whom they had been introduced. In another study, speech-anxious individuals recalled less information about the environment in which they made a speech than did non-speech-anxious persons (Daly, Vangelisti, & Lawrence, 1989). In yet another, socially anxious persons had more difficulty recalling information presented just prior to their turn to speak in front of a group (Bond & Omar, 1990). Hope, Heimberg, and Klein (1990a) also found evidence of disrupted recall of socially transmitted information.

Hope et al. (1990a) asked high and low socially anxious undergraduate women to take part in a conversation with an undergraduate man (actually a research assistant). As the interaction began, participants were put in a situation of either high or low social-evaluative threat. In the high-threat condition, participants were told that the experiment concerned how women make impressions on men and that their behavior in the conversations would be videotaped and later rated by the man. In the low-threat condition, the man was the focus of evaluation. Participant and assistant were asked to converse and get to know one another but told to follow a structured list of topics, as required by the research. After the conversation was completed, the participants were asked to complete a 12-item questionnaire assessing their memory of the background and interests of the assistant. High socially anxious students recalled less information about the assistant than did low-anxious students, and they were more likely to recall incorrect information, as well. Anxious participants' recall tended to be most impaired in the high-threat condition. We also examined the frequency with which participants provided no answers to recall-test items. In the high-threat condition, socially anxious students made more omission errors than low-anxious students. Interestingly, however, the pattern was reversed in the low-threat condition. That is, low-anxious students showed poorer recall in the low-threat condition than did the high-anxious students. Maybe in that condition they just did not care!

Perspective Taking in Social Phobic Imagery and Recall

D. M. Clark and Wells (1995; Stopa & Clark, 1993) assert that when a person with social phobia perceives that he or she may fail to make a desired impression on others, his or her attention shifts to detailed self-observation and self-monitoring. The information generated in this process may be used to infer how the person appears to others and what those others think of him or her. This line of reasoning also suggests that cognitive activity in the form of imagery may be as important to the person with social phobia as are cognitive self-statements.

Hackmann, Surawy, and Clark (1998) compared the reports of spontaneous images of 30 individuals with social phobia and 30 nonanxious controls. Participants were asked to recall a recent social situation in which they had experienced anxiety and to report whether an image had passed through their minds at their most anxious moment. They were then asked to evoke the image and rate whether the predominant perspective was " 'one of viewing the situation as if looking out through their eyes, observing the details of what was going on around them' (the field perspective), *or* 'one in which they were observing the self, looking at the self from an external point of view' (observer perspective)" (1998, p. 6). Clinicians also rated images for emotionality.

More participants with social phobia (77%) than controls (47%) reported experiencing images in social situations at least "sometimes." The images of people with social phobia were more negative and more likely to be viewed from the observer perspective. Hackmann et al. (1998) provide several examples of clients' images, which typically involved the visual portrayal of how they might appear to others in catastrophic social situations. For example:

> *Client D's* predominant fear was that other people would see he *looked nervous*. He described the image he experienced while eating in a restaurant as follows: I am rushing through the restaurant trying to get past people, knocking them over, it's crowded and other people are looking confused. Where's he gone? What's happening? I look hot and sweating, silent.
> *Client F's* predominant fear was that people would think he was *stupid, inarticulate, and boring*. He described the image he experienced during an episode at work as follows: Picture of me looking guilty, nervous, anxious, embarrassed. It's my face—features distorted, intensified, big nose, weak chin, big ears, red face. Slightly awkward body posture, turning in on myself. Accent more pronounced. I sound stupid, not articulate or communicating well. (p. 9, emphasis in original)

A. Wells, Clark, and Ahmad (1998) examined memories for anxiety-evoking social and nonsocial situations. When asked to form an image of a recent social situation in which they felt really anxious and uncomfortable, individuals with social phobia were more likely than normal controls to rate the image as being from an observer's perspective. However, when asked to form an image of a recent nonsocial situation in which they felt really anxious and uncomfortable, both groups rated their images as from a field perspective.

A. Wells and Papageorgiou (1999) found that only clients with social evaluative concerns (individuals with social phobia or agoraphobia) reported an observer perspective for images when recalling anxiety-provoking social situations. Individuals with blood or injury phobias and normal controls reported a field perspective for memories of both social and nonsocial situations. Interestingly, only individuals with social phobia demonstrated a shift from a field perspective when recalling nonsocial situations to an observer perspective when recalling social situations; all other groups reported the same perspective for memories of both social and nonsocial situations. In summary, these studies suggest that, when asked to recall a recent anxiety-provoking social situation or images experienced during these situations, individuals with social phobia reported taking an observer perspective.

The study of perspective taking in social phobic imagery is just beginning, but it promises to be an important area of future research. Research in social psychology over many years has demonstrated that observer and field perspectives are related to differences in attributions about the actor in the image (Watson, 1982). The field perspective is most likely to be associated with attributions for behavior to situational factors, whereas the observer perspective is associated with attributions to traits of the observed individual (Frank & Gilovich, 1989). If the observer perspective is taken by a person with social phobia who by definition does not like what he sees of himself in a social situation and who then makes a negative trait attribution to account for it, the image may be a contributing factor to his continuing anxiety and impairment. In fact, this is essentially what we found in a recent study of memory perspective in individuals with social phobia and normal controls (Coles, Turk, Heimberg, & Fresco, 2001). Participants were asked to recall social situations in which they had experienced low, medium, or high anxiety. As the anxiety experienced in the recalled situation increased, participants with social phobia were increasingly likely to take the observer perspective, but this was not the case for control participants. Also, as the anxiety experienced in the recalled situation increased, attributions made by participants with social phobia for their performances became more internal, stable, and global, whereas the attributions of control participants showed the opposite pattern.

5

A Cognitive-Behavioral Formulation of Social Phobia

with Ronald M. Rapee and Cynthia L. Turk

In the last several chapters, we have shared with you most of what we know about social phobia, from basic information about its prevalence to the many varieties of cognitive biases and errors in thinking that may characterize the persons who suffer from it. In this chapter, we try to bring some of this material one step closer to real life by looking closely at Joe, a client with social phobia; his experiences that may have contributed to the development of his disorder; the difficulties he had in adjusting to adult life; and the cognitive biases and logical errors that made it difficult for him to function well in everyday life.[1] In so doing, we rely heavily on our prior work on the etiology of social phobia (Juster et al., 1996a) and on the experiences of persons with social phobia when confronted with demands for social interaction or performance in front of others (Rapee & Heimberg, 1997; Turk, Lerner, Heimberg, & Rapee, 2001). Many of the topics discussed in previous chapters appear in our presentation of Joe. Here, we demonstrate how several of these factors may interact with each other in the experience of the person with social phobia.

Ronald M. Rapee, PhD, is Professor, Department of Psychology at Macquarie University, Sydney, Australia.

Cynthia L. Turk, PhD, is Associate Director of the Adult Anxiety Clinic of Temple University, Philadelphia, Pennsylvania.

The Client

Joe is 37 years old. He is the eldest of three children born to a family of Italian descent and brought up in a tight-knit blue-collar neighborhood in the city. He has lived his entire life within a few blocks of the house in which he was born and in which his mother still resides, and he spends most of his leisure time at his mother's home. His mother, now in her 60s, is alive and in good physical health. However, she has a history of episodes of probable major depression. In between episodes, she would appear to have been quite an anxious person herself, and Joe describes her both as one might describe a person with generalized anxiety disorder ("a world-class worrywart") and as a person with social phobia ("always shy and withdrawn," "terribly concerned about what everyone thought about her and the rest of the family," "never felt loved or accepted in the community"). Joe's father passed away more than 10 years ago. Before his death from a heart attack and other complications of high blood pressure, he had had a history of intermittent problems with alcohol abuse and with controlling his temper. In his younger years, Joe was subjected to his father's constant criticisms directed either at him or at his mother.

Joe was educated in the city's public schools and graduated from high school. He did well, but not as well as his teachers thought he could. He wanted to go on to university studies, but he was too frightened to venture out on his own. He had always had a problem talking to his teachers and speaking up in class. Doing so at college, in large classes with other students looking on, was more than he could expect of himself. After he finished high school, he took evening classes at the local community college for a while but found that too stressful and gave it up. He got a job, with his father's help, in the local butcher shop, which was owned by one of his father's boyhood friends. He worked mostly in the back of the shop, but during other employees' lunch breaks or at busy times, he would have to wait on customers. Most of the time, he kept to himself, talking little to the other employees (although he wanted to be friends with them), and he spent much of each day worried that he might have to help a customer with an order.

Joe had some good friends whom he had known since childhood. A few still lived in the old neighborhood, and they would sometimes get together to watch a ball game or play cards. On those occasions, Joe tended to drink too much because it made him feel more comfortable. Most of his friends, however, no longer lived in the neighborhood, as their personal fortunes had taken them to different neighborhoods or even different cities; he would see them only when they would visit their families for holidays or special occasions. A few of his childhood friends had become quite successful. Although Joe was very happy for them, he avoided getting together with them, because he felt like a failure around them.

Joe had never been married, although he had dated a few women over the years. He could not talk to women without getting extremely anxious, and his anxiety would show itself to others in a tendency to blush brightly, to tremble, and to avert his gaze. His relationships with women typically began at social events or at bars, because he felt quite a bit more relaxed after a couple of drinks.

Typically, the women that Joe dated lost interest in him when they saw him sober and anxious, and he had never had a long-term relationship.

Joe came to the clinic when he realized that he was drinking more and more and that it was causing him trouble. Although he was less anxious interpersonally as a result of his drinking, he was starting to be late for work, to have headaches in the morning, and to show other signs of dependent drinking. He was also feeling depressed almost all the time. Joe first sought treatment for his problem drinking at the local rehabilitation facility, but he soon found that the requirement for participation in its confrontational group program made his social anxiety intolerable. Unlike the staff at the rehabilitation facility, who saw Joe's alcoholism as the source of his other difficulties, we conceptualized Joe's social anxiety as the primary problem. In short, he drank because it relieved his social anxiety, although his drinking caused other problems and seemed to take on a life of its own. He was dysphoric more days than not because he had little in his life that was rewarding. He went to work and spent the day doing his job and worrying that he would make a mistake or otherwise embarrass himself in front of others. He had little social life other than the occasional get-together with old friends, and he spent most of his leisure time either alone in his apartment or at his mother's house.

With the help of clinic staff, Joe set a number of goals for himself during the process of diagnosis and assessment. He desired to become more comfortable in and increase the frequency of (1) casual conversations with other employees at work; (2) casual conversations with women, with the ultimate goal of working on the development of dating relationships without reliance on alcohol; (3) situations in which he had to do something in front of others, such as helping customers, working while other people were in the store and might be watching him, or speaking up in a group; and (4) dealing with other people's expressions of anger. In addition to social phobia, Joe also met criteria for diagnoses of dysthymic disorder and alcohol dependence.

The Development of Joe's Social Anxiety

Although it is hard to say anything definitively about the development of an emotional or behavioral disorder, Joe appears to have come by his social anxiety in a number of ways. He apparently had a significant genetic loading for social phobia, as evidenced by examination of his family tree. His mother was quite socially anxious, as noted, as were several other relatives from her side of the family. She had always described her own mother as a social recluse, although it was unclear whether this was a result of social anxiety or of other factors. Her brother appears to have had rather severe problems with social interaction anxiety, as had the children of one of her sisters. Joe had a brother and a sister, both of whom were socially anxious but in more limited ways than Joe was.

Joe's mother's social anxiety may also have contributed to Joe's anxiety in other ways. She was herself quite anxious making casual conversation with others, and she was hesitant to have Joe play with other children in their home because it placed demands on her to interact with the mothers of the children. She was additionally concerned that if any of the other parents came to her house, they would find out what a "bad mother and housekeeper" she was or that they would see her husband drinking and gossip about their family. Although she was a warm and caring person at heart and more than willing to devote her time and energy to her children, she avoided organized activities (e.g., little league baseball) because she did not think she would be able to make conversation with the other parents for hours at a time. Not surprisingly, Joe did little with other children, coming home immediately after school each day. This fit Joe's natural inclinations quite well, as it seemed that he was not one who liked to take any kind of risk or to seek out new experiences on his own, and he often appeared quite content to engage in solitary play. Understanding Joe's feelings of social anxiety, Joe's mother would also occasionally permit him to stay home from school on days when he had to make a presentation in class or if he had been bullied by a classmate at school the previous day. Joe's inhibited personality and his mother's social anxiety "conspired" to make social interaction with other children something very foreign to Joe and to increase the likelihood that he would feel out of place in normal everyday social situations. This interaction between the child's natural temperament and the mother's tendency to overprotect is a common characteristic of families of anxious children (Hudson & Rapee, 2000).

Joe's father may have contributed to the mix in a different way. It was hard to determine whether Joe also received a genetic loading for social phobia from his father's side of the family (as his father had rarely talked about such things with Joe), but it seems that he may have received a genetic loading for alcohol dependence. We do know that Joe's father was highly critical of Joe and set very high standards for his son's performance in school and other areas of life. Joe's grades were generally a bit above average, but his father wanted more. Joe's grandfather had been a military man who believed that failure to achieve was a result of lack of discipline, and Joe's father had learned this well. Thus he rarely let up on Joe for fear that he would be undisciplined. He was always critical of Joe and would vent his frustrations at his son's failure to excel in outbursts of extreme anger. Whatever Joe did was never good enough. If Joe tried harder and did better, his father expected more. Joe told us more than once that he felt that he had never pleased his father in anything he had done, and it was one of his great sorrows that, because his father had passed away, he would never be able to do so.

Joe's experiences with peers were also potential contributors to his later social anxiety. He would tremble and his voice would quiver if he had to answer a question in class, and his classmates teased him mercilessly for displaying this frailty. We now know childhood teasing to be associated with anxiety and depression in adult life (Roth, Coles, & Heimberg, in press). Because he was not involved in many activities outside his home, he had little opportunity to engage in games or sporting events with other children. Not surprisingly, he felt uncomfortable and awkward in team sports. He was so self-conscious that he was forever making throwing errors and mental mistakes. Joe hated recess as a child because he either spent the time standing alone at the fringe of the schoolyard or played games, thereby subjecting himself to further teasing by his peers. Leaving the schoolyard in tears, something Joe did often, also served to further perpetuate the teasing.

Learning from Experience

Of course, Joe learned a lot from his parents and peers. From his mother, he learned that one should be afraid of other people. He learned that people have opinions about you that matter and that it is most important that other people not form bad opinions of you. He also learned from her, that it was OK to shy away from social invitations, to initiate little, and to stay home and remain isolated. He did not learn from her, or from experiences that are facilitated by most parents, the proper ways to behave in social situations, and he grew up with precious little experience with them.

While his mother taught him the virtues of withdrawal and nonparticipation, Joe's father and his peers taught him that whatever he did was not good enough. Joe's father reinforced the teachings of his mother that the opinions of others are extremely important and, by his own behavior toward Joe, that other people are constantly evaluating you and concluding that you fall short of the mark. In effect, Joe learned that he did not have what it takes to satisfy the standards that he believed his father held for him. When Joe started school, his childhood peers became additional sources of negative learning. He was teased on a regular basis for his shortcomings as a public speaker and as an athlete. He learned that his best efforts typically earned him no respect and that his mistakes were seriously punished.

Developmental experiences such as these must influence the person's view of the world in which he lives. Joe, like many other persons with social phobia, came to develop a set of beliefs about transactions with others that were extremely negative. These beliefs were the direct outgrowths of his experiences as a child and may or may not have been distorted at that time. Nevertheless, Joe came to believe that interactions with other people are dangerous to the extreme, and he carried this belief with him into later life. Social interactions or situations in which Joe might become the center of attention held little prospect for enjoyment and mutual fulfillment. Instead, he saw them as opportunities for yet another helping of humiliation and embarrassment. With beliefs like this, why would anyone want to put himself or herself at the mercy of others?

Joe learned other things as well. He learned that other people would tease him and set standards for him that he could not meet. He also learned that other people did not seem to have the same troubles that he did. He saw other children speak up in class with no particular problem. In fact, there were a couple of students in his class who liked to speak in public so much that they just would not shut up! He also learned that there were plenty of kids who did not always make fools of themselves on the playground. So what did they have that Joe lacked? This type of social comparison can be extremely harmful to the person with social anxiety. It leads him or her to the conclusion that negative social outcomes can be avoided by others but not by oneself. With this type of belief, Joe felt that he was all alone, with nothing to protect him from the slings and arrows of other children's name calling and social rejection.

To summarize in the terms of Juster et al. (1996a), Joe came to believe that social situations are dangerous. He also learned that these dangers could be avoided by other children, but that he was not capable of behaving to a standard that would allow him to do so. With this generic set of beliefs, Joe then went on to do what all human beings do, that is, make attempts to predict the outcomes of situations. What sort of predictions might Joe make about any upcoming social encounter? It is an opportunity for embarrassment, for humiliation, for rejection, for loss of status, for all things bad, for nothing good.

Confronting Feared Social Situations

With knowledge of Joe's experiences as a child and developing person, let us examine his experiences as an adult with social phobia more closely. To do so, we rely on the cognitive-behavioral formulation of social anxiety developed by Rapee and Heimberg (1997), which is displayed in the form of a flowchart in Figure 5.1. For present purposes, we focus on Joe's report of a situation that occurred shortly before he presented for treatment in which he was introduced to a woman at a local singles' group. He found her to be very attractive and wanted to get to know her better. However, because he had recognized by this time that he had to get a hold on his drinking behavior, he stayed away from the bar. Joe's report of his experiences in this situation were more illuminating than his report of other situations because his senses were not clouded by alcohol.

In Figure 5.1, we schematize what we believe happens in the experience of a person with social anxiety in a social situation. We suggest that when socially anxious persons perceive that they might be negatively evaluated, a cascade of psychological events is unleashed. These events have the effect of decreasing the person's sense of efficacy and safety in the situation, stoking the fires of anxiety and further fueling the person's negative judgments, over and over again in a cyclical pattern. In the paragraphs to follow, we define each of the components of the flowchart and apply them to Joe's experience at the social club.

The Perceived Audience

For socially anxious individuals, and Joe is no exception, the perception of an audience starts a chain of cognitive, behavioral, and emotional events with which

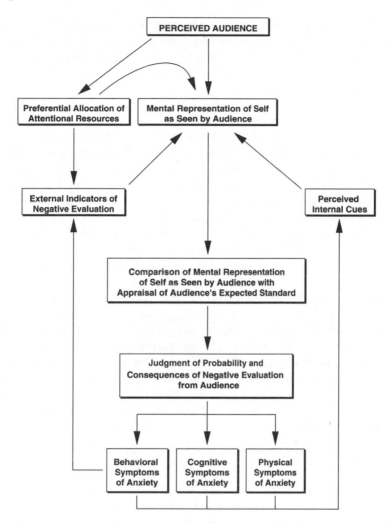

FIGURE 5.1. A model of the generation and maintenance of anxiety in social/evaluative situations. From "A Cognitive-Behavioral Model of Anxiety in Social Phobia," by R. M. Rapee and R. G. Heimberg, 1997, *Behaviour Research and Therapy, 35,* p. 743. Copyright 1997 by Elsevier Science. Reprinted by permission.

they are all too familiar. What constitutes a threatening audience varies among socially anxious individuals, although the main point is that it is a person or group who has the opportunity to negatively evaluate the person. For some individuals, the feared audience may be colleagues watching them give a formal presentation. For others, it may be strangers who might incidentally observe them walking down the street, sitting on a bus, or eating in a cafeteria. Alternatively, it may be an authority figure, romantic interest, or group of people who may judge them during an interaction. We talk about the *perceived* audience because this person does not actually have to be watching and evaluating the person with social phobia. The only thing that matters is that the person with social phobia thinks that he or she may be being evaluated.

For Joe, the audience was a woman named Pam. Joe's buddy from the old neighborhood, an outgoing fellow named Frank, persuaded Joe to go with him to a meeting of his social club. After the business of the club was completed at this weekly gathering, the regulars and some of their friends would hang out together, usually drinking and always trying to have a good time and make plans for the following weekend. Frank introduced Pam to Joe, said a couple of facilitative things, and then disappeared, presumably to look after his own social calendar. Pam, a 32-year-old divorced single mother, had just returned to the social scene after an extended absence. Although she wanted to get back into the swing of things quickly, she felt hesitant and awkward herself (as she told Joe some time later). Although usually at ease in social settings, she felt little confidence in this one. However, Joe did not perceive her discomfort, seeing only that she was a beautiful and desirable woman. Of course, this made Pam a very threatening audience because, as Joe stated, "Good-looking women don't want to talk to losers." In fact, Joe had actually started to worry about how he might appear to the women at the social club as soon as Frank had invited him to come along. Although he did not know the audience would be Pam, there was no doubt in his mind that he would experience an evaluative and judgmental audience. These situations are inherently evaluative, but Joe quickly turned a casual conversation into a high-stakes game, and it was his fragile self-esteem that he stood to lose.

The Mental Representation of the Self as Seen by the Audience

Once the audience has been perceived, socially anxious individuals construct a mental representation of how their behavior and appearance are likely to be viewed by the audience, and this forms the basis for much of their later concern about how they will be evaluated. Joe started to think about how he might appear to Pam. His image of how he might appear to her was more important than his own view of how he might appear, because it was her evaluation of him that was most threatening. Unfortunately, this image of how he would be viewed by Pam was negatively distorted because, having been constructed by a socially anxious person, it was based on largely faulty information.

Joe constructed his mental representation of how he might appear to Pam on the basis of how he believed he had appeared to other women in the past. However, he had never asked any of these women how they had perceived him, and he had little information about their more subtle reactions because he was looking at the floor most of the time. Instead, his mental representation of how he might appear to Pam was based on a recurrent and anxiety-evoking image that Joe had whenever he was in similar situations, an experience that appears quite common among persons with social phobia (Hackmann, Clark, & McManus, 2000). In that recurrent image, he saw himself as a young teenager in one of his middle school classes, sitting near "the girl of my dreams." He tried to speak to her as the class period ended, but he could not get a word out. He blushed and walked away as quickly as he could. However, in Joe's mind, the horror of this image was greatly magnified. He saw himself stammering, trying to speak. In the image, the girl asked him if something was the matter, and he blushed such a bright shade of crimson that everyone in the room could (and did) see. The other students stopped talking and stared in silence as he tried and tried to speak. After an eternity of deafening silence, he ran out of the room, pushing other students out of the way as he escaped. As he was running down the hall, he heard the other students laughing at him.

Thus Joe's mental representation of how he might appear to Pam was more a representation of his anxiety than of anything that had to do with Pam's view of him. As the conversation progressed, Joe adjusted his negatively biased image of how Pam perceived him. These adjustments were based on Joe's moment-to-moment reactions to his physical state (e.g., "My heart is pounding; I can barely hear myself think"), evaluations of his own behavior and appearance (e.g., "I'm not dressed right; I look like I don't fit in"), and his perceptions of Pam's reactions (e.g., "She's looking all around. She thinks I'm a loser"). An already negative image of how he might appear to Pam was repeatedly adjusted in a more and more negative direction.

Preferential Allocation of Attentional Resources

As previously discussed, socially anxious individuals preferentially allocate attentional resources toward detecting social threat in the environment. That means that any reaction from the audience that could be construed as negative will be detected with great efficiency. However, not all that is negative comes from without, and socially anxious persons also allocate attentional resources to monitor and adjust their mental representation of how they are perceived by the audience. In effect, they attempt to simultaneously monitor the environment for evidence of negative evaluation, check their appearance and behavior for flaws that might elicit negative evaluation from others, *and* attend to and engage in the social tasks at hand. Of course, social interaction is difficult enough without having to pay attention to so much at the same time, and little attention remains for the detection of positive reactions from others. Furthermore, it is hard to juggle so many balls in the air without dropping some, and performance may realistically suffer. For instance, it may be hard for the socially anxious person to remain focused on the topic of conversation when so much is going on, and the other person may not feel listened to.

Joe's reactions to Pam provide a good example of how attention biased toward the negative can influence a person's evaluation of the situation. Starting with a negatively biased representation of how he might appear to Pam, he was highly vigilant for any information that would confirm this negative image (e.g., "She's looking all around. She thinks I'm a loser"). The moment-to-moment adjustments noted earlier were likely to be almost exclusively negative given the much greater likelihood that he would register negative information than positive information. Joe also paid a great deal of attention to his own discomfort and his imagined awkward appearance. In turn, this focus reinforced his negative mental representation.

Comparison of the Mental Representation of Oneself with Appraisal of the Audience's Expected Standard

In addition to monitoring their mental representation of how they are perceived by the audience, persons with social phobia also project the performance standard expected by the audience. That is, how well do they think the audience expects them to perform? How well must the person do in order to keep the audience satisfied? The degree to which socially anxious individuals believe their behavior meets the expectation of the audience can fluctuate based on changing perceptions of the audience, the demands of the social situation, and their own behavior.

Joe projected that Pam would hold a high standard for him even before they spoke a word to each other. As soon as he decided that she was very attractive, he determined that she would have higher standards than most and that he would have a great deal of difficulty meeting her standards. After all, he was just an average-looking guy, and surely a beautiful woman would want to be with a handsome gentleman. Any further attribution of positive characteristics to the audience should raise the bar even higher, and as they talked further, he noted that she was a sensitive person who seemed to like other people and who cared deeply for her kids. Whereas others may have used these data to suggest that Pam was probably not the most negative or critical person in the room, Joe reacted differently. With each positive attribute that he noted, he just assumed that she would expect more and more from him.

Judgment of the Probability and Consequences of Negative Evaluation from the Audience

The importance of the socially anxious person's comparison of his image of how he might appear to the audience with the standard he believes the audience holds for him lies in what he decides. The more he believes that his behavior and appearance fall short of his estimate of the audience's expectations, the more likely negative evaluation and its accompanying painful consequences are predicted to be. Of course, our discussion to this point strongly suggests that the socially anxious person will judge the probability and cost of negative evaluation by the audience to be high. Application of this aspect of the model to Joe's circumstances is straightforward. Joe believed, on the basis of memories and recurrent images of his past behavior with women, that he would not do well. On the basis of his own evaluation of Pam as a beautiful, sensitive, and caring person, he was certain that he would not live up to her high standards. Of course, this "failure" was perceived by Joe as another in a string of social failures that underscored his inadequacies and that support his belief that he does not have what it takes to have even a casual relationship with a woman, much less an intimate one. Thus Joe concluded that he would not be able to impress Pam, that she would not have any interest in him, that she was representative of all women he found attractive, and that he would be alone for the rest of his days, quite a load to place on the outcome of one conversation.

Anxiety Symptoms

COGNITIVE SYMPTOMS OF ANXIETY

Of course, Joe's mental experiences as he and Pam talked to each other were extremely deflating, and this was reflected in his conscious thoughts. He reported a stream of thoughts that were all emotionally loaded: "Here we go again," "I'm such a loser," "She's gorgeous. What would she want with a stiff like me?" "What can I talk to her about?" "How long will she stand here before she gets totally bored with me?" and "What's the use?"

BEHAVIORAL SYMPTOMS OF ANXIETY

An appraisal that negative evaluation is a likely and costly outcome may produce a desire to flee the social situation. Joe certainly experienced a strong desire to leave the social club (and to stop at the bar for a double on the way out the door), but he did not. Even if a socially anxious person persists in the feared social situation, however, he may engage in a variety of subtle behaviors, referred to previously as safety behaviors (Wells et al., 1995). These behaviors may include avoiding eye contact, standing on the outside of a crowd, or minimizing participation in a conversation. Unfortunately, these behaviors frequently have the effect of reducing effective social performance. Consequently, socially anxious individuals may receive verbal and nonverbal feedback from the audience that their performance is inferior. Joe engaged in a number of these behaviors (avoiding eye contact, not talking about himself, standing in a stiff military posture). These subtle avoidance behaviors had the added effect of increasing Pam's own anxiety and had a negative effect on her reaction to Joe.

PHYSICAL SYMPTOMS OF ANXIETY

Socially anxious individuals often report physiological arousal when exposed to feared situations, and many of the symptoms they endorse (e.g., blushing, muscle twitching, sweating) may be observed by others. Socially anxious individuals tend to overestimate the visibility of their anxiety, to catastrophize about how negatively others will react to their anxiety, and to become focused on those symptoms that they believe hold a high potential for eliciting negative evaluation from others. Joe reported that he blushed "bright crimson," that his voice quivered and his hands shook during his conversation with Pam. Joe also reported a rapidly pounding heart, which he believed was a signal of impending loss of control over his behavior.

Perceived Internal Cues

Internal anxiety cues (cognitive and some physiological and behavioral symptoms of anxiety) are used as sources of information that feed back into the mental representation of the self as seen by the audience. As mentioned, Joe reported a stream of negative thoughts during his conversation with Pam. He took these thoughts as true indications of the quality of his conversational performance and of Pam's lack of interest in him. His racing and pounding heart was yet another indication that he was not doing well. He was aware that he was having difficulty looking her in the eyes and took this as more evidence of his inadequacy. Of course, these evaluations cycled back to negatively influence his mental representation of how he appeared to Pam. Unfortunately, however, as he thought he looked worse and worse to her, he thought that he must be falling farther and farther below her expectations for him, and his predictions of bad outcomes were reinforced. This is the vicious cycle of social phobia.

External Indicators of Negative Evaluation

Behavioral symptoms of anxiety and, in some cases, social skills deficits may function to reduce effective social performance and result in negative verbal or nonverbal feedback from the audience. This may be true, as well, for overt signs of physiological arousal. Importantly, social feedback is often indirect and ambiguous. Given an information processing bias toward detecting and possibly remembering threatening social information, socially anxious individuals will readily incorporate possible external indications of negative evaluation into their ongoing and long-term mental representation of themselves. For instance, when Pam yawned, or whenever their conversation slowed down, Joe worried that things were going poorly. When she encouraged him to loosen up and relax a little, he took this invitation to mean that she thought quite badly of him, and his mental representation of how he appeared to Pam took another hit.

After the Situation Concluded

What happens after an anxiety-evoking social encounter for persons with social phobia? It appears that they engage in repeated processing of the event, but this processing is hardly adaptive (Rachman, Grüter-Andrew, & Shafran, 2000). Because they have seen the threat as extreme and have selectively attended to any circumstances that suggest the great potential for negative evaluation, they may feel compelled to play the situation over and over again in their minds. This mental playback serves the seemingly positive but elusive goal of trying to learn from the negative experience or at least to undertake some sort of damage control, whether reality suggests that this is necessary or not.

It is likely that the person will call up a visual image of the situation as he or she has experienced it. It will probably be viewed as if through the eyes of another person, because this is the vantage point which is of most concern to the person with social phobia. It is quite likely, as the person has never actually viewed his or her behavior from that perspective, that the image will be negatively biased. That is, Joe would most likely focus on the imagined negative aspects of the interaction and ignore any positive aspects. Regardless of the actual quality of one's behavior, it may thus be judged as lacking (remember that persons with social phobia rate their own performances more harshly than independent observers do) or as failing to meet the presumed standard held by other persons. The likely outcome is that the person with social phobia will conclude that his or her behavior has been inadequate to the extreme and will become worried that the same outcomes will be repeated in the future. Our good friend Joe played the conversation with Pam over and over in his mind and decided that he should never have let Frank drag him to the club in the first place and that he had embarrassed himself too badly with Pam to be able to go back even if he wanted to.

Comment

Joe's story is a compelling but not uncommon one. It is not so different from the stories that many of our clients with social phobia have to tell. What makes it important is that it demonstrates a number of the problematic cognitive, physiological, and behavioral processes that fuel the experience of social phobia and brings our discussions of these topics in the previous chapters to life. Joe's story also suggests several points of intervention in the treatment of social phobia and gives us some notion of what effective treatments for social phobia should include. From our perspective, effective treatments for social phobia should address several aspects of the disorder. These would include:

- Negative beliefs about social situations and other people
- Negative beliefs about the self

- Negative predictions about the outcomes of social situations
- Anticipatory anxiety
- Attentional focus on social-threat cues
- Avoidance of feared situations
- Negative evaluation of performance after the situation has passed

These are the targets that Cognitive-Behavioral Group Therapy for social phobia, the treatment protocol we share in Part II of this book, is designed to modify.

Note

1. Joe is, in actuality, a composite of several clients who have come to our clinics over the years. Although he is typical in all respects, we chose to present this composite client so as to highlight the several aspects of the cognitive-behavioral formulation of social phobia in the context of a single case.

6

Assessment of Social Phobia

with Cynthia L. Turk

In this final chapter of Part I, we describe self-report and clinician-administered instruments, as well as behavioral and cognitive assessment methods, for the clinician who attempts to understand the difficulties experienced by a client with social phobia. We also briefly mention measures from other domains that are important in the comprehensive assessment of social phobia.

Repeated assessment is an important aspect of the cognitive-behavioral treatment of social phobia described in Part II of this book, and detailed analyses of the specifics of the client's social phobia are described in Chapter 8 ("The Treatment Orientation Interview"). However, we strongly recommend that psychometric assessment be undertaken with all clients before the initiation of treatment. In initial clinical interviews, shame and fear of negative evaluation may lead clients to give descriptions of their problems that do not fully reflect the severity or pervasiveness of their anxiety and avoidance. Administration of psychometrically sound self-report and clinician-rated measurement devices facilitates the assessment of fear and avoidance in a broad range of social situations within a relatively brief time frame. Furthermore, pretreatment scores on validated measures of social anxiety provide a baseline against which progress can be objectively assessed.

We also recommend behavioral and cognitive testing prior to treatment. Behavior tests provide objective information about how anxious the client becomes during social interaction, performance, or observational situations. They also provide an objective index of the quality of the client's social behavior and help the therapist to estimate how likely the client's efforts are to be met with a positive response in the real world. This objective information cannot be replaced by the self-report of the client, given that socially anxious individuals describe their social behavior as more inadequate (e.g., Rapee & Lim, 1992; Stopa & Clark, 1993) and their anxiety as more obvious (e.g., Alden & Wallace, 1995) than do independent judges. Cognitive assessment measures provide valuable information about the extent of bias or distortion in the client's view of the world, an obviously important piece of data for the cognitive-behavioral therapist.

In our review, we strive for a balance between discussion of clinical utility and the tedium of psychometric details. For readers who desire more scholarly overviews of literature on the psychometric assessment of social phobia, we suggest reviews by D. B Clark et al. (1997), Cox and Swinson (1995), Hart, Jack, Turk, and Heimberg (1999), or McNeil, Ries, and Turk (1995b). McNeil et al. (1995b) deal especially thoroughly with behavioral and physiological assessment. Also, Elting and Hope (1995) provide a more thorough review of cognitive assessment strategies. Readers who seek an overview of the assessment of social phobia with a more clinical emphasis should consult the relevant chapter by Hope, Turk, and Heimberg (in press). Because of space considerations, we do not review structured diagnostic interviews, but see Hart et al. (1999) and Cox and Swinson (1995).

Self-Report Assessment

Social Interaction Anxiety Scale and Social Phobia Scale

The Social Interaction Anxiety Scale (SIAS) and Social Phobia Scale (SPS) (Mattick & Clarke, 1998) are the two self-report scales that we find the most valuable for the assessment of social phobia. Therefore, we present them for your use in Figures 6.1 and 6.2. We have presented the 20-item version of the SIAS, which is the version that appears in most published studies. The Mattick and Clarke 1998 version of the SIAS contains only 19 items and differs from the 20-item version only by the elimination of the reverse-scored item, "I find it easy to make friends of my own age."

The SIAS and SPS were designed to capture two distinct types of social fears: the fear of interacting in dyads and groups and the fear of being observed and scrutinized by others, respectively (Mattick & Clarke, 1998). Although social interaction anxiety and scrutiny/observation fears frequently co-occur, this is not always the case. Some individuals may feel quite comfortable doing a formal presentation in an area of expertise but feel very anxious about their ability to respond spontaneously and appropriately during a conversation. Other individuals may feel comfortable talking to others informally but feel extremely anxious about their ability to deliver an effective, informative speech or complete a task in front of others because of their fear of making a mistake or showing signs of anxiety. Factor analytic studies

FIGURE 6.1. The Social Interaction Anxiety Scale. Reprinted with the permission of Richard P. Mattick.

For each question, please circle a number to indicate the degree to which you feel the statement is characteristic or true of you. The rating scale is as follows:

0 = Not at all characteristic or true of me
1 = Slightly characteristic or true of me
2 = Moderately characteristic or true of me
3 = Very characteristic or true of me
4 = Extremely characteristic or true of me

	Not at all	Slightly	Moderately	Very	Extremely
1. I get nervous if I have to speak with someone in authority (teacher, boss).	0	1	2	3	4
2. I have difficulty making eye contact with others.	0	1	2	3	4
3. I become tense if I have to talk about myself or my feelings.	0	1	2	3	4
4. I find it difficult mixing comfortably with the people I work with.	0	1	2	3	4
5. I find it easy to make friends of my own age.	0	1	2	3	4
6. I tense up if I meet an acquaintance in the street.	0	1	2	3	4
7. When mixing socially, I am uncomfortable.	0	1	2	3	4
8. I feel tense if I am alone with just one person.	0	1	2	3	4
9. I am at ease meeting people at parties, etc.	0	1	2	3	4
10. I have difficulty talking with other people.	0	1	2	3	4
11. I find it easy to think of things to talk about.	0	1	2	3	4
12. I worry about expressing myself in case I appear awkward.	0	1	2	3	4
13. I find it difficult to disagree with another's point of view.	0	1	2	3	4
14. I have difficulty talking to attractive persons of the opposite sex.	0	1	2	3	4
15. I find myself worrying that I won't know what to say in social situations.	0	1	2	3	4

(continued)

FIGURE 6.1. (continued)					
	Not at all	Slightly	Moderately	Very	Extremely
16. I am nervous mixing with people I don't know well.	0	1	2	3	4
17. I feel I'll say something embarrassing when talking.	0	1	2	3	4
18. When mixing in a group, I find myself worrying I will be ignored.	0	1	2	3	4
19. I am tense mixing in a group.	0	1	2	3	4
20. I am unsure whether to greet someone I know only slightly.	0	1	2	3	4

support this conceptual distinction between social interaction fears and scrutiny/ observation fears (Habke, Hewitt, Norton, & Asmundson, 1997). When the items from the SIAS and SPS were factor analyzed together, social interaction fears loaded on a single large factor, whereas scrutiny/observation fears loaded on multiple smaller factors (Safren, Turk, & Heimberg, 1998).

Multiple studies have demonstrated that the SIAS and SPS have good psychometric properties. Both scales have been found to have good internal consistency and high test–retest reliability among clients with social phobia (Heimberg, Mueller, Holt, Hope, & Liebowitz, 1992; Mattick & Clarke, 1998). They have also demonstrated a strong relationship with self-report and clinician-administered measures of social anxiety (Mattick & Clarke, 1998; Heimberg et al., 1992). However, as would be expected, the SIAS has been consistently more highly associated with other measures of social interaction anxiety than the SPS, and the SPS has been more highly associated with measures of performance anxiety than the SIAS. The SIAS has also been more highly related to measures of neuroticism and uncontrollable worry, whereas the SPS has been more highly related to fear of anxiety symptoms and to panic symptoms (E. J. Brown et al., 1997; Norton, Cox, Hewitt, & McLeod, 1997).

Most important, individuals with social phobia score significantly higher on both scales than individuals with other anxiety disorders and than community controls (E. J. Brown et al., 1997; Mattick & Clarke, 1998). In our research on these scales, we have determined that scores of 34 on the SIAS and 24 on the SPS do a very good job of identifying persons with clinically severe social anxiety (E. J. Brown et al., 1997; Heimberg et al., 1992) and a score of 42 on the SIAS is likely to accurately identify persons with generalized social phobia (Mennin, Fresco, & Heimberg, 1998).

The SIAS and SPS also predict cognitive and behavioral responses in threatening social and performance situations. In one study, higher SIAS scores among clients with social phobia were associated with fewer positive thoughts and more negative thoughts following a conversation role-play task. Higher SPS scores were associated with early termination of a speech role-play task (Ries et al.,

FIGURE 6.2. The Social Phobia Scale. Reprinted with the permission of Richard P. Mattick.

For each question, please circle a number to indicate the degree to which you feel the statement is characteristic or true of you. The rating scale is as follows:

0 = **Not at all** characteristic or true of me
1 = **Slightly** characteristic or true of me
2 = **Moderately** characteristic or true of me
3 = **Very** characteristic or true of me
4 = **Extremely** characteristic or true of me

	Not at all	Slightly	Moderately	Very	Extremely
1. I become anxious if I have to write in front of other people.	0	1	2	3	4
2. I become self-conscious when using public toilets.	0	1	2	3	4
3. I can suddenly become aware of my own voice and of others listening to me.	0	1	2	3	4
4. I get nervous that people are staring at me as I walk down the street.	0	1	2	3	4
5. I fear I may blush when I am with others.	0	1	2	3	4
6. I feel self-conscious if I have to enter a room where others are already seated.	0	1	2	3	4
7. I worry about shaking or trembling when I'm watched by other people.	0	1	2	3	4
8. I would get tense if I had to sit facing other people on a bus or a train.	0	1	2	3	4
9. I get panicky that others might see me faint or be sick or ill.	0	1	2	3	4
10. I would find it difficult to drink something if in a group of people.	0	1	2	3	4
11. It would make me feel self-conscious to eat in front of a stranger at a restaurant.	0	1	2	3	4
12. I am worried people will think my behavior odd.	0	1	2	3	4
13. I would get tense if I had to carry a tray across a crowded cafeteria.	0	1	2	3	4
14. I worry I'll lose control of myself in front of other people.	0	1	2	3	4

(*continued*)

FIGURE 6.2. (*continued*)

	Not at all	Slightly	Moderately	Very	Extremely
15. I worry I might do something to attract the attention of other people.	0	1	2	3	4
16. When in an elevator, I am tense if people look at me.	0	1	2	3	4
17. I can feel conspicuous standing in a line.	0	1	2	3	4
18. I can get tense when I speak in front of other people.	0	1	2	3	4
19. I worry my head will shake or nod in front of others.	0	1	2	3	4
20. I feel awkward and tense if I know people are watching me.	0	1	2	3	4

1998). Finally, both measures have been found to be sensitive to the effects of cognitive-behavioral treatment of social phobia (Cox, Ross, Swinson, & Direnfeld, 1998; Heimberg et al., 1998; Ries et al., 1998). Medium to large effect sizes have been reported for both the SIAS and the SPS after 12 weeks of cognitive-behavioral treatment (Cox et al., 1998; Ries et al., 1998).

Social Phobia and Anxiety Inventory

One of the best validated measures of social phobia is the Social Phobia and Anxiety Inventory (SPAI; S. Turner et al., 1989a), which assesses somatic, cognitive, and behavioral responses to a variety of interaction, performance, and observation situations. The SPAI contains 45 items, 21 of which require multiple responses (109 responses are required in total). For example, for the item that begins "I feel anxious when stating an opinion to . . . ", the client indicates how frequently situations involving "strangers," "authority figures," the "opposite sex," and "people in general" elicit anxiety (0–6 Likert-type scale). In addition to items that assess social phobia, the SPAI includes an Agoraphobia subscale that assesses anxiety in situations commonly feared by agoraphobic persons (e.g., waiting in line). A Difference score, which is intended to index social anxiety independent of the concerns common to agoraphobic clients, is calculated by subtracting the Agoraphobia subscale score from the Social Phobia subscale score. The SPAI collects a large amount of very specific information that can be useful in treatment planning. On the other hand, the time and effort required to administer the SPAI pose relative drawbacks.

The SPAI has demonstrated adequate internal consistency with both college students with social phobia (S. Turner et al., 1989a) and outpatients with social phobia, both before treatment and after treatment (Cox et al., 1998). It has also been shown to have good test–retest reliability over a 2-week period among undergraduates with social phobia (S. Turner et al., 1989a).

Undergraduates with social phobia score significantly higher on the SPAI than nonanxious undergraduates (Beidel, Turner, Stanley, & Dancu, 1989c; S. Turner et al., 1989a). Additionally, clients with social phobia had more elevated scores on the SPAI than clients with panic disorder, panic disorder with agoraphobia, or obsessive–compulsive disorder (S. Turner et al., 1989a). In one study (Peters, 2000), the SPAI was superior to the SPS and SIAS in discriminating between social phobia and panic disorder with and without agoraphobia.

S. Turner et al. (1989a) recommend a score of 80 for differentiating between clients with social phobia and those with other anxiety disorders and a score of 60 for flagging possible cases of social phobia for additional assessment. Individuals with generalized social phobia score significantly higher on the SPAI than individuals with specific social fears (Ries et al., 1998; S. Turner et al., 1992).

Several studies have examined the validity of the SPAI. It correlates significantly with other self-report measures of social anxiety (e.g., Herbert, Bellack, & Hope, 1991; Ries et al., 1998). Herbert and colleagues (1991) reported that the SPAI was correlated with anxiety ratings during a role-play test, but not with measures of trait anxiety or depression. SPAI scores were also associated with daily ratings of distress in social encounters (Beidel, Borden, Turner, & Jacob, 1989a) and closely matched ratings made by significant others (S. Turner, Stanley, Beidel, & Bond, 1989b).

The SPAI has also demonstrated sensitivity to treatment-related change (Beidel, Turner, & Cooley, 1993). Medium to large effect sizes have been reported after 12 to 16 weeks of cognitive-behavioral treatment (Cox et al., 1998; Ries et al., 1998; Taylor, Woody, McLean, & Koch, 1997).

One topic of debate has been whether the Social Phobia subscale or the Difference score is the better measure of social phobia symptomatology. The creators of the instrument prefer the Difference score largely because it controls for symptoms of agoraphobia and has been shown to provide a clearer differentiation between social phobia and panic disorder and/or agoraphobia (Beidel & Turner, 1992; S. Turner et al., 1989a). In contrast, Herbert and colleagues (Herbert et al., 1991; Herbert, Bellack, Hope, & Mueser, 1992a) suggest that the Social Phobia subscale score is more parsimonious because it does not require the assumption that endorsement of items on the Agoraphobia subscale indicates fear of panic attacks rather than fear of negative evaluation (e.g., fear of waiting in line may be due to observational concerns). Additionally, recent research suggests that panic symptoms may be an important aspect of the clinical picture for many individuals with social phobia (Jack et al., 1999). These findings highlight the complexity of the relationship between social phobia and panic symptomatology and perhaps argue for examining both domains independently, without making *a priori* assumptions about the relation of one to the other. Finally, other researchers have suggested that administering the Social Phobia subscale alone may be more practical and time efficient because it is shorter and highly correlated with the Difference score ($r = 0.92$; Ries et al., 1998).

One unique aspect of the SPAI is that separate versions of the scale have been developed for the assessment of children (Beidel, Turner, & Fink, 1996; Beidel, Turner, & Morris, 1995) and adolescents (D. B. Clark et al., 1994). The SPAI is available from Multi-Health Systems, Inc. (1-800-456-3003; *www.mhs.com*).

Social Phobia Inventory

The Social Phobia Inventory (SPIN; Connor et al., 2000) is a new instrument for the assessment of social phobia. There is, in fact, only one published study to date, but it warrants our attention because it is being used with increasing frequency in pharmaceutical industry studies of new medications for social phobia. The SPIN includes 17 items that are rated on a 0 ("not at all") to 4 ("extremely") Likert-type scale. Based on the clinician-administered Brief Social Phobia Scale (Davidson et al., 1991, 1997; see upcoming section), it also contains subscales for the assessment of fear, avoidance, and physiological arousal related to social phobia.

The initial published study suggests that the SPIN has sound psychometric properties (Connor et al., 2000). The total scale demonstrated good test–retest reliability, although the retest intervals were quite brief, and further assessment is required. Internal consistency was excellent, and the SPIN discriminated well between persons with social phobia and those without social phobia but with other psychiatric disorders, as well as between persons with social phobia and nonpsychiatric controls. A score of 19 appears to be a sound cutoff for the identification of clinical cases as determined by receiver operating characteristics analyses. The SPIN also demonstrated sensitivity to the effects of drug therapy.

The subscales seem to have reasonable psychometric characteristics, as well. However, the correlations among the subscales were not reported, and the subscale structure does not seem to map well onto the factor structure of the scale. Further research is needed before the subscales can be meaningfully employed.

In a recent study that speaks to the validity of the SPIN, three items from the scale ("Being embarrassed or looking stupid are among my worst fears"; "Fear of embarrassment causes me to avoid doing things or speaking to people"; "I avoid activities in which I am the center of attention") were administered to 9,375 clients at two health maintenance organizations (Katzelnick et al., 1999). Several of these clients later received a diagnosis of generalized social phobia on the basis of a structured diagnostic interview administered by telephone (8.2% of those interviewed). The data analysis revealed that clients who scored 6 or higher in response to the three SPIN items were highly likely to meet diagnostic criteria for generalized social phobia. In fact, the 3-item SPIN screener demonstrated 88.7%

sensitivity and 90% specificity for the detection of generalized social phobia in this sample. Certainly, the SPIN deserves further attention in the assessment of social phobia. The SPIN is available from Dr. Jonathan R. T. Davidson, Department of Psychiatry and Behavioral Sciences, Duke University Medical Center, Durham, NC 27710.

Fear Questionnaire (Social Phobia Subscale)

The Social Phobia subscale of the Fear Questionnaire (FQ-Social; Marks & Mathews, 1979) is a 5-item measure that assesses fear-motivated avoidance of being observed, performing, being criticized, and talking to authorities. Items are rated on a 9-point Likert-type scale (0 = "would not avoid it," 8 = "always avoid it"). It has demonstrated adequate test–retest reliability in a sample of phobic clients (Marks & Mathews, 1979) and adequate internal consistency in a large sample of clients with anxiety disorders (Oei, Moylan, & Evans, 1991b). It is also correlated with other instruments for the assessment of social phobia and social anxiety (e.g., Herbert et al., 1991; Mattick & Clarke, 1998). Clients with social phobia achieve higher FQ-Social scores than those with panic disorder, agoraphobia, or generalized anxiety disorder (Cox, Swinson, & Shaw, 1991; Oei et al., 1991b). The FQ-Social has differentiated between social phobia subtypes in some studies (E. J. Brown et al., 1995; Gelernter et al., 1992) but not in others (Heimberg et al., 1990c; Holt et al., 1992a). It has also demonstrated sensitivity to treatment effects in several studies (e.g., Heimberg et al., 1990b; Mattick & Peters, 1988; Mattick, Peters, & Clarke, 1989). However, it produced a smaller effect size than the SPAI in one study (Taylor et al., 1997). Because the FQ-Social contains only 5 items, the breadth of the content domain of social phobia assessed is limited. Its importance lies mostly in the fact that it is the oldest and most widely used of any of the scales employed in the assessment of social phobia and facilitates comparisons across newer and older studies. The FQ appears in the original paper by Marks and Mathews (1979) and has been reprinted in the clinical sourcebook edited by Fischer and Corcoran (2000).

Clinician-Administered Measures

Liebowitz Social Anxiety Scale

The Liebowitz Social Anxiety Scale (LSAS; Liebowitz, 1987) is probably the most frequently used clinician-administered instrument designed for the assessment of social phobia (see Figure 6.3). The LSAS separately evaluates fear and avoidance of 11 social interaction and 13 performance situations using a 4-point Likert-type scale. It contains 4 subscales: Fear of Performance, Avoidance of Performance, Fear of Social Interaction, and Avoidance of Social Interaction. Total Fear and total Avoidance subscale scores can also be derived. Summing the fear and avoidance ratings for all 24 items yields an overall total score. For the fear ratings, the anchors are 0 = none, 1 = mild–tolerable, 2 = moderate–distressing, 3 = severe–disturbing. For the avoidance ratings, the anchors are 0 = never (0%), 1 = occasionally (1–33%), 2 = often (33–66%), and 3 = usually (67–100%).

The LSAS has several strengths. As a clinician-administered instrument, it allows the interviewer to ensure that the client understands each item, to challenge inconsistencies in the client's report, and to draw from clinical experience and judgment in finalizing ratings. Furthermore, although research has shown that all of the Fear and Avoidance subscales of the LSAS are highly correlated in clinical samples (Heimberg et al., 1999), some clients do exhibit little avoidance despite severe fear, and the LSAS provides the opportunity to capture and explore such discordance.

The LSAS total score and subscale scores have been shown to have excellent internal consistency (Heimberg et al., 1999). As expected, the total score and subscale scores have been found to correlate substantially with self-report measures and other clinician-rated measures of social anxiety and avoidance (Heimberg et al., 1999). Furthermore, the Fear of Social Interaction and Avoidance of Social Interaction subscales have been shown to be more strongly related to measures of interaction anxiety than to measures of performance or observational anxiety (Heimberg et al., 1992, 1999). Conversely, the Fear of Performance and Avoidance of Performance subscales have been shown to be more strongly related to other measures of performance and observational fears than to measures of interaction anxiety (Heimberg et al., 1992, 1999). Research also suggests that the total score and subscale scores are more highly related to other measures of social anxiety than to measures of other constructs such as depression (Fresco et al., 2001; Heimberg et al., 1999). Using a receiver operating characteristics analysis, Mennin et al. (in press) concluded that a total score of 30 was adequate to identify persons with a diagnosis of social phobia and that a total score of 60 was adequate to identify persons with generalized social phobia. Importantly, the LSAS has demonstrated sensitivity to change following both pharmacological and cognitive behavioral treatment (e.g., Heimberg et al., 1998).

Recent research suggests that the LSAS may also be used as a self-report instrument. In a study in which the LSAS was administered twice an average of 13 days apart—once by a clinician and once as a self-report measure—the total score and subscale means and standard deviations were quite similar for both administration formats for clients with social phobia and for normal controls (Fresco et al., 2001). Furthermore, the self-administered LSAS demonstrated good internal consistency, convergent validity, and discriminant validity, consistent with the clinician-administered version. However, anecdotally, this appears to be the case only when the self-report version of the LSAS is accompanied by detailed instructions about the approach the client should take to making ratings. The instructions we have used with the self-report version of the LSAS are:

FEAR OR ANXIETY   AVOIDANCE
0 = None   0 = Never (0%)
1 = Mild   1 = Occasionally (1–33%)
2 = Moderate   2 = Often (33–67%)
3 = Severe   3 = Usually (67–100%)

	ANXIETY (S)	ANXIETY (P)	AVOID (S)	AVOID (P)
1. Telephoning in public (P)				
2. Participating in small groups (P)				
3. Eating in public places (P)				
4. Drinking with others in public places (P)				
5. Talking to people in authority (S)				
6. Acting, performing, or giving a talk in front of an audience (P)				
7. Going to a party (S)				
8. Working while being observed (P)				
9. Writing while being observed (P)				
10. Calling someone you don't know very well (S)				
11. Talking with people you don't know very well (S)				
12. Meeting strangers (S)				
13. Urinating in a public bathroom (P)				
14. Entering a room when others are already seated (P)				
15. Being the center of attention (S)				
16. Speaking up at a meeting (P)				
17. Taking a test (P)				
18. Expressing disagreement or disapproval to people you don't know very well (S)				
19. Looking people you don't know very well in the eyes (S)				
20. Giving a report to a group (P)				
21. Trying to pick up someone (P)				
22. Returning goods to a store (S)				
23. Giving a party (S)				
24. Resisting a high-pressure salesperson (S)				
Total Performance (P) Subscore				
Total Social Interaction (S) Subscore				
TOTAL SCORE				

FIGURE 6.3. The Liebowitz Social Anxiety Scale. From "Social Phobia," by M. R. Liebowitz, 1987, *Modern Problems in Pharmacopsychiatry, 22,* p. 152. Copyright 1987 by S Karger Ag, Basel, Switzerland. Reprinted by permission.

1. This measure assesses the way that social phobia plays a role in your life across a variety of situations.
2. Read each situation carefully and answer two questions about that situation.
3. The first question asks how anxious or fearful you feel in the situation.
4. The second question asks how often you avoid the situation.
5. If you come across a situation that you ordinarily do not experience, we ask that you imagine "what if you were faced with that situation," and then rate the degree to which you would fear this hypothetical situation and how often you would tend to avoid it. Please base your ratings on the way that the situations have affected you in the last week.

One caveat about the LSAS is in order, and a similar caution applies to the SPS. In a recent confirmatory factor analysis of the LSAS with a large sample of clients with social phobia, the 2-factor model (i.e., social interaction and performance) was not supported for ratings of either fear or avoidance (Safren et al., 1999). Separate exploratory common factor analyses of fear and avoidance items yielded four factors: (1) Social Interaction, (2) Public Speaking, (3) Observation by Others and (4) Eating and Drinking in Public. Like the SIAS, the LSAS subscales for social interaction anxiety and avoidance appear to be unifactorial. However, like the SPS, the performance anxiety and avoidance subscales of the LSAS appear to be multifactorial, and these subscale scores should be used with appropriate caution.

Brief Social Phobia Scale

The Brief Social Phobia Scale (BSPS; Davidson et al., 1991, 1997) is a clinician-administered scale that is being used with increasing frequency in studies of the pharmacological treatment of social phobia. It includes ratings of fear and avoidance of seven social situations and severity of four physiological symptoms. Items on all three subscales are rated on 0–4 Likert-type scales.

The reliability of the BSPS appears good. Davidson and colleagues reported satisfactory test–retest reliability (Davidson et al., 1997) and excellent interrater reliability (Davidson et al., 1991). Furthermore, the internal consistency was satisfactory for the overall scale, as well as the fear and avoidance subscales. The physiological subscale demonstrated poor internal consistency, however, and should be used with caution.

In a factor analysis, the three-factor structure of the BSPS was not supported. Davidson and colleagues (1997) arrived at a six-factor solution, with some items loading on multiple factors. All fear and avoidance items loaded on the first factor, all physiological items loaded on the second factor, and several fear and avoidance items accounted for the remaining four factors, suggesting that it may be best to rely on the BSPS total score rather than the scores on specific subscales. The BSPS has been shown to be significantly correlated with self-report social phobia scales, as well as the LSAS (Davidson et al., 1991), and has demonstrated sensitivity to drug treatment (Davidson et al., 1997). The BSPS appears in the original paper by Davidson et al. (1991).

Cognitive Assessment

Brief Fear of Negative Evaluation Scale

Although developed prior to the inclusion of social phobia in DSM-III, the Fear of Negative Evaluation Scale (FNE; Watson & Friend, 1969) has been widely used in the assessment of social phobia. Its popularity stems largely from the fact that it assesses the core cognitive construct in social phobia. The FNE consists of 30 items in a true/false format. The newer brief version of the scale (BFNE; Leary, 1983a; see Figure 6.4) contains 12 items, uses a 5-point Likert-type format (1 = "not at all characteristic of me"; 5 = "extremely characteristic of me"), and correlates highly with the original scale ($r = .96$).

In some studies, clients with social phobia have been found to score higher on the original FNE than clients with other anxiety disorders (Gelernter et al., 1992; Stopa & Clark, 1993), although they scored higher than only clients with simple phobia in others (Oei, Kenna, & Evans, 1991a; S. Turner, McCanna, & Beidel, 1987). Individuals with generalized social phobia have obtained higher scores on the FNE than individuals with nongeneralized social phobia (E. J. Brown et al., 1995; Gelernter et al., 1992; Holt et al., 1992a). Change in fear of negative evaluation has been shown to be a significant predictor of endstate functioning in two studies (Mattick & Peters, 1988; Mattick et al., 1989).

The FNE appears to be sensitive to change following treatment, although these changes are typically small in magnitude (Heimberg, 1994). The BFNE, with its 5-point Likert-type format, may ultimately prove to be more sensitive, although it was less sensitive to treatment-related change than the SPAI in one study (Taylor et al., 1997).

An examination of item content may suggest another possible concern. Several items appear to confound the assessment of anxiety and cognition (e.g., "I become tense and jittery if I know I am being judged by my superiors"). Thus the FNE scales may be relatively insensitive to differences in the magnitude of cognitive change produced by various interventions. However, in the absence of better measures of the important construct of the fear of negative evaluation, they will certainly continue to be used. The FNE appears in the original paper by Watson and Friend (1969), and the BFNE appears in the article by Leary (1983a). Both have been reprinted in the clinical sourcebook edited by Fischer and Corcoran (2000).

Social Interaction Self-Statement Test

The Social Interaction Self-Statement Test (SISST; Glass et al., 1982) is a thought-endorsement measure. It contains 15 positive (facilitative) and 15 nega-

Read each of the following statements carefully and indicate how characteristic it is of you according to the following scale. Circle a number to indicate how characteristic the statement is of you.

1 = **Not at all** characteristic of me
2 = **Slightly** characteristic of me
3 = **Moderately** characteristic of me
4 = **Very** characteristic of me
5 = **Extremely** characteristic of me

	Not at all	Slightly	Moderately	Very	Extremely
1. I worry about what other people will think of me even when I know it doesn't make a difference.	1	2	3	4	5
2. I am unconcerned even if I know people are forming an unfavorable impression of me.	1	2	3	4	5
3. I am frequently afraid of other people noticing my shortcomings.	1	2	3	4	5
4. I rarely worry about what kind of impression I am making on someone.	1	2	3	4	5
5. I am afraid that others will not approve of me.	1	2	3	4	5
6. I am afraid that people will find fault with me.	1	2	3	4	5
7. Other people's opinions of me do not bother me.	1	2	3	4	5
8. When I am talking to someone, I worry about what they may be thinking about me.	1	2	3	4	5
9. I am usually worried about what kind of impression I make.	1	2	3	4	5
10. If I know someone is judging me, it has little effect on me.	1	2	3	4	5
11. Sometimes I think I am too concerned with what other people think of me.	1	2	3	4	5
12. I often worry that I will say or do the wrong things.	1	2	3	4	5

FIGURE 6.4. The Brief Fear of Negative Evaluation Scale. From "A brief version of the Fear of Negative Evaluation Scale," by M. R. Leary, 1983, *Personality and Social Psychology Bulletin, 9,* p. 373. Copyright 1983 by the Society for Personality and Social Psychology. Reprinted by permission of Sage Publications.

tive (inhibitory) self-statements relevant to one-on-one interactions with the opposite sex. However, pronouns are often modified to make the instrument relevant to other situations, such as public speaking and same-sex interactions. Items on the positive self-statement scale (SISST-Positive) address optimistic anticipation of the interaction and coping, and items on the negative self-statement scale (SISST-Negative) concern self-deprecation and fear of negative evaluation. Participants are asked to endorse how often they experienced each thought on a 5-point Likert-type scale (1 = "hardly ever had the thought"; 5 = "very often had the thought"). The instructions for the original scale ask the participant to rate the frequency of these thoughts immediately prior to participating in a role play of a social interaction. However, both Dodge et al. (1988) and Zweig and Brown (1985) have developed versions of the SISST that ask participants to rate the frequency of thoughts experienced in typical social situations.

The SISST was initially developed in a college student sample (Glass et al., 1982), and the split-half reliability of both subscales was adequate. SISST-negative was positively related to anxiety ratings and negatively related to skill ratings made by the participant, a role-play confederate, and an observer immediately after a role play. SISST-Positive was less consistently related to these measures. Socially anxious individuals scored higher on SISST-Negative and lower on SISST-Positive than non–socially anxious individuals.

Dodge et al. (1988) examined the validity of the SISST with clients with social phobia. Compared with clients with primary public speaking fears, clients with primary interaction fears obtained higher scores on SISST-Negative but not on SISST-Positive. Dodge et al. (1988) found SISST-Negative and SISST-Positive to be significantly correlated and, therefore, conducted partial correlation analyses controlling for the other scale. When doing so, SISST-Negative was related to measures of social anxiety and depression, but SISST-Positive generally was not. Similarly, SISST-Negative was related to the percentage of negative thoughts generated after a role play, but SISST-Positive was not. Neither scale was related to positive thoughts generated after the role play, to heart rate prior to or during the behavior test, or to clinician ratings of phobic severity. Becker, Namour, Zayfert, and Hegel (2001) evaluated the specificity in a sample of 277 clients seeking treatment for anxiety. Both SISST-Negative and SISST-Positive discriminated between clients with social phobia and those with other anxiety disorders.

There are a number of advantages and disadvantages to using an endorsement measure such as the SISST. Endorsement instruments are brief, easy to administer and score, and allow for comparisons across studies and persons. They may have clinical utility for individuals who have difficulty spontaneously reporting thoughts. However, they do not capture the idiosyncratic nature of a client's thoughts and may have demand characteristics that pull for responses that reflect how the client was generally *feeling* rather than what he or she was actually *thinking* during the situation. The SISST has been reprinted in the clinical sourcebook edited by Fischer and Corcoran (2000).

Thought Listing

The goal of production methods used in the assessment of social phobia is to produce a representative sample of the client's thoughts in anticipation of, during, and/or after exposure to feared social stimuli. Probably the most commonly used production method is thought listing, which requires clients to write down all of the thoughts that they can recall having during a particular period of time (Cacioppo et al., 1979). In the clinical setting, thought listing may be facilitated by asking clients to imagine themselves in a fear-evoking situation, to participate in a role play of a threatening social interaction, or to watch a videotape of themselves engaged in a role play. In contrast to endorsement methods, production methods capture the idiosyncratic nature of the client's thoughts.

Thought listing records can be used in a variety of ways. They may serve as a starting point for cognitive restructuring activities in cognitive-behavioral treatment for social phobia, as is often the case in CBGT. Alternatively, they can be coded and quantified in various ways in order to assess severity and index change following treatment. Probably the most frequently used approach to coding has been to have independent judges classify the thoughts as positive (e.g., facilitative, happy), negative (e.g., inhibitory, anxious), or neutral. However, other dimensions, such as the target of the thought (i.e., self or other), may also be utilized (Hofmann, 2000).

As noted in Chapter 3, R. Schwartz and Garamoni (1989) proposed that the relative balance between positive and negative thoughts is especially important to adjustment and mental health. According to the States of Mind (SOM) model, an asymmetrical balance of positive thoughts (P) to the total of positive plus negative thoughts (P + N) that approximates .62 is considered optimal. Prior to treatment, the SOM ratio of individuals with social phobia is characterized by a preponderance of negative thoughts (Bruch et al., 1991) and is associated with more self-reported anxiety during a role play and higher scores on measures of social anxiety (Heimberg et al., 1990a). However, following successful treatment, these individuals have SOM ratios similar to what is considered optimal by the SOM model. Hofmann (2000) also recently demonstrated that successful cognitive-behavioral treatment of social phobia is associated with a reduction in the number of negative self-focused thoughts reported after a behavioral test.

Information Processing Tasks

To date, information processing tasks have been used mostly to examine the nature of social phobia and less frequently to measure social phobia severity or treatment outcome. In fact, of the many tasks described in Chapter 4 of this volume, only the modified Stroop color-naming task has been examined in relation to treatment outcome. Clients who showed a positive response to treatment of social phobia also showed a reduction in color-naming latencies for social-threat words, whereas nonresponding clients did not (Mattia et al., 1993). However, there are good reasons to adapt these tasks for clinical assessment. If they do, in fact, tap into basic cognitive processing and/or processes not immediately accessible to awareness, these measures would provide indices of progress that may be less confounded by clients' desire to appear in a positive light to their therapists or by momentary fluctuations in mood. Software programs are increasingly available that make the programming of these tasks straightforward.

Behavioral Assessment Tests

Although clinicians commonly use informal observation of behavior to make inferences about how clients behave outside of sessions, a more systematic evaluation of client behavior is useful. In Behavioral Assessment Tests (BATs), clients with social phobia confront fear-eliciting social situations in a controlled environment, typically in a role-play task. BATs provide an opportunity for firsthand observation of quality of social performance, visibility of anxiety symptoms, avoidance behaviors (e.g., refusing to engage in the BAT), and escape behaviors (e.g., leaving the situation prematurely). As we noted earlier in this chapter, observation of clients' behavior in a BAT cannot be replaced by the clients' own reports of behavior in the natural environment, because clients are just not very good observers of the quality of their own behavior. In addition, ratings of anxiety can also be easily collected before, during, and after the BAT (see Coles & Heimberg, 2000; Herbert et al., 1992b), and it is a simple matter to ask clients to record their thoughts after the BAT is concluded (Bruch et al., 1991; Heimberg et al., 1990a).

The most common types of situations for BAT role plays are a conversation with a same-sex or opposite-sex stranger, a conversation with two or more people, and a speech to a small audience. BATs may either be standardized (the same situations are role played by all clients) or individualized to meet the needs of a specific client. Standardized role plays allow for the observation of differences across clients in the same situation. In contrast, individualized BATs may more precisely target the idiosyncratic fears of the client and incorporate specific stimuli that occur frequently in that client's life. For example, an individualized BAT could require a client to present materials relevant to his or her real-life job to confederates in a role play of a staff meeting. Of course, individualized role plays are an important part of the activities of cognitive-behavioral treatment for social phobia.

There are two general levels of behavior analysis commonly used in BATs: molar versus molecular analyses. The molar approach targets the overall performance of the individual. For example, in a public speaking task, a rater or the clinician might assess the person's overall skill in speaking formally to others. The molecular approach, most commonly used in social skills research, attempts to break down the observed behavior into components. In a public speaking task, a molecular approach might target specific behaviors, such as eye contact or gestures. One assessment protocol for BATs, the Social Performance Rating Scale (Fydrich, Chambless, Perry, Buergner, & Beazley, 1998), uses five separate ratings in midlevel behavior assessment: vocal quality, gaze or eye contact, visible discomfort, speech length, and conversation flow. Each of these scales combines multiple molecular ratings. For example, voice quality includes ratings of tonal quality, clarity, pitch, and volume.

Although BATs have been used extensively in research on social phobia, relatively little attention has been devoted to their psychometric properties. Interrater and test–retest reliability are the most likely to be reported. For example, impromptu speech tasks have been shown to demonstrate high one-week test–retest reliability for both self-ratings of anxiety level and length of speech time (Beidel, Turner, Jacob, & Cooley, 1989b). BATs have also been shown to be sensitive to pre- and posttreatment differences and to differentiate between clients receiving cognitive-behavioral treatment and clients in a credible placebo-control condition (e.g., Heimberg et al., 1990b). Rating systems with good psychometric properties are available for behavioral assessment techniques (e.g., Fydrich et al., 1998), but they have not been widely used. More research is warranted to explore which procedures enhance the reliability and validity of BATs for social phobia.

Adjunctive Measures

In addition to social anxiety instruments, we routinely administer measures that tap other constructs. There are several important areas that should be examined among clients with social phobia. Here we focus briefly on depression, general anxiety, disability, and quality of life.

Depression

It is not uncommon for socially anxious individuals to experience a dysphoric or depressed mood secondary to the impairment associated with social anxiety. Therefore, we administer the Beck Depression Inventory (BDI; Beck, Rush, Shaw, & Emery, 1979) or BDI-II (Beck, Steer, & Brown, 1996), which assess symptoms of depression, including the affective, cognitive, behavioral, somatic, and motivational components, as well as suicidal intent. In a recent study of the BDI among clients with social phobia in our clinic, the BDI exhibited good internal consistency and retest reliability (Coles, Gibb, & Heimberg, 2001). It also correlated significantly more strongly with other measures of depression than with measures of either social or nonsocial anxiety. See Beck, Steer, and Garbin (1988) for a more general review of the psychometric characteristics of the BDI. The BDI-II is available from The Psychological Corporation (1-800-872-1726; *www.psychcorp.com/catalogs/paipc/psy092apri.htm*).

General Anxiety

Clients with social phobia often have anxieties far beyond their social concerns. There are four different measures that we sometimes find useful in assessment of our clients. The first of these is the State–Trait Anxiety Inventory (STAI; Spielberger, Gorsuch, Lushene, Vagg, & Jacobs, 1983), which provides measures of the general tendency to react to situations with anxiety (trait anxiety), as well as the degree of anxiety that the person may be experiencing at the moment (state anxiety). However, the trait scale of the STAI has been criticized because it is sometimes highly correlated with depression. Bieling, Antony, and Swinson (1998) recently conducted factor analytic studies of the trait anxiety scale and have developed separate anxiety and depression subscales that are potentially quite useful. The STAI is available from Mind Garden Inc. (650-261-3500; *www.mindgarden.com*) and a computerized version of the STAI for Windows™ is available from Multi-Health Systems, Inc. (information given earlier in this chapter).

The Beck Anxiety Inventory (Beck, Epstein, Brown, & Steer, 1988; available from the Psychological Corporation; *www.psychcorp.com/catalogs/paipc/psy093bpri.htm*) provides an index of the number of somatic symptoms of anxiety the person experiences. The Anxiety Sensitivity Index (Reiss, Peterson, Gursky, & McNally, 1986; available from IDS Publishing, 614-885-2323) assesses belief in the dangerousness of the symptoms of anxiety. High anxiety sensitivity has frequently been related to the experience of panic attacks, and anxiety sensitivity is elevated among clients with social phobia who experience panic attacks (Jack et al., 1999). The Penn State Worry Questionnaire (in Meyer et al., 1990, and Molina & Borkovec, 1994) assesses the uncontrollable and pathological worry that is often associated with generalized anxiety disorder but that is also elevated in many clients with generalized social phobia.

Disability

Because clients with similar levels of social anxiety may have very different levels of functional impairment, we also administer disability measures. A variety of disability measures are available (see Mendlowicz & Stein, 2000). Two measures designed for use with clients with social phobia are the Liebowitz Self-Rated Disability Scale and the clinician-rated Disability Profile (both in Schneier et al., 1994). Both assess current and lifetime impairment across a number of domains (e.g., educational attainment, romantic relationships, friendships, activities of daily living). The Liebowitz Self-Rated Disability Scale also assesses alcohol abuse, drug abuse, and mood dysregulation. Preliminary research suggests that these scales have adequate psychometric properties (Hambrick, Heimberg, & Turk, 2001; Schneier et al., 1994). In addition to ascertaining the overall severity of client disability, the scales can be used clinically by examining items on an individual basis in order to determine the domains most affected by the client's symptoms.

Quality of Life

Perhaps the best standard by which to judge the impact of a treatment is in terms of its effect on the client's overall sense of well-being. Therefore, we also administer the Quality of Life Inventory (QOLI), a self-report measure that assesses the extent to which clients perceive themselves as satisfied in the areas of their lives that they deem important to their happiness (Frisch, 1994). The Quality of Life Inventory appears to have good psychometric properties, and normative data are available (Frisch, 1994; Frisch, Cornell, Villanueva, & Retzlaff, 1992). QOLI scores are improved after cognitive-behavioral treatment for social phobia (Safren et al., 1997a), and these gains are maintained for at least six months after treatment (Eng, Coles, Heimberg, & Safren, 2001). The Quality of Life Inventory is available from NCS Assessment (1-800-627-7271 ext. 5151; *www.assessments.ncspearson.com/assessments/tests/qoli.htm*).

II

COGNITIVE-BEHAVIORAL GROUP THERAPY FOR SOCIAL PHOBIA: A TREATMENT MANUAL

7

An Overview of Cognitive-Behavioral Group Therapy for Social Phobia

Cognitive-behavioral group therapy (CBGT) works to break the vicious cycle of social anxiety described in Chapter 5 through the integration of cognitive restructuring and exposure techniques, both in the therapy office and in the client's world beyond it. CBGT has three primary components: in-session exposure to feared social situations, cognitive restructuring, and homework assignments for *in vivo* exposure and self-administered cognitive restructuring. In-session exposures form the hub of the protocol, with the cognitive interventions occurring before, during, and after each exposure. After the first few sessions, homework typically follows from the situation targeted during the in-session exposure. As in the session, clients are asked to engage in cognitive restructuring activities before, during, and after each assigned *in vivo* exposure.

Exposure to feared situations serves to disrupt the cycle of social anxiety in several ways (Hope et al., 2000). First, it short-circuits avoidance of anxiety-provoking social situations and allows the client to experience the natural reduction in anxiety that comes with staying in the situation long enough on repeated occasions (i.e., habituation). Second, exposure allows the client to practice behavioral skills in situations that may have been long avoided (e.g., asking someone for a date, being assertive). Third, exposure gives the client the opportunity to test the reality of his or her dysfunctional beliefs (e.g., "I won't be able to think of anything to say if I join my coworkers for lunch").

In-session exposures allow this process to begin in a protected environment, under the observation and control of the therapists. In this less threatening setting, clients can approach feared situations that are provided at the proper intensity. In-session exposures also provide clients an opportunity to practice their cognitive restructuring skills and experience success in an approximation of the real situation before they tackle it as part of a homework assignment. Of course, exposure to the feared situation in homework assignments facilitates the transfer of learning to where it matters most, the client's life outside the therapy session. The ultimate goal of homework assignments, and of CBGT as a total package, is for the client to become his or her own cognitive-behavioral therapist, equipped to adaptively confront anxiety-provoking situations in the present and into the future.

Cognitive restructuring also plays an important role in breaking the cycle of social anxiety (Hope et al., 2000). Cognitive restructuring provides a direct challenge to clients' beliefs, assumptions, and expectations. Clients are asked to evaluate whether these cognitions really make sense or are helpful and to entertain more realistic and adaptive ways of viewing feared situations. These techniques should supplement and support changes in cognition that follow from exposure to feared situations and increase the probability that clients' negative thinking will not override a successful exposure experience. As the client's assessment of the danger inherent in social situations becomes more realistic, physiological symptoms of anxiety often diminish as well. Furthermore, addressing the client's cognitions often frees up additional attentional resources and allows the client to increase focus on the social task and potentially improve performance. Changing dysfunctional beliefs also helps decrease anticipatory anxiety and avoidance and increase the client's ability to take credit for successes, which, in turn, gives the client the opportunity to experience the naturally occurring positive reinforcement available from other people. Lastly, cognitive restructuring teaches clients to think adaptively about their experiences after they have transpired rather than to enter into a cycle of rumination that might otherwise turn victory into defeat.

Thus CBGT combines in-session exposure, cognitive restructuring, and homework assignments to help clients overcome their anxiety and get more satisfaction in their transactions with themselves and others. In this section, we provide an overview of CBGT procedure. CBGT can be loosely divided into four parts: (1) an initial treatment orientation interview, (2) Sessions 1 and 2, (3) Sessions 3 through 11, and (4) the final (12th) session.

The Treatment Orientation Interview

This interview has several specific goals, which are fully delineated in the next chapter. Importantly, it allows the client to become acquainted with one of the therapists, thereby serving to provide a familiar face at the first meeting of the group. The client is introduced to the Subjective Units of Discomfort Scale (SUDS), which will be used throughout the treatment to quantify the client's anxiety experience. The therapist helps the client to develop explicit treatment goals and a Fear and Avoidance Hierarchy that represents situations to be targeted in therapy. The techniques of CBGT are described to the client, his or her questions are answered, and reading materials are assigned in advance of the first treatment session.

Sessions 1 and 2

The first two sessions set the stage for the remaining sessions and provide basic training in cognitive restructuring (see Chapters 9 and 10). Among the several tasks of the first session are: (1) presentation and discussion of the cognitive-behavioral model of social phobia and the rationale for cognitive-behavioral treatment, (2) initial training in cognitive restructuring, focusing on the identification of automatic thoughts, and (3) assigning homework to keep a diary of automatic thoughts during the following week. The second session further emphasizes the development of basic cognitive restructuring skills. Therapists use the automatic thoughts recorded for homework to introduce the concept of thinking errors and to highlight thinking errors common in the thoughts of persons with social phobia. Therapists also introduce clients to the process of disputing automatic thoughts and developing rational responses. The second session ends with the assignment of homework to label and dispute thinking errors in identified automatic thoughts.

Sessions 3 through 11

Sessions 3 through 11 are the heart of CBGT. Armed with cognitive restructuring skills learned in the initial sessions, clients confront personally relevant feared situations in in-session exposures (see Chapter 11). In a sense, the group becomes a theater in which feared situations are dramatically enacted, starting with situations of moderate difficulty and working toward more difficult situations as treatment progresses. An important aspect of CBGT is the integration of in-session exposures and cognitive restructuring (see Chapter 12). Once a client is chosen to participate in an exposure, automatic thoughts regarding the situation are elicited, thinking errors are labeled and disputed, and an alternative rational response is developed. The client is helped to evaluate his or her goals for the exposure and to make sure that these goals are observable, behavioral, and achievable. Throughout the exposure, therapists prompt the client each minute for his or her SUDS ratings, which play an important part in later cognitive restructuring activities. Repetition of rational responses at these times helps the client to focus his or her attention and apply cognitive coping skills during in-session exposures.

Each exposure continues until the client's anxiety begins to decrease or level off and behavioral goals are met (typically about 10 minutes). Cognitive debriefing following the exposure may include review of goal attainment and effective use of rational response(s) and other cognitive coping skills, analysis of the evidence provided by the experience that may undermine the client's belief in his or her automatic thoughts and bolster belief in the rational response, and examination of the pattern of SUDS ratings (i.e., how variations in experienced anxiety relates to events and/or thoughts during the exposure). Personalized homework assignments are developed for each client (see Chapter 13). The therapists and clients work together to develop assignments that will allow the client to confront situations similar to those practiced in the group. Clients are strongly encouraged to utilize cognitive restructuring skills before, during, and after their homework exposures.

Session 12

The first half of the final session allows time for additional exposures and associated cognitive restructuring activities (see Chapter 14). The second half is devoted to reviewing each client's progress over the course of treatment. Therapists also work with clients in identifying situations that may still be problematic and rational responses that may be useful in these situations and in setting goals for continued work after the termination of formal treatment.

Setting Up the Group

In this section, we consider several issues that have to do with the general structure of CBGT. These topics include the characteristics of the therapists and clients who will participate in the group, number and length of sessions, and the setting in which the group will be conducted.

Therapists

In our research program, therapists have been selected from the ranks of clinical and counseling psychologists and advanced doctoral students in clinical or counseling psychology. However, the specific professional discipline with which a therapist identifies is less important than the therapist's knowledge, demeanor, and experience. Several therapist characteristics are desirable. First, they should have sufficient experience in the role of therapist that they can devote their full attention to the clients and the conduct of group activities without undue anxiety or self-consciousness. Because the clients will look to the therapists as experts and as persons who can help them overcome their own anxieties, it is important for therapists to appear reasonably relaxed. Second, they should have a thorough knowledge of social phobia and of how clients may respond in a group setting. Third, they should be familiar with the basic principles of group dynamics and the fostering of group cohesion. Fourth, and most obviously, they should be intimately familiar with cognitive-behavioral theory and the procedures of CBGT.

We recommend that CBGT groups be conducted by two cotherapists. Although we have conducted single-therapist groups on occasion, the utilization of cotherapists may be more effective. Single therapists may find it difficult to simultaneously monitor the clinical state of each of the clients and to become involved in group activities. In-session exposures may require therapists to serve multiple functions including, but not limited to, role playing, monitoring the anxiety experienced by the target client, and counting the number of behaviors performed by the target client who is attempting to achieve a specific behavioral goal. Although these functions can often be assigned to other clients in later sessions, they will typically fall to the therapists initially. This heavy load can rapidly fatigue a single therapist and reduce his or her clinical effectiveness.

It is also best if there is one therapist of each gender. Obviously, this will provide the greatest flexibility for the therapists to tailor in-session exposures to the needs of the target client, as clients' fears will often involve interactions with the opposite sex or with mixed-sex groups. In addition, clients who present with extreme fears of interaction with individuals of the opposite sex may simply be afraid to interact with a therapist of the opposite sex and may find the group much less threatening if there is a same-sex therapist available.

Clients

Our experience suggests that the ideal group size for CBGT is six clients. This number is small enough to allow frequent individualized attention. With six clients, each client can become the focus of the group's effort at least once every other session. With each additional client, this becomes increasingly more difficult to accomplish. Six clients also provide some insurance against inevitable dropouts and missed sessions. Starting a group with fewer clients may increase the probability that group size may drop too low for effective administration of group procedures or that the remaining group members may become disenchanted.

The next issue concerns the mix of clients who participate in a CBGT group. Clients vary on a number of important characteristics, including gender, locus of fear, and severity of symptoms. Groups should include roughly equal numbers of men and women. With a group size of six, we recommend that there not be fewer than 2 men or 2 women. This balance is especially important for clients whose fears concern heterosexual interaction, as generalization of treatment gains should be facilitated by interaction with a variety of persons of the opposite sex. For those clients, initial in-session exposures will probably involve interactions with the opposite-sex therapist, but later in-session exposures should include all other opposite-sex group members.

Persons with social phobia may fear interacting with anyone in any circumstance, or they may fear more specific situations, such as public speaking, eating, drinking, or writing in public, or using public restrooms. All of these feared situations involve being the center of attention or being negatively evaluated in some manner, and it has been our experience that clients with very different profiles of fears may still relate well to each other's concerns. Thus clients with different fears may be mixed in the same group with several benefits. Clients with fears of public speaking, for instance, may find it relatively easy to play the role of the other person in an in-session exposure for a client with fears of social interaction. Clients with a variety of fears may serve as audience members for public-speaking-fearful clients with little threat to themselves. However, it may be difficult for social-interaction phobics to help each other in this manner early in treatment. Thus a group made up exclusively of interaction phobics may be problematic. Similarly, it is often a problem if there is a single client whose fear is very different from those of the rest of the group members. It has been our strategy to attempt to balance the group on this dimension, striving for a mix of clients with generalized fears of social interaction and clients with fears of more specific social situations.

Finally, clients with social phobia may differ a great deal in the severity of their symptoms or the degree of impairment in functioning they experience. It is typical that all clients will experience a great deal of anticipatory anxiety about the group experience. They may each decide (without evidence) that they are the "worst" or the "sickest" or that they will not be accepted by the rest of the group. If one client is, in fact, significantly more impaired than the other group members, his or her fears may well be realized. This demoralizing situation may be avoided by attempting to enroll clients of similar severity in any particular group.

Group Sessions

Our CBGT groups have been conducted for 12 to 24 weekly sessions of varying duration, sometimes with monthly booster sessions for a period of 6 to 7 months after the termination of weekly sessions. Currently, groups meet for twelve 2½-hour weekly sessions, and this format has proven quite workable. With a group of six, 2½-hour sessions have provided the maximal opportunity to provide individualized attention to as many clients as possible without excessive mental or emotional fatigue on the part of the clients. Longer sessions may wear clients down and actually produce an increase in anxiety for those whose work time comes at the end of the session. Shorter sessions lead to a rushed attempt to get from one client to another and should be avoided. Although we have seen little difference in efficacy of groups that meet for 12 sessions compared with those that meet for 14 or 15, groups that have met for 24 sessions may warrant further study. Our preliminary experience with 24-week groups in the course of an ongoing study is that they may help clients to "lock in" and expand on the gains they have achieved by the end of 12 weeks. However, it can sometimes be difficult to retain clients for the duration of a 24-week group. The jury is still out on the utility of booster sessions. Finally, an interval of one week between sessions appears to be the minimum period to allow clients adequate time for home practice.

Our groups have been conducted in a living-room setting with comfortable sofas and easy chairs for clients to sit on. Enough spots are provided so that clients may determine their own boundaries of personal space. Temperature should be adequately controlled for client comfort. Although these details may not appear worth mentioning, we believe they may be very important for the proper management of clients with social phobia. If clients are crowded together, their concerns about being evaluated by the nearest group members may increase, and a similar effect may occur if they find themselves squirming around on uncomfortable chairs. Temperature control may be very important for clients who fear that their anxiety will make them sweat in front of others. Increasing the comfort of the group setting will reduce the degree to which clients are distracted by these seemingly irrelevant details.

One piece of equipment is essential to the proper conduct of CBGT. This is an easel or chalkboard. We prefer an easel because pages from earlier sessions can be retained, making it easy to access previously covered material if needed. Over the course of group exercises or in-session exposures, therapists will elicit automatic thoughts and help clients to develop rational responses to use in combating their anxiety. When clients become anxious, their ability to remember rational responses is impaired, but it can be supplemented by referring to responses that have been recorded for their use. Specific procedures are described in later chapters.

When constructing a CBGT group, refer to this checklist:

- Two therapists, 1 male and 1 female.
- Six clients, balanced for gender, feared situations, and degree of impairment.
- 12 sessions, 2½ hours' duration.
- A comfortable group setting.
- A chalkboard or easel.

Assessment of Fear of Negative Evaluation

In our research program, we assess clients' level of concern about negative evaluation by others each week. For this purpose, we administer the 12-item Brief Fear of Negative Evaluation Scale (BFNE; Leary, 1983a) at the beginning of each session, including the first. A copy of the BFNE appears in Chapter 6 (Figure 6.4). A stack of questionnaires and pencils are placed on the coffee table in the group room, and clients complete the BFNE as they arrive for the session. With little intrusion on group time, we are thus able to examine on a weekly basis an objective index of this construct that is so central to social phobia.

8

The Treatment Orientation Interview

At the Adult Anxiety Clinic of Temple University, all potential clients are assessed with the Anxiety Disorders Interview Schedule—Lifetime Version for DSM-IV (ADIS-IV-L; DiNardo, Brown, & Barlow, 1994) and a comprehensive questionnaire battery consisting of measures described in Chapter 6. The ADIS-IV-L provides comprehensive diagnostic information about social phobia and the other anxiety disorders, depression, and a number of other psychiatric problems that may interfere with the course of cognitive-behavioral group treatment for social phobia (e.g., alcohol or substance abuse). Thereafter, an additional interview is conducted, which we call the "treatment orientation interview." The treatment orientation interview serves a variety of purposes, many of which have to do with the particulars of specific research studies, which are not included here. However, the interview serves a variety of clinical purposes as well:

1. To discuss with the client the specific diagnoses that were derived from the ADIS-IV-L interview, as well as the findings of the other assessments; to determine whether group treatment is appropriate for the client at this time; and to discuss referrals for treatment elsewhere if appropriate.
2. To further delineate the specifics of the client's social phobia if necessary.
3. To complete the Individualized Fear and Avoidance Hierarchy.
4. To train the client in the use of the Subjective Units of Discomfort Scale (SUDS), which will be used repeatedly in the group.
5. To develop a contract between the client and the interviewer about which aspects of the client's social phobia should be addressed in the group.

6. To familiarize the client with the specific group procedures (in-session exposures, cognitive restructuring, homework assignments).
7. To address the client's fears about participating in a group and to discuss the several potential advantages that group treatment may possess over individual treatment.
8. To prepare the client to begin group treatment sessions.

Clients for Whom Cognitive-Behavioral Group Therapy May Not Be Appropriate

Some clients will be poorly suited to any specific intervention procedure. In the practice of group treatment, however, it is not only important that the treatment fits the client but also that the client's presence in the group does not disrupt its functioning or retard the progress of other group members. Clients who are extremely verbose, loud, hostile, demanding of attention, or lacking motivation are poor candidates for any group, as are clients who are so profoundly disturbed that they are unable to tune in to whatever is going on around them. Issues of group composition, differences in severity of social phobic symptoms, and differences in focus of fear were discussed in Chapter 7. However, clients may present additional concerns that should be addressed in the treatment orientation interview. Positive answers to any of the following questions should lead to consideration of other treatment options, tailored to the individual case:

Is the client so extremely anxious that the treatment group itself represents an overwhelming anxiety-provoking stimulus? We have been repeatedly surprised at the willingness of our clients to participate in group treatment. Although almost all express significant discomfort at the mention of the group, they rarely refuse to participate, and we rarely exclude them because we are worried that they may be overwhelmed by their anxiety. That said, the occasional client whose anxiety is severe to the extreme may have difficulty tolerating the anxiety that is generated simply by sitting in the group session. This client may have difficulty concentrating on (and therefore understanding) the treatment rationale or the concepts that are taught in the first two sessions. Similarly, extreme anxiety may compromise the client's ability to monitor automatic thoughts, and these clients may protest that they do not think, that they simply get anxious and their hearts beat. They may attempt to control their anxiety by minimizing participation or avoiding group sessions. They may also be less likely to attempt homework assignments, and, in the worst case, they may terminate treatment prematurely. Thus, if the client's anxiety about being in a group is so severe that he or she would be unlikely to benefit from the situation, it is may be best to pursue individual treatment options as alternatives to group treatment or as precursors to it.

Clients whose anxiety about being in group is high but not so high as to be disorganizing (admittedly a judgment call) need not be excluded from group treatment. They may find that their anxiety about the group abates as they become more familiar with the therapists and other clients. They may become less embarrassed about sharing their anxious thoughts when other group members do so. In addition, specific intervention procedures are available to help these clients become increasingly comfortable in the group setting. These strategies are outlined in Chapter 12.

Is the client experiencing substantial depression? Depression is a common side effect of social phobia, and the mere presence of unhappiness or an occasional drop in mood is not a cause for concern. However, if substantial depression is present, a decision should be made as to whether the client is ready for group treatment or for any treatment directed at social phobia at this time. The decision to treat one problem or the other is made after a careful functional analysis of the relationship between the client's anxiety and depression and consideration of the relative severity of each. When social anxiety precedes depression, further analysis may reveal that depressive symptoms have progressed from a history of increased avoidance, isolation, and deprivation of social reinforcement or occupational attainment. Although it seems intuitive that treatment of social phobia would result in reduced depression, other factors need to be considered as well.

If the client is significantly depressed, he or she may experience symptoms of lethargy, inertia, low motivation, and hopelessness. He or she may be unable to find the energy for the various group and homework tasks or to attempt many of them. He or she may interpret slow progress as yet another in a long line of failures and personal inadequacies. Hopelessness may also have a negative effect on other group members during the critical early sessions. Depression of this nature has been associated with less satisfactory outcomes of CBGT (Chambless, Tran, & Glass, 1997). Active suicidal thinking associated with any meaningful degree of intent requires attention before a client can be considered a candidate for CBGT.

Does the client suffer from a concurrent anxiety disorder? This need not lead to automatic exclusion of a client from CBGT. However, if the other anxiety disorder is of greater severity, it may be most appropriate to treat it first. This is particularly the case for clients with panic disorder, who may be significantly afraid of their physical symptoms and only secondarily concerned about the evaluations of others. CBGT is not designed to be a treatment for panic disorder, and because cognitive-behavioral treatments for panic disorder (e.g., D. M. Clark, 1997; Craske & Barlow, 2000) have shown good success, the client should be referred to one of them. CBGT does appear to be efficacious for clients with social phobia who have panic attacks that occur primarily in feared social interaction and performance situations (Scott, 2000).

If a client receives concurrent diagnoses of social phobia and another anxiety disorder, but these are of equal severity and degree of interference in the client's life, we find it a reasonable strategy to leave the decision to the client. Such was the case for a client who presented with social phobia and a specific phobia of dentists. Upcoming dental work made the specific phobia more salient to this client, and he chose to pursue treatment for his dental phobia in advance of participating in our treatment program.

Does the client currently rely on anxiolytic medications to control the physiological symptoms of anxiety? Many clients with social phobia will be taking one or more psychotropic medications when they present for treatment. Some will be taking medication to control their social anxiety, and others will be taking medications for depression or other comorbid conditions. Research has demonstrated that several pharmacological treatments are efficacious for social phobia (for a review, see Scott & Heimberg, 2000). Nevertheless, some clients experience little or only partial symptom relief from their medication and pursue psychological treatment with the hope of experiencing additional improvement. Other clients are satisfied with the symptom relief provided by their medication but dislike being on a medication and hope that therapy will allow them to eventually discontinue pharmacotherapy.

Several outcomes are possible when psychosocial and pharmacological treatments for social phobia are combined: (1) the medication may interfere with the client's ability to benefit from cognitive restructuring and exposure (e.g., insufficient anxiety is aroused during exposures); (2) the medication may enhance the effectiveness of cognitive-behavioral interventions (e.g., anxiety is reduced to a level that allows the client to attend to and learn more from the exposure); or (3) no appreciable gains (or losses) are seen with the combination of psychotherapy and medication. Lack of research on this issue prevents us from drawing any definitive conclusions about the consequences of combining CBGT with an ongoing medication treatment. The possibility that different types of medication may interact with cognitive-behavioral therapy in different ways further complicates the matter.

We do not require clients to discontinue their medications prior to starting CBGT (unless dictated by a specific research protocol). However, we do ask clients to stabilize their dosage before starting treatment and to refrain from changing their dosage or trying any new medications during cognitive-behavioral treatment. Clinically, we want clients to attribute positive changes in their symptoms to the work they are doing in therapy rather than changes in their medication regimen. Individuals who take medication on an "as needed" basis are asked to refrain from taking it before group sessions or exposure homework assignments.

Clinical experience suggests that some clients who are highly dependent on benzodiazepines may not benefit substantially from cognitive-behavioral treatment, or, if they do benefit, they may be at increased risk for relapse. They seem unlikely to tolerate the anxiety that is an inherent component of in-session exposures and homework assignments. They may feel more inclined than other clients to take an extra dose of their medications to reduce anxiety before group sessions or before *in vivo* exposures. As a result, these exercises are unlikely to seem "real enough" to them, little relevant cognitive activity may occur, and clients may paradoxically wonder what is wrong with the treatment. These outcomes might be expected to have a negative effect on the client's motivation or on that of other group members. Also, a client who maintains medication use but does improve is quite likely to attribute that improvement to the drug rather than to his or her own efforts. Withdrawal from medication may then produce a significant increase in symptoms. Although similar experiences have been reported among clients with panic disorder (e.g., Otto, Pollack, & Sabatino, 1996), research in that area has taken a somewhat different approach. A number of studies have investigated whether cognitive-behavioral treatment can assist the client in discontinuing treatment with high-potency benzodiazepines while maintaining and consolidating treatment gains (e.g., Bruce, Spiegel, & Hegel, 1999; Otto et al., 1993). Results of these studies have been quite promising and suggest that a similar strategy may be viable for social phobic clients with a strong benzodiazepine habit who present for cognitive-behavioral treatment.

Other classes of medications may not be as problematic as the benzodiazepines for the person with social phobia, although little research is available to guide our decision making here. Nevertheless, it is not unreasonable for a client to be quite hesitant to give up his or her current means of coping with anxiety before the benefits of cognitive-behavioral treatment have been realized. Therefore, it may be prudent to take an intermediate course. Rather than exclude all clients who take antianxiety medications, attempting new behaviors without medication (or at progressively decreasing dosages) may become a primary treatment goal.

It is not possible for us to provide a thorough review of pharmacotherapy for social phobia or of how to combine cognitive-behavioral and pharmocological treatments for social phobia in a productive way. The reader is referred to the chapter by Liebowitz (2000) in the Client Workbook for an up-to-date discussion of the various medications in current use for the treatment of social phobia and issues that may arise in the implementation of combined treatment strategies.

Does the client suffer from concurrent substance use? Although limited space does not allow us to thoroughly discuss the impact of substance use on treatment for social phobia, the specific matter of alcohol use deserves comment. As reviewed earlier, many individuals with social phobia also have alcohol use problems. Thus it is not uncommon to encounter this type of client in clinical practice. As in the case of depression, it is important to perform a functional analysis to determine how the client's alcohol use is related to his or her social anxiety. Because social anxiety predates difficulties with alcohol use in the large majority of cases, many clients with social phobia may have learned to use alcohol as a means of coping in social situations. Common sense would suggest that in such cases, treatment for social phobia would ameliorate drinking problems. However, not all individuals with social phobia who have drinking problems are good candidates for CBGT. Clients must be able to commit to *not* drinking either during group or during out-of-session exposure exercises and must have the self-regulatory skills necessary to follow through on such proclamations. Drinking during exposures limits their ability to engage in cognitive tasks and can lead them to (paradoxically) attribute both successes and failures to the alcohol. Furthermore, drinking in social settings (including the group) and then driving home can be very dangerous. Clearly, a careful analysis of drinking behavior must take place before admitting clients into CBGT. In some cases, particularly when criteria for alcohol dependence are met, it may be prudent to refer clients for treatment for their alcohol use problems prior to their entering treatment for social phobia.

Discussion of the Specifics of the Client's Social Phobia

One of the primary goals of the treatment orientation interview is to discuss the client's specific social fears. This discussion has several purposes. First, it facilitates the development of rapport between the client and the interviewer (especially if the treatment orientation interviewer was not the same person who administered the intake/diagnostic interview). Second, if the interviewer is also to be one of the group therapists, it reduces clients' concerns that they will go into a group in which no one knows about them or their problems. At least one familiar person will be there at the initial group session. Third, it allows the client and therapist to share detailed and specific information about the client's phobia that will be necessary for designing individualized treatment strategies. Fourth, it facilitates the completion of the Individualized Fear and Avoidance Hierarchy. Fifth, it aids in the process of contracting for specific behavior change goals.

In this discussion, we focus on delineating as many situations as possible in which anxiety is problematic. All relevant situations are examined, and an attempt is made to:

1. Describe the anxiety response in detail, including cognitive, behavioral, and physiological aspects.
2. Isolate the stimuli that signal the anxiety response.
3. Look at variations in the situation and how they may affect the client's anxiety.

It may be enough for a diagnosis of social phobia to know that a person fears embarrassment or scrutiny in public speaking situations and that he or she is impaired by these fears. However, this information is *not* adequate for the design of cognitive-behavioral interventions, including the central techniques of CBGT (in-session exposures, cognitive restructuring, homework assignments). Several more pieces of information are necessary. For instance, a male client with a fear of public speaking reported that:

1. He experiences rapid heartbeat, sweating, and dry mouth when in public speaking situations.
2. He worries that others will see his anxiety and negatively evaluate him.
3. He believes that the quality of his behavioral performance will deteriorate as he becomes focused on how nervous he is.
4. He experiences intense anxiety when asked to talk in staff meetings at work or while giving formal sales presentations.
5. He is much less anxious when speaking to groups of friends or when making a point at a PTA meeting.
6. His anxiety is less if he feels more comfortable with the material being presented.
7. He finds it easier to answer questions than to make a presentation without interruption.
8. His anxiety increases when his supervisor or other superiors are present.
9. He becomes more anxious when people disagree with his points.
10. He becomes more anxious if presenting from a standing position.

As will be seen in later chapters, this information is critical for the proper design of in-session exposures and homework assignments, and the earlier it becomes available, the less likely therapists will be to design inadequate exposures or to spend group time engaged in this sort of data collection.

The Individualized Fear and Avoidance Hierarchy

When the preceding discussion is complete, it is useful to both client and interviewer to make a written list of the client's feared situations. To accomplish this, we help the client create an Individualized Fear and Avoidance Hierarchy. The client is asked to rank order his or her 10 most feared situations. In actuality, clients do not tend to report 10 distinct functionally unrelated situations; rather, they report variations on two or three situations. In addition, we ask our clients to provide two ratings for each listed situation: degree of fear or anxiety (Subjective Units of Discomfort Scale; next section) and degree of avoidance, each on 0–100 scales (with 100 representing the most extreme fear/anxiety and avoidance). A completed example for the client with public speaking fears described in the previous section appears in Figure 8.1.

The Individualized Fear and Avoidance Hierarchy not only serves to organize and summarize the findings of the previous discussion but also provides a guide for sequencing in-session exposures during CBGT. Its use in that context is described in later chapters. Beginning cognitive-behavioral therapists may wish to consult Chapter 4 of the Client Workbook which includes several examples and questions that may be used to assist the client in developing the Fear and Avoidance Hierarchy.

The Subjective Units of Discomfort Scale (SUDS)

In the construction of the Fear and Avoidance Hierarchy, the client provides 0–100 SUDS ratings for each situation. The use of the SUDS continues during group sessions, as clients are requested to rate their anxiety each minute during in-session exposures. However, as indicated by its name, this scale is quite subjective, and the meaning of specific scale values may differ from client to client. In addition, certain clients may create problems in the use of the scale by giving only very low ratings, suggesting they may feel a sense of failure or fear the reaction of the therapists or group if they were to report higher numbers. Other clients may report consistently high numbers, thus conveying a sense of their need for help. Because clients will inevitably compare their own ratings with those provided by other group members, some degree of standardization is in order.

Our procedure is as follows. First, scale points of 0 (no anxiety, calm, relaxed) and 100 (very severe anxiety, worst ever experienced) are defined. A specific situation corresponding to a rating of 100 is elicited from the client. Second, definitions of scale values of 25, 50, and 75 are provided, and specific examples of each scale value from the client's personal experience are again elicited. This procedure is easily integrated with the construction of the Fear and Avoidance Hierarchy and yields a personalized series of anchor points that is kept in the therapists' group file so that a client may refer to it as needed or therapists may use it to provide corrective feedback. An example of a completed "SUDS Sheet" appears in Figure 8.2.

Contracting about Specific Targets for Treatment

It does not follow that a client will wish to confront a specific fear just because it exists. In fact, this is often not the case at all. A common example is the client with generalized social fears who comes to treatment when a change in a job-related situation puts him or her in a role involving training others or in which public speaking is required. This client may be socially avoidant, have few friends or potential romantic contacts, and so forth. However, the immediacy of his or her job situation makes it the only situation he or she cares about. Similarly, we have seen doctoral students who have become quite anxious at the prospect of the oral defense of their theses or dissertations, upcoming conference

Situation	SUDS	Avoidance
#1 most difficult situation is *Giving a formal presentation about a new product; material is new and unfamiliar; audience is large; supervisor is present; standing during presentation*	100	100
#2 most difficult situation is *Same as 1, but more familiar and comfortable with the material; audience smaller*	90	90
#3 most difficult situation is *Giving a report at a regular weekly staff meeting; supervisor present; coworker who has disagreed with client in the past also present*	90	90
#4 most difficult situation is *Same as 3; disagreeable coworker absent*	80	60
#5 most difficult situation is *Giving a formal presentation on familiar material when client knows supervisor will be absent*	70	40
#6 most difficult situation is *Disagreeing with another coworker at a staff meeting*	60	80
#7 most difficult situation is *Presenting a report at a staff meeting and answering questions about it*	50	50
#8 most difficult situation is *Sitting at a conference table with coworkers, sharing opinions on a new project*	40	40
#9 most difficult situation is *Giving a presentation to a group of sales trainees*	30	10
#10 most difficult situation is *Expressing an opinion at a meeting of the Parent–Teacher Association (PTA)*	20	50

Rating Scales for Individualized Fear and Avoidance Hierarchy

Subjective Units of Discomfort Scale (SUDS)

0	10	20	30	40	50	60	70	80	90	100
No anxiety, calm, relaxed		Mild anxiety, alert, able to cope			Moderate anxiety, some trouble concentrating			Severe anxiety, thoughts of leaving the situation		Very severe anxiety, worst ever experienced

Avoidance

0	10	20	30	40	50	60	70	80	90	100
Never avoid		Avoid once in awhile			Avoid sometimes			Usually avoid		Always avoid

FIGURE 8.1. A completed Fear and Avoidance Hierarchy for a client with a fear of public speaking.

presentations, or the need to give colloquia when interviewing for academic jobs. At such times, they simply are not interested in more broadly based treatment, "need" it or not. Therefore, it is important to know that a client fears a specific situation *and* that he or she wishes to make it a target for treatment.

Our practice is to query the client about each fear listed on the Individualized Fear and Avoidance Hierarchy. If the client wishes to work on it, so be it. If not, the reasons for this decision are discussed, and the situation may be bypassed. However, in the course of this discussion, it is useful to assess whether the client's lack of interest stems from fear of being overwhelmed by the situation

---

SUBJECTIVE UNITS OF DISCOMFORT

0	50	100
No anxiety		Maximum anxiety

Record at least one specific situation for each anxiety level listed below.

SUDS rating	Definition
0	Client is totally relaxed, on the verge of sleep. *Sitting at the beach, watching and listening to the waves.*
25	Client experiences mild anxiety. Anxiety does not interfere with performance (able to think of things to say, etc.). *Telling a joke or story to friends at a party.* *Stating my position on an issue at a PTA meeting.*
50	Anxiety becomes uncomfortable. Concentration is adversely affected, but the client continues on. *Presenting a report at a staff meeting and answering questions about it when I am familiar with the material I am presenting.*
75	Anxiety becomes increasingly uncomfortable, and client becomes preoccupied with symptoms of anxiety. Client finds it extremely difficult to concentrate and entertains thoughts of escaping the situation. *Giving a formal sales presentation to other salespeople in the company, no supervisor is present.*
100	The highest anxiety that the client has ever experienced. *Giving a formal sales presentation about a new product to a large group of middle managers including my supervisor.*

FIGURE 8.2. A completed Subjective Units of Discomfort Scale (SUDS) Definition Form for a client with a fear of public speaking.

or a strong belief that he or she is simply not up to the challenge. Situations of this nature may be deferred for consideration after the client has shown some degree of improvement in the first several sessions of CBGT. Remaining situations constitute the initial "contract" between the client and the group.

Introduction to Group Procedures

Clients are provided with an overview of what will happen in the treatment group. The procedures (in-session exposures, cognitive restructuring, homework assignments) are named, a rationale for their effectiveness is presented, and a description of how they have been effectively applied to other clients is provided. As much of this information is also presented in the group during Session 1, specific descriptions appear in Chapter 9. In the treatment orientation interview, however, the interviewer can present this information in a more individualized manner and also describe potential application to the client's personal concerns.

Part of the interviewer's job is to instill hope that the person will be able to make significant changes as a result of treatment. In fact, positive outcome expectancies are associated with more favorable CBGT outcomes (Chambless et al., 1997; Safren, Heimberg, & Juster, 1997b). We typically tell clients that CBGT is an empirically supported treatment and that studies have shown that, of individuals completing the 12 weeks of group therapy, approximately 75–80% are rated by independent clinical interviewers as having experienced meaningful reductions in their social anxiety. We also emphasize that attending group regularly, doing homework, and being open to new ways of looking at the world, other people, and oneself are factors that substantially influence whether or not someone becomes a "treatment responder" and that these factors are to a large degree under the client's control.

It is almost certain that clients will become anxious over the prospect of working on their specific fears in the group setting. This fear stems from two issues. First, because the group asks clients to talk about and expose themselves to personally relevant situations, it also asks them to become the center of the group's attention for extended periods of time. Second, as in the cognitive-behavioral treatment of all anxiety disorders, they will be asked to do the very things they fear, and they may be afraid of the anxiety that this implies. Straightforward discussion of these issues with the client is often sufficient to allay these fears and reduce the client's indecision over whether or not to attend the initial session.

The Advantages of Group Treatment

A discussion of group procedures naturally leads to a discussion of why we have selected the group modality, usually in the form of a request for individual treatment or an expression of anxiety over being in the group. Sank and Shaffer (1984) present a list of advantages of group over individual treatment that we have adapted and found useful:

1. *Learning that others have similar problems*: Many individuals with social phobia, because they are anxious about talking to others, may never have talked with anyone else about their anxiety and may believe that they are the only ones so afflicted. The group can provide a powerful corrective experience by putting the client in contact with similar others.
2. *Vicarious learning*: The group format allows the client to learn from other clients who are using the skills they are learning.
3. *Peer learning*: Clients may learn from others who closely resemble them but who are learning to cope with and overcome obstacles. Coping models, who experience anxiety but persist in the face of it, may be perceived as more relevant to the client than "fearless" models.
4. *Learning through helping others*: Group treatment provides the client with an opportunity to help others overcome their problems. Clients can thereby become a support system for each other in meaningful ways during and after the group therapy program.
5. *Encouragement through observation of others' successes*: The client will initially doubt his or her ability to overcome anxiety. However, seeing someone else succeed can serve to increase positive expectations.
6. *Fostering independence*: The group format encourages clients to rely on each other rather than to develop extreme dependence on an individual therapist.
7. *Public commitment*: By the act of joining the group, the client makes public his or her intention to change.

To this list we add that, for clients with social phobia, the group provides an opportunity to directly confront a phobic stimulus, to test out concerns about the perceptions of others, and to take advantage of the presence of others to create a variety of therapeutic simulations.

Ground Rules

Next, we discuss with the client what is expected of him or her as a member of the group. Attendance, promptness, and completion of homework assignments are stressed. However, the two issues that receive the greatest attention are confidentiality and participation in the group by helping other clients work on their specific fears. As these issues are reiterated in the initial group session, further discussion is deferred until Chapter 9.

Preparing the Client to Begin Group Treatment Sessions

At this point, it is appropriate to send clients home with a reading assignment to further ready themselves for the CBGT experience. Specifically, they may be asked to read and study the first three chapters of the Client Workbook (Homework assignments described in Chapters 2 and 3 of the Client Workbook need not be completed at this time.). These chapters include information on the etiology of social phobia, the nature of anxiety, the specific components of cognitive-behavioral therapy, and so forth, and may serve to reinforce concepts raised in the treatment orientation interview and prepare the client for further discussion of these ideas in the first few sessions of the group. Clients can be asked to read these chapters and bring questions to the first group session. Particularly important are sections of Chapter 1 entitled "How Do I Know if This Program Is for Me?" which asks several questions about the impact that social phobia has had on the client's life; "Will This Program Work for Me?" which describes a bit about the history of CBGT and what improvement in treatment means; and "What Can I Do to Get the Most Out of This Program?" which describes the approach that clients might best take toward their treatment. Specifically, it is recommended to clients that they:

1. Seriously invest effort and energy in the process of change.
2. Do the prescribed exercises carefully and practice, practice, practice!
3. Persevere if treatment does not seem to produce immediate results.
4. Be kind to themselves, celebrate the progress that they make while trying to minimize the tendency to be self-critical.
5. Be willing to try new ways of dealing with their social anxiety.

9

Session 1

MATERIALS

- Pens or pencils
- Name tags
- Clipboards to use as writing surfaces
- Copies of the Brief Fear of Negative Evaluation Scale (Figure 6.4)
- Group Confidentiality Contract (Figure 9.1)
- Copies of the Reaction to Treatment Questionnaire (Figure 9.3)
- Copies of the Form for Monitoring Automatic Thoughts (Figure 9.4)
- A newsprint easel
- A marker pen
- Audio- or videocassette recorder and tape (for self-study or supervision)
- This manual

TOPICS

- Introductions
- Review of ground rules for group membership
- Sharing of individual problems and goals
- Presentation of the cognitive-behavioral model of social phobia
- Discussion of the components of treatment
- Assessment of expectancies for treatment outcome
- Initial training in cognitive restructuring
  - Introduction to automatic thoughts
  - Eliciting automatic thoughts about group treatment
- Homework assignment for Session 1: Monitoring and recording automatic thoughts

This manual provides a great deal of detail about the conduct of group sessions, especially Sessions 1 and 2. In our experience, it is best for therapists to be very familiar with the manual but to have it available and refer to it on an as-needed basis during sessions. Also, the several therapists' dialogues that appear throughout this manual should be taken as exemplars rather than scripts to be followed verbatim. ***Therapists should never read these scripts directly from the manual***, but instead, they should be familiar with the intended content and express it in their own words. Boxes like this one are provided throughout the remainder of the manual to highlight key points for therapists' attention.

The first session is a critical one in the life of the group. It is the first time that the clients, several of whom may be morbidly afraid of meeting new people, speaking in front of a group, or even being in a group, will be assembled. Clients may have experienced considerable anticipatory anxiety about the group and about the initial session, and several may have been able to think of little else for days. Although we have been repeatedly surprised at clients' ability and willingness to speak up in this initial session, therapists should be consistently mindful of the anxiety-provoking potential it holds. Therefore, therapists should be ready to carry much of the load during this session and should be more accepting of clients' hesitance to participate than would be the case in later sessions.

Introductions

Therapists begin by introducing themselves to the group. Introductions should include a bit of personal information and are used to lay the groundwork for group cohesion. For instance, a therapist may start the introductions in the following way:

THERAPIST 1 (T1): Thanks to everyone for coming tonight. We are all setting out on a journey together, to work together to overcome the anxiety that each of us feels in our lives. Before we can set out on our trip, let's get to know our fellow travelers a little bit. Each of us will introduce ourselves in turn and share something about ourselves as we do so. Let me begin. I'm John Friedman. I am a clinical psychologist and have been working with clients with social phobia for the last several years. When I'm not here working with clients, I keep myself busy with my family or with several hobbies. I like to jog and I spend a lot of time surfing the Web, but the truth is that I am a major sports junkie!

Remember, I want each of us to share something of ourselves so that we can get used to talking in front of everyone else—but at this point people should feel free to say as much or *as little* as they want. The minimum should be your name and one thing that has nothing to do with anxiety. That will help us to get to know each other as people.

THERAPIST 2 (T2): Hi, my name is Elaine Starkey. I met most of you at the individual interviews we held before the group. I'm a doctoral student in the clinical psychology program here at the university, and I've been working in the anxiety clinic for the last two years. When I'm away from school and work, I like to go to the theater and I just love to eat out at gourmet restaurants when I can afford it. How about each of you? Remember, it's OK to just say a little bit, but do say something—your name and one thing about you. Then just stop, take a deep breath, and let someone else take a turn.

It is best not to go around the room in order during the introductions or other group activities. These situations are uncomfortable for many, but especially so for the last group member in the circle, whose anticipatory anxiety may rise to uncomfortable levels. It is also best to wait for group members to begin to introduce themselves without calling on particular people so that the clients do not fall into the habit of waiting to be called on before speaking.

Each client takes a turn and says as much or as little as desired. If a person is unable to say anything at all, the therapists should gently and empathically introduce the client to everyone and mention something they know about him or her. Thereafter, *name tags* should be distributed to all clients and therapists and should be worn for the first several sessions to avoid the embarrassment or anxiety that clients may experience if they are unable to recall the name of another group member.

Ground Rules for Group Membership

The following rules and guidelines should be discussed with the group members. Therapists may wish to distribute a written copy. These rules (and several procedures used in the first two sessions of the CBGT protocol) have been adapted from the excellent and ageless work of Sank and Shaffer (1984).

Attendance

T1: This is not school, and you are not required to attend. Life's distractions can often get in the way, as can feelings of anxiety about coming to session. But we strongly encourage you to attend *every* session. We do this for two reasons. First, if your attendance is sporadic, we will have less opportunity to devote the group's effort to you. You simply can't benefit if you don't come. Second, if you are not here, you can't help the other group members work to overcome their anxiety. We can all best support each other if we all come. If you must miss a session, please call in advance and let us know.

Promptness

T2: Please make every attempt to get here on time. Your promptness will keep us from delaying the start of the session or repeating ourselves when you come in late. Also, if you are prompt and other group members are late, you may feel penalized for your efforts and angry at the latecomer. Arriving here on time shows respect for your fellow group members and for yourself as well. However, if you know you will be late, don't let your anxiety keep you from coming. Once again, please call in advance and let us know.

Homework Assignments

T1: Homework assignments are tasks that we will ask you to complete between our weekly sessions. They are designed to help you practice the coping skills you will learn here outside the group and are essential to your progress. You may be asked to read something, think about something and write it down to bring to group, or do something and report on how it went. It is critical to your progress and to your relationship with the other group members that you follow through on your homework, even if it causes you some real anxiety.

Once you have agreed to do something, do it. If you are pretty certain that you are not going to do it, if you are worried that it will cause more anxiety than you are willing to tolerate, or if you just think that it is not a good thing to do, please say so, and we will work out something that we can all be happy with. If it doesn't go well, that's OK because we can work on it more in the group.

Group Participation

T2: It is always easiest to sit back and become part of the scenery, to withdraw, to watch, rather than take an active part. It may feel safer to be low key and quiet, but you will make much more progress in treatment if you actively take part. As you volunteer to work, help out in work we do for the other group members, and put your two cents' worth into discussions, you will be treating your fears of speaking before a group. If you don't, you miss the chance.

Confidentiality

T1: (*Pass around Group Confidentiality Contract; see Figure 9.1.*) The form that is being passed around represents a pact that we must all make with

---

Confidentiality Contract for Social Phobia Groups

1. This instrument is a contract for confidentiality among the members of this group whose purpose is the reduction of social anxiety among its members.

2. Each member of the group acknowledges the need to keep personal information shared in the group private.

3. For the purpose of this group, any information shared by a group member about himself or herself should be considered personal and private information.

4. In order to become a group member and maintain membership in the group, each person must agree to protect this private information. Information gathered about other members of the group cannot be shared with anyone else. That information shall remain with the group members and not be transmitted or communicated to any other person.

5. If you agree to abide by these restrictions, please acknowledge your agreement by signing in the space below.

Signature   Date

_____   _____

_____   _____

_____   _____

_____   _____

_____   _____

_____   _____

FIGURE 9.1. Confidentiality contract for social phobia groups.

each other. In this group, we will be talking about some pretty sensitive issues. At the beginning, we'll be doing this in front of a group of people we don't really know. That's never an easy thing to do because we don't yet know who we can trust. This form is a contract, an agreement to treat each other with respect. As therapists, we are bound by professional ethics and legal requirements—we will not talk about the people or activities in this group to any outsider in a way by which any group member may be identified. Group members don't have the same ethical or legal requirements. So we make a contract—to talk about group members by name only while in the group, to not betray each others' right to stay low key and private about their participation in a therapy group. This is not to say that you can't talk to anyone about your experiences—you are entirely free to do so. Just protect the privacy of everyone else. We call this *confidentiality*.

In most settings, during the intake interview, clients would have been told about limitations to confidentiality such as may be required in situations involving mandated reporting of child abuse, danger to self, or duty to warn. However, if there is doubt about clients' understanding of these issues, we recommend revisiting the nature of the limitations of confidentiality during the first group session.

T2: (*Read Group Confidentiality Contract aloud.*) Are there any questions about the contract? (*If so, respond to questions, then say:*) Good. Everyone should sign the contract as it passes around the room. Also, let me say one other thing about confidentiality. Another aspect of protecting confidentiality has to do with what happens when we bump into each other on the street. If we [therapists] run into any group member in a public place, we will not acknowledge you, we will not say "Hi" to you, unless you speak first. This is not because we are ignoring you or don't want to see you. It gives *you* control of the situation. If you are with your boss, you simply may not want to introduce him or her to your therapist. If you want to chat, just let us know, and we will.

Sharing of Individual Problems and Goals

Once again each client is asked to speak briefly, this time on his or her reasons for being in the group, that is, what the concerns are for which he or she has sought treatment, how these fears have affected his or her life, and what he or she hopes to accomplish during treatment. Each participant is called on by the therapists. This should be done in an order different from that in which they previously introduced themselves, because many clients experience an increasing surge of anxiety while waiting for their turn to speak.

Therapists should provide liberal assistance to clients who may find themselves quite anxious speaking before the group about their self-perceived inadequacies and weaknesses. Any client who is too anxious to speak at length should be given ample room to speak only briefly, but all clients should be asked to contribute something to this exercise. Many clients may never have shared these aspects of themselves with another human being and may truly believe that they are the only ones who feel this way or that they are more seriously impaired than anyone else. The purpose of this exercise is to demonstrate the similarity among clients and to build group cohesion, not to provide an exposure experience.

Although it is not necessary for clients to speak in detail, therapists might prompt a client with some of the following if they observe that he or she is floundering or highly anxious:

1. What is your greatest fear or the situation that causes you the greatest concern?
2. What happens to you when you think about facing your feared situation (anticipatory anxiety)?
3. What happens to you when you are actually in the feared situation?
4. What physical symptoms and thoughts do you experience in the situation?
5. What do you feel like after the situation has ended?
6. What would you like to be able to do that your anxiety keeps you from doing?

Clients will show a diversity of symptoms and eliciting situations. They may differ considerably in the amount of impairment they experience. However, all clients will have commonalities with other group members. Many clients will spontaneously point out similarities and differences between their symptoms and experiences and those described by other group members. We typically ask these clients to address comments to each other in order to facilitate the development of relationships among the group members rather than having them report the similarities they notice directly to the therapist. Therapists should facilitate this process using as little prompting as the anxiety of the group members will allow. Although differences should not be ignored, the therapists should strive to highlight similarities as a means of bringing the group members closer together. In facilitating this discussion, therapists may point out:

1. Similarities among pairs of clients in presenting problems, that is, that they wish to overcome anxiety in the same situations.
2. Similarities among clients in their cognitive, physiological, and behavioral symptoms.
3. Similarities among clients in their concerns about negative evaluation and scrutiny by others.

Presentation of the Cognitive-Behavioral Model of Social Phobia

In this segment of Session 1, we begin to develop a common understanding of social phobia among the group members and to provide clients with a framework for understanding the reasons that they will be asked to participate in specific group activities in later sessions. A script of a lecture follows that highlights the notion that social anxiety is a mostly learned response based on negative beliefs and predictions about the outcomes of social situations and consisting of cognitive, physiological, and behavioral components. Therapists should be certain to include all major concepts in their presentation but should not present it verbatim. Therapists should provide clients with the opportunity to ask clarifying questions and provide multiple examples relevant to the specific clients in the group.

Current cognitive-behavioral models (e.g., D. M. Clark & Wells, 1995; Rapee & Heimberg, 1997) are quite a bit more sophisticated than the more generic model presented here. However, in the current context, a very simple and straightforward approach is called for. Therapists should avoid the temptation to "jargonize" or to provide too much detail at this moment. The anxious clients are better served by a succinct presentation that begins a process of reconceptualizing their social phobia than they are by a lecture that presents more detail than can be processed in a highly anxious state.

T1: Now we know what everyone is concerned about and what we want to accomplish during treatment. Next we want to talk about social phobia, what it is all about, and, in a few minutes, what we will do about it. There are many reasons why someone develops social phobia. I'm sure that this is something that each of you has spent a lot of time thinking about, and you each have probably developed your own theories about it. What do you think?

Assist clients in generating a list of the usual suspects: inherited disorder, difficult family environment during formative years, parental divorce or absence, traumatic events, learning from watching anxious parents or siblings, being teased or rejected by peers, childhood illness, and so forth. List these on the easel. Do not engage in detailed discussion of each client's personal traumas at this time, but maintain a focus on the cognitive-behavioral model. These issues are summarized in Chapter 3 of the Client Workbook.

T2: Social phobia runs in families. However, scientists do not believe that there is a specific gene for social phobia. In fact, geneticists say that less than a third of social phobia is genetically determined, and most of the rest is a direct result of the experiences that people have after they are born.

Thus, while biology may have given us a push in a particular direction, for the most part, **WE HAVE LEARNED TO BE ANXIOUS IN SOCIAL SITUATIONS AS A RESULT OF OUR EXPERIENCES**. That's really good news because it means that there is a really good chance that *WE CAN LEARN NEW WAYS* **AND** *UNLEARN THE OLD WAYS*. We can learn to replace anxiety with increased confidence and a bit of calm in the situations that are now such a problem.

Write on the easel:

___

SOCIAL PHOBIA IS A LEARNED RESPONSE. WE CAN LEARN NEW WAYS.

___

Let's think for a minute about what it is that we have learned that is so harmful to us. Think back on your own experiences or the kinds of things we just discussed. What does a person learn about social situations from these kinds of events? What might a person come to believe about social situations?

___

Assist clients in generating beliefs that may logically follow from the negative social, familial, and environmental circumstances discussed previously. Lead the group toward the conclusion that reasonable people would conclude that social situations are:

- Likely to be dangerous (i.e., they are likely to result in punishing outcomes).
- Unlikely to be worth the risk (i.e., they are unlikely to result in rewarding outcomes).

Record these beliefs on the easel. Further develop this theme by asking **"But you see other people who seem to do fine in social situations, don't you? Social situations do not appear dangerous for them."** Use clients' responses to generate the further negative beliefs that:

- If one can perform perfectly in a social situation, things may turn out OK.
- Other people can do this, at least some of the time.
- The clients lack what it takes to do so.

___

T1: **NO WONDER SOCIAL SITUATIONS SEEM SO HORRIBLE!!!!!!** Let's take this a step further. Look at the easel and think about these beliefs. Get into them for a minute; think about them as if they are true. Now think about the next time you have to do something you are afraid of, maybe giving a committee report at work, giving a reading at church or synagogue, interviewing for a job, or anything else relevant. With these beliefs, how would you predict the situation would turn out?

___

Record on the easel negative predictions that the clients generate. These should include, among other things, that social situations result in:

- Embarrassment   • Rejection   • Drops in self-esteem
- Humiliation   • Loss of status

___

T2: **THESE BELIEFS AND PREDICTIONS CAN ONLY LEAD TO BAD CONSE-QUENCES. YOU COME INTO THE SITUATIONS ALL PRIMED FOR DISASTER!!!!! IT JUST ISN'T FAIR!!!!!!**

The Three Components of Anxiety

T1: So do you see how someone might be set up to be anxious in social situations by these beliefs and predictions? These ways of looking at the world are certain to make us anxious, right? OK, but what is anxiety anyway? (*Solicit client responses.*) It's an emotion, and a very unpleasant one for sure. But it's easier to understand if we break it down into its parts. The three parts of the anxiety response are known to health professionals as the **cognitive, physiological, and behavioral components of anxiety.** (*Write on easel.*) In plain language, these are what you **think**, what you **feel** in your body, and how you **behave**. It is very important for you to get to know the specifics of your anxiety response.

T2: Let's look first at the **COGNITIVE COMPONENT OF ANXIETY.** When you are in one of those situations that make you anxious, or just waiting for one to happen, your mind is not empty. In fact, it is usually working overtime, right? What do you think about in those situations?

Therapists should obtain a sample of five to six thoughts from the group. Examples might include the following: "I know I'm going to get anxious," "I won't be able to think of anything to say," "What if they don't like me?," or "I'm just not good enough to. . . . "

If some clients protest that they are not thinking in these situations but that they experience their minds as blank, suggest that they have not yet learned to be attuned to their anxious thoughts and that this will be a focus of treatment. Facilitate their participation in this discussion by pulling for their thoughts with alternative questions, such as "What goes through your head?" "What are you worried might happen?" or "What are you afraid of in this situation?" If appropriate, point out that responses to these additional probes are typically representative of what persons with social phobia actually think about during or in anticipation of feared situations.

T1: OK, let's try to work from a specific example. Imagine that you are at a party where there are some people that you would really like to meet . . . pick someone who might really be important to you—someone from your job, someone you are attracted to, or an important person whom you admire. You see the person standing alone at the snack table, looking lost, so you decide to go over and make small talk. As you do, you start to get anxious and. . . .

Each of you focus on what's going on inside your head. Don't try to evaluate it, change it, or pretty it up. What kinds of thoughts were running through your heads?

Solicit examples and write on easel. These will probably include such thoughts as:

- "I'll get tongue-tied."
- "He'll be able to see how nervous I am."
- "I won't be able to get a word out."
- "She won't like me (respect me) because she'll see I'm nervous."
- "I'll look foolish (silly, dumb, like a jerk, etc.)."

T2: When these thoughts occurred to you, did you:

- Question them?
- Evaluate them?
- Wonder if they were true or accurate?
- Accept them as if they were facts?

If you accepted them without questioning or if you treated them as absolute facts, what effect did they have on you? (*Solicit reactions.*)

T1: Did you treat these thoughts like facts? If so, they are examples of what we call **AUTOMATIC THOUGHTS,** or **ATs**. ATs are negative, illogical thoughts about yourself, others, the world, or the future. They are called automatic thoughts because they often seem to come into your mind automatically and seem like they are true. However, ATs are the moment-to-moment reflections of the negative beliefs and predictions you have developed about social situations, and they can be very harmful. Learning to identify and change your ATs is a major step to learning to manage your social anxiety.

Write the definition of automatic thoughts on the easel:

ATs are negative, illogical thoughts about yourself, others, the world, or the future.

Now let's review the ATs again, but treat them as if you are the other person, that is, I'm walking up to you and I'm the one who's nervous. What would you say to me if you knew what I was thinking?

Solicit responses—prompt the idea that the person would be supportive rather than rejecting. This suggests that there is more than one way to view a situation and that therefore it is not safe to assume that ATs are true just because they "feel right."

T2: Now let's look at the **PHYSIOLOGICAL COMPONENT**. Each of you experiences physical symptoms of anxiety when you enter social situations. (*Draw examples from earlier client descriptions and write on easel; generate additional symptoms if appropriate.*) The symptoms are your body's way of gearing up to protect itself from dangerous situations. For instance, the rapid beating or pounding of your heart is really an attempt to get oxygen to your muscles faster so that your body can protect itself. Muscle tension is your body getting ready for quick action. But what are your bodies getting ready for? **SOCIAL SITUATIONS ARE NOT DANGEROUS**! Remember, we mistakenly learned that social situations are dangerous as a result of our experiences, but this is not the case.

Imagine for a moment: A caveman wanders out of his cave and finds himself face-to-face with a saber-toothed tiger. What happens to him? His gets a rush of adrenaline, which mobilizes him to either fight the tiger or to run away. He experiences many of the same symptoms that you do in social situations. His heart beats fast and hard, his muscles tense, and so forth. But his responses work for him because his life is at stake. Whatever you may think when you are about to panic in a social situation, **your life is not at stake—you have just learned from your experiences to react that way**. The problem is that you get all aroused, but unlike the caveman, **you have nothing to fight**! There is no way to get rid of your arousal so it just goes on and on and on. Can you think of other examples like this (someone cuts you off in traffic and you have to make a sudden stop; a loud noise, etc.)? What might happen to your physical symptoms if you could come to believe that social situations are not dangerous? (*Solicit responses.*)

T1: The last part of the anxiety response is the **BEHAVIORAL COMPONENT**. One effect of anxiety is that it **DISRUPTS** your behavior. You may not be able to think of anything to say, or you may stutter and stammer. You may laugh a lot because you are nervous, you may not be able to look other people in the eye, you may not be able to stand still, or your hands or body or face may tremble.

A second, and more harmful, behavioral aspect of anxiety is **AVOIDANCE**. When you are anxious (or expect to be), you do something, you behave in some way to control the anxiety. You may **AVOID** the situation by doing something like skipping class, not calling someone for a date, not starting a conversation, or maybe choosing a job that won't put you into a social situation that you fear. You can also avoid anxiety by making sure that you have had a few drinks or by using drugs before doing something that scares you. What kinds of effects do you think **AVOIDANCE** has on you?

Therapists should elicit a variety of responses from group members and write them on the easel. Make sure to include the following effects of avoidance:

1. Avoidance reduces anxiety and provides immediate relief, but
2. Avoidance keeps you from getting what you want,
3. Avoidance keeps you from having a chance to get over your anxiety,
4. Avoidance reduces your confidence that you can handle the situation the next time, and
5. Avoidance makes you feel less able to cope in general.

Therapists should also elicit from the group the notion that reducing avoidance is an important piece of learning to manage one's social anxiety.

How the Components of Anxiety Interact with Each Other in Social Situations

T2: Let's review for a minute. The **ANXIETY RESPONSE** has three components. These are the (*write on easel*):

(P) **PHYSIOLOGICAL COMPONENT**   = what your body feels
(B) **BEHAVIORAL COMPONENT**   = what you do
(C) **COGNITIVE COMPONENT**   = what you think

The three components all feed into each other and keep anxiety going in a vicious cycle. Let's look at how this may happen in an anxiety-provoking situation. Let's say that you are interviewing for a job that you really want. You are waiting in the reception area for the interviewer to call you into his or her office. (*Refer to Figure 9.2; draw the figure on the easel as you talk your way through the example.*) You think to yourself "I've **got** to do good on this interview" (C), and the cycle begins. As you think that thought, you can feel your body rev up! Your heart begins to race, your muscles tense, and you begin to feel sweaty and clammy (P). As you become aware of these physiological symptoms, you think to yourself, "Oh, I'm so nervous. I just know I'm going to mess up, say the wrong thing or something" (C). The tension is building, and you can't sit still. You start to pace, wring your hands. You check your watch every few seconds (B). Clock watching leads you to think, "What's keeping him? He must really not want to see me. I'll never get this job" (C). You feel yourself getting more and more aroused to the point where you begin to feel nauseous (P)! You tell yourself, "I'm so nervous, I can't do it" (C). You start to leave (B), but you know you want the job, so you force yourself to stay. But you still think, "I can't handle it" (C). You decide to leave (B). The anxiety goes away as you leave the building, but then you think, "What's the matter with me? Other people can handle this. I'm just no good" (C).

Although we have described this exercise with the therapist presenting a monologue, an alternative that may be very effective is to conduct it in a

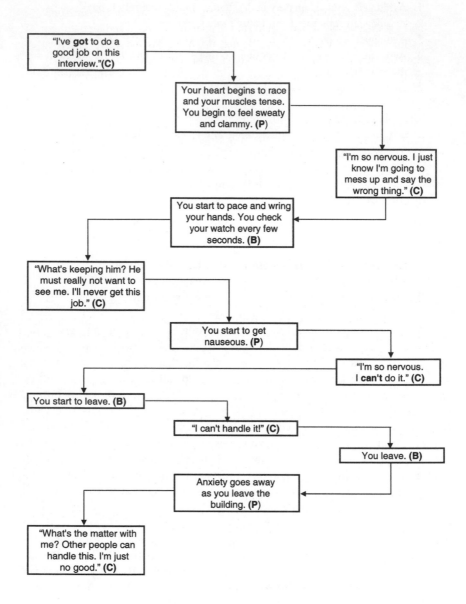

FIGURE 9.2. Interaction of the cognitive (C), physiological (P), and behavioral (B) components of social anxiety in a person awaiting a job interview.

more interactive format. One of the therapists may present the situation and ask the clients, "What would start happening to you?" and let them go as long as possible. At various points, the therapists may give different prompts such as, "What would be going on in your body?" "Ever do something like wipe the palms of your hands on your pants in a situation like that?" or "Would you start thinking about how the interviewer might react to you? What would you be worried about?" Therapists may then record clients' responses on the easel, labeling each new item as a B, C, or P and drawing arrows each step of the way (Figure 9.2 may be regarded as a guide to doing this rather than a specific version of the situation that should be portrayed). Therapists may specifically raise the notion that the person decides to leave the interview and then probe for short- and long-term consequences from the clients as the way of ending the exercise.

Discussion of the Components of Treatment

T2: All three components of the anxiety response are important, and they interact with each other to increase your feelings of anxiety and helplessness, so it is important to do something to treat each component. So our treatment includes several techniques that are designed to reduce the three components of the anxiety response.

The three primary treatment techniques are **IN-SESSION EXPOSURES**, **COGNITIVE RESTRUCTURING**, and **HOMEWORK ASSIGNMENTS**. These techniques have been explained to each of you individually, but now you can more clearly understand what they are designed to do.

IN-SESSION EXPOSURES involve acting out situations of specific relevance to each of you, here in the group, creating as much of the real thing as possible. (Give some examples of possible in-session exposures that might be employed with this group of clients). In-session exposures have positive effects on two components of the anxiety habit, the **physiological** and **behavioral components**. They help the physiological component because you will experience arousal in the situation but stay with it instead of coping with it however you might have before. This means:

- No avoiding
- No escaping
- No withdrawing
- No use of drugs or alcohol

The inevitable result is that your body's natural processes will bring the anxiety down—an important thing for you to see. In-session exposures will also help the behavioral component because you will be doing whatever you need to be doing while the arousal runs its course.

Let me say one other thing before we go on. I can see on your faces that the idea of doing these exposures is scary. It will make you anxious to do them, but remember several things. First, it is important to face your fear, and it is necessary to help you get better, but we won't just throw you into these situations and leave you to suffer. We will start with situations that are not your most feared ones, and as you gain confidence, we will work our way up to situations that are more difficult for you. We will also be teaching you skills to reduce your anxiety while you are doing these exposures. That brings us to the **COGNITIVE PART OF TREATMENT**.

T1: **COGNITIVE RESTRUCTURING**. With a name like that, it's got to help the cognitive component of anxiety, right? We'll help you pick out your ATs, analyze them, and question them. You'll learn to treat them like scientific hypotheses and even design experiments to test them out.

After you gain some skill at identifying ATs, we'll have you prep yourself with a cognitive restructuring routine before in-session exposures. Then after exposures, you will do a cognitive analysis of what happened—a "cognitive debriefing," so to speak. Then we'll be getting all the components of the anxiety response at the same time.

T2: The third part of treatment is **HOMEWORK ASSIGNMENTS**. What we've said so far is all fine in the clinic. What we have to do is get you into action in real life—out there in the front lines. So we'll ask you to do things between sessions. It may be something specific to your individual problem—to attempt something you have been avoiding—or it may be something we will all be working on together—like monitoring automatic thoughts. Whatever it is, homework is the link between the group meeting and the rest of your life. **Doing it daily** can help you conquer all the components of anxiety and help you move closer to enjoying the things in life you may be missing.

At this point, expect a number of questions from clients who may be anxious about the treatment procedures. These questions typically reflect their anxiety about participation in in-session exposures or whether or not they will be able to complete homework assignments without being overwhelmed. Answer all questions completely before moving on. In doing so, focus on the graduated and collaborative approach to selection of in-session exposures and homework assignments, the clients' ability to learn and apply new skills, and the support clients will receive from the therapists and other group members.

Assessment of Expectancy for Treatment Outcome

In the next segment of this session, we assess clients' reactions to the treatment that has been described to them. This has been done to assure that different treatment conditions in our research studies produce similar positive expectancies for change and are viewed as equally credible by the clients. However, these procedures also have considerable clinical utility, and we recommend their inclusion in all CBGT groups. We ask clients to complete a brief questionnaire called the Reaction to Treatment Questionnaire (RTQ; see Figure 9.3). The RTQ is a slightly modified version of the measure originally described by Holt and Heimberg (1990) and includes a section on the credibility of the treatment (developed by Borkovec & Nau, 1972), a section asking clients to assess the effectiveness of the treatment for reducing anxiety in several social and performance situations (originally derived from the work of Amies, Gelder, & Shaw, 1983), and a series of questions asking clients to rate how anxious they expect to be in the future. Additional information about the RTQ is available in Holt and Heimberg (1990). After the RTQ is completed, therapists look them over briefly. If all appear optimistic, it is important to say so. However, given the finding by Safren et al. (1997b) that clients with low RTQ scores do not do as well in treatment, it is important to discuss in the group any responses that are reserved, cautious, or negativistic. Clients should be advised of the obvious importance of keeping an open mind about treatment and the strong possibility that halfhearted efforts may undermine treatment response.

Initial Training in Cognitive Restructuring

The remainder of Session 1 and the entirety of Session 2 are devoted to training of group members in the cognitive restructuring skills they will need for the conduct of later in-session exposures and homework assignments. Structured exercises and homework assignments are used to help group members achieve several goals:

1. Develop an awareness of the frequency of their own maladaptive thinking.
2. Develop the skills for identifying errors in their own thoughts.
3. Develop an awareness of the connection between the occurrence of distorted thinking and anxiety.
4. Reconceptualize their thoughts as hypotheses to be tested rather than facts to be accepted.
5. Develop the skills for challenging and changing their own thoughts.

Introduction to Automatic Thoughts: How Automatic Thoughts Influence Emotions and Behavior

The goal of the first restructuring exercise (which is based on Sank and Shaffer [1984]) is to demonstrate that negative automatic thoughts exist and that alterna-

Reaction to Treatment Questionnaire

Name _____ Date _____

On a scale from 1 (low) to 10 (high), please rate your reaction to the explanation of your group treatment. Indicate your rating by circling the appropriate number.

1. How logical does this treatment seem to you?

1	2	3	4	5	6	7	8	9	10
Not logical									Very logical

2. How confident are you that this treatment will be successful in reducing your social anxiety?

1	2	3	4	5	6	7	8	9	10
Not at all confident									Very confident

3. How confident would you be in recommending this treatment to a friend with social anxiety?

1	2	3	4	5	6	7	8	9	10
Not at all confident									Very confident

4. How successful do you feel this treatment would be in decreasing different fears?

1	2	3	4	5	6	7	8	9	10
Not at all successful									Very successful

You may or may not be fearful in the following situations. If you were fearful in them, how confident would you be that this treatment would eliminate your fear? (Circle the number that corresponds to your level of confidence.)

5. Writing in public

1	2	3	4	5	6	7	8	9	10
Not at all confident									Very confident

6. A first date

1	2	3	4	5	6	7	8	9	10
Not at all confident									Very confident

7. Giving a speech

1	2	3	4	5	6	7	8	9	10
Not at all confident									Very confident

8. Being introduced

1	2	3	4	5	6	7	8	9	10
Not at all confident									Very confident

9. Eating in public places

1	2	3	4	5	6	7	8	9	10
Not at all confident									Very confident

10. Meeting people in authority

1	2	3	4	5	6	7	8	9	10
Not at all confident									Very confident

11. Being observed by others

1	2	3	4	5	6	7	8	9	10
Not at all confident									Very confident

12. Being teased

1	2	3	4	5	6	7	8	9	10
Not at all confident									Very confident

13. Using the telephone

1	2	3	4	5	6	7	8	9	10
Not at all confident									Very confident

14. How severe is your social anxiety today?

1	2	3	4	5	6	7	8	9	10
Not at all confident									Very confident

15. How severe do you expect your social anxiety to be immediately following treatment?

1	2	3	4	5	6	7	8	9	10
Not at all confident									Very confident

16. How severe do you expect your social anxiety to be 1 year after treatment?

1	2	3	4	5	6	7	8	9	10
Not at all confident									Very confident

17. How severe do you expect your social anxiety to be 5 years after treatment?

1	2	3	4	5	6	7	8	9	10
Not at all confident									Very confident

FIGURE 9.3. The Reaction to Treatment Questionnaire. Portions of this measure have been adapted from "Credibility of Analogue Therapy Rationales," by T. D. Borkovec and S. D. Nau, 1972, *Journal of Behavior Therapy and Experimental Psychiatry, 3*, p. 258. Copyright 1972 by Elsevier Science. Adapted by permission.

tive ways of viewing any situation are possible. A therapist presents a situation that could plausibly have happened to him or her and that generated significant distress or anxiety. The situation is described, and the therapist presents a listing of the ATs that occurred to him or her. Group members are asked to help the therapist evaluate the validity of these thoughts by asking questions about each AT and examining the answers to these questions. Rational responses to each of the thoughts are generated as well. Again, the primary goal is for clients to understand that both automatic thoughts *and* alternative thoughts exist. It is not necessary (or likely) that they will come to strongly accept the validity of the rational responses at this early point in treatment.

T1: Cognitive restructuring is a self-help technique that you can all use to manage your anxiety reactions. The basic idea is that events do not cause our emotions and behaviors—our thoughts about events do.

T1 should do the following while making the above statement:

1. Write on the easel: **Events → Emotions and Behaviors**
2. Draw a bold line through this phrase: ~~**Events → Emotions and Behaviors**~~
3. Then write on the easel: **Events → Thoughts → Emotions and Behaviors**

T2: If we can change our thoughts, we can change our emotions. We can break into that vicious cycle of anxiety we discussed before. The first step is to identify these automatic thoughts. When you feel anxious, you should stop and ask yourself, "What am I saying to myself?" or "What is going through my mind right now?" Once you've discovered your AT (e.g., "I'll look like a fool"), **question it**! Am I certain about this? Is there another possibility? What is my evidence? Your answers to these questions will be much more reasonable than your original ATs! This is not a cure-all, but with this questioning approach, you should soon gain a degree of control over your emotional responses. You may then be able to respond to the situation more thoughtfully and rationally.

By the way, we are not selling "the power of positive thinking." You will not simply be trading in a negative thought for a positive one. You will begin to recognize and examine your assumptions about life and the pursuit of happiness and then question and evaluate them. The goal is to get rid of the automatic negative thinking and replace it with thoughts that are more objective and reasonable.

T1: Let's look at an example of some ATs. I want to present you with a situation of mine. I think it is one that most of us can relate to.

It is not necessary for therapists to use the specific situation presented here. Sank and Shaffer (1984), who originated this exercise, used a situation in which the therapist tells of an upcoming trip to a professional meeting and becoming distressed over what might happen while he or she is away. We have left it to the discretion of the therapists to determine whether they can perform more effectively using a canned situation or whether they would prefer to devise one of their own. We have used situations concerning upcoming class presentations, job interviews, parties, and other social events with no apparent difference in effectiveness.

T2: A few weeks ago, I attended a meeting of psychologists to present a speech about the research on social phobia we have conducted here at the anxiety clinic. I usually feel pretty good about giving talks, but on the morning of the talk, I began to feel very uncomfortable. As time passed, I became more and more anxious and tense. I began to feel the tension I always feel in my neck and shoulders and around my eyes. My heart began to race and I even got a little short of breath. I was really upset by this because I had a lot to do to get ready for the talk and I was wasting my time being anxious. So I started to **get cognitive** with myself. I found several ATs floating around in my head—they all had to do with my concerns about the speech and how I would come off to the members of the audience (all other psychologists and professionals, including some of the "biggies" in the field). Any guesses?

Here they are in all their glory. (*Write on easel; leave room at bottom of sheet.*)

1. "I'll be so nervous I won't be able to talk."
2. "I'll make a bad impression; I'll look stupid."
3. "I won't be able to get my point across to the audience."
4. "They won't like my research and will decide I'm a lousy researcher."
5. "I'll lose career opportunities because I'll look so bad."

T1: One way to help [cotherapist] **get rational** here is ask her questions about the situation and her ATs. What questions could you ask [cotherapist] to help her think about the situation differently?

Therapists should present each of the ATs listed on the easel and assist group members in questioning each one. Any questions offered by group members should be recorded on the easel, and T2 should respond to them.

If group members have difficulty generating questions, the following can be offered (and written on the easel if appropriate):

1. How would an objective observer view your situation?
2. What is the evidence in support of your thought?
3. What is the evidence against your thought?
4. Is there an alternative explanation?

If a client offers an alternative thought rather than asking a question, one of the therapists might reframe it as a question. For example, if a client offers, "If they did not like your research, they would not have invited you to speak," a therapist might suggest, "So you would ask [cotherapist], 'Are there reasons to believe that they might like your research?' "

After clients have questioned each of T2's ATs, therapists should ask the group to come up with a statement or two to summarize the alternative perspectives that have been generated. These should be recorded on the easel, with modifications as needed, and should be explicitly labeled by therapists as "rational responses." Group members should then be asked to consider how T2 might have reacted differently to her presentation if she had been able to keep the rational responses in mind.

To assist therapists in this exercise, we provide possible rational responses to each of the ATs:

Automatic thought: "I'll be so nervous I won't be able to talk."
Rational response: "It's time to get cognitive here. I have given many talks before. Have nerves ever caused me to lose my ability to talk? No, I may be nervous, but I've always been able to talk before."

Automatic thought: "I'll make a bad impression; I'll look stupid."
Rational response: "Again, how many talks have I given? Have I made a bad impression before? Sometimes, but I give a lot of talks, and people keep inviting me to do them. I need to give it my best shot, and things should work out OK. What does 'stupid' mean, anyway? I'm just using this label to beat myself up, and I need to stop that."

Automatic thought: "I won't be able to get my point across to the audience."
Rational response: "Yes, I will. I'm pretty organized in my presentations. If my statements are not always clear, my slides will help the audience understand. If they don't, they can ask questions, and I can take

it as an opportunity to learn from them and improve my speaking skills."

Automatic thought: "They won't like my research and will decide I'm a lousy researcher."

Rational response: "Think so? What is my evidence for that idea? It is possible that they won't like my research, but it has been well received at other times. Even if they don't like it and they do think I'm a lousy researcher, this is only their opinion, and they're entitled to it."

Automatic thought: "I'll lose career opportunities because I'll look so bad."

Rational response: "I've already established that I won't look so bad, right? So, its unlikely that this will happen. If it does, does it pay to focus on this and make myself miserable? Remember, I've done all right in my career so far."

Eliciting Automatic Thoughts Regarding Group Treatment[1]

Because most group members will have mixed feelings about participating in a group, this presents a common ground for a group exercise on automatic thoughts. The group members are now asked to generate their own ATs about being in group treatment (i.e., negative reactions to being in a group, pessimistic predictions about ultimate outcome, etc.). The following instructions should be given:

T1: To bring the concept of ATs even more to life, please think about your reactions to being in this group. For now, please focus on any negative thoughts you may have had in regard to yourself or the progress you expect to make. If you have any trouble generating ATs, think how anyone embarking on group treatment might think.

On occasion, we have had groups who universally deny negative thoughts about treatment. Of course, if this is truly the case, the exercise is doomed. However, it is more likely that the clients are hesitant to make negative statements about the treatment or are afraid of rejection by the therapists or other group members if they truly speak their minds. If ATs do not flow quickly from the clients, it is useful to suggest that clients look for thoughts that begin with "I'm . . .," " "I'm going to . . .," or "He or she will think. . . . " Furthermore, thoughts that contain emotion words (e.g., *ner-*

vous, anxious, scared, worried) or negative labels (e.g., *stupid, incompetent*) are also good candidates. The following questions, suggested by Hope et al. (2000), may also be useful:"

"What doubts do I have about whether this program will work for me?"
"What worries do I have about the in-session exposures?"
"What doubts do I have that I will be able to make real, lasting change?"
"What doubts do I have that the therapists will really be able to understand and help me?"

Solicit group members' responses. Remember that they may have significant difficulty at this point in stating ATs in a useful manner. Gently transform questions into statements. Record responses on the easel. ATs generated by group members will probably be variations of the following thoughts:

1. "My problems are worse than everyone else's."
2. "I won't be able to talk in front of all these people."
3. "If I speak up, I'll sound stupid."
4. "If the others find out what I'm really like, they won't like me."

These ATs and others provided by group members can now be handled as in the previous exercise. However, clients are likely to struggle more with the effort to restructure their own ATs than is typically the case in the first exercise. It is important for therapists to avoid the tendency to move in too quickly and save them from this struggle. It is best to guide them along the way and give them the opportunity to experience firsthand the impact that cognitive restructuring may have on their feelings. Sample rational responses for the ATs listed previously might look like this:

Automatic thought: "My problems are worse than everyone else's."
Rational response: "I can't know this so early and I may never know how severe everybody else's problems are. Also, the difficulty of someone's problems is such a relative thing. Even if my problems are more difficult to solve, it doesn't mean that I can't do well for myself here."

Automatic thought: "I'll never be able to talk in front of all these people."
Rational response: "It's unlikely that I won't be able to speak in this group. Actually, this is a safe situation in which to take risks. I may actually be more talkative here than in most group situations. Even if I'm not the most talkative person here, I can see that there is going to be much to learn and I can benefit a lot by listening well."

Automatic thought: "If I speak up, I'll sound stupid."

Rational response: "I have no reason to believe that I'll sound stupid and much evidence to believe that I won't. I'm also not here to win any intelligence contests. I'm here to learn and I can do that best by participating. So, it is actually less 'stupid' to speak up than to hold my tongue."

Automatic thought: "If the others find out what I'm really like, they won't like me."

Rational response: "I don't know whether or not everyone would like me if they knew me well. Everyone doesn't need to like me for me to be happy. If there are some parts of me that I would like to change, I can work on them. I don't have to show all to everyone, but this group is a safe place to find out how others react to me. It's a good opportunity to practice being myself and see how others react."

This exercise moves group members one step closer to using these techniques to counter their own illogical thinking in personally meaningful situations. However, some may regard the eliciting of ATs about membership in a group as courting trouble. Sank and Shaffer (1984) argue persuasively that this exercise can be most helpful in building rapport and in establishing the therapists as persons who will deal with issues and who will not attempt to sidestep criticism. Furthermore, it provides the opportunity to respond to objections and to enlist the aid of both objectors and other group members in rebutting these criticisms.

Homework Assignment for Session 1: Monitoring and Recording Automatic Thoughts

To facilitate the cognitive restructuring exercises in Session 2, the group members should collect a sample of ATs that occur to them in the course of their daily lives. Instruct clients that anxiety should be viewed as a signal for them to pay close attention to what they are saying to themselves. Most group members will encounter sufficient numbers of anxiety-provoking situations in their daily lives that this will not be difficult, and it is not necessary to suggest that they purposefully enter stressful situations that they currently avoid. Group members should be provided with a self-monitoring log to record their ATs (see Figure 9.4), and the procedure for recording should be briefly reviewed. They should record a brief description of the situation, write down the content of their automatic thought(s) exactly as the thought occurred to them, and specify the emotion that was associated with the thought(s). Clients should be encouraged to bring in a sample of at least 5 to 10 ATs that are associated with the experience of anxiety in situations or in anticipation of them.

Monitoring Your Automatic Thoughts

Date _____   Name _____

1. Situation (*Briefly describe the anxiety-provoking situation.*)

2. Automatic Thoughts (*List the thoughts you have about this situation.*)

3. Emotions you feel as you think these thoughts (*Check boxes that apply.*)

❑ Anxious/nervous   ❑ Frustrated   ❑ Irritated   ❑ Ashamed

❑ Angry   ❑ Sad   ❑ Embarrassed   ❑ Hateful

Other:_____

FIGURE 9.4. Form for monitoring automatic thoughts. From *Managing Social Anxiety: A Cognitive-Behavioral Therapy Approach* (Client Workbook) (Figure 5.3, p. 79), by D. A. Hope, R. G. Heimberg, H. R. Juster, and C. L. Turk, 2000. Copyright 2000 by Graywind Publications. Reprinted by permission.

It is important to instruct clients about when to record their thoughts. It is always best to fill out the form as soon as possible after the conclusion of the target event. If this is not possible for whatever reason, clients should make every effort to complete the form prior to retiring for the night. This is especially important for clients who tend to play situations over and over again in their minds. Delayed recording by these clients may be especially vulnerable to distortion.

Some group members may be sufficiently avoidant that they may go through the week with little experience of anxiety or negative thinking. In order to make sure that these clients also have ATs to contribute, suggest to group members that, if no situations occur in the first four to five days of the week, they should set aside a period of 15 to 30 minutes and visualize a situation that is listed on their Fear and Avoidance Hierarchy (see Chapter 8) as if it were really happening and attempt to tune in to their negative thinking. ATs that occur to them in this context can then be entered on the self-monitoring log.

Clients may also be instructed to read and study Chapter 5 in the Client Workbook, which should serve to reinforce the major content covered in this session.

Note

1. Adapted from *A Therapist's Manual for Cognitive Behavior Therapy in Groups* (pp. 73–75), by L. I. Sank and C. S. Shaffer, 1984, New York: Plenum. Copyright 1984 by Kluwer Academic/Plenum Publishers. Adapted by permission.

10

Session 2

MATERIALS

- Pens or pencils
- Name tags
- Clipboards to use as writing surfaces
- Copies of the Brief Fear of Negative Evaluation Scale (Figure 6.4)
- Copies of the List of Thinking Errors (Figure 10.1)
- Copies of the List of Disputing Questions (Figure 10.3)
- Copies of the Cognitive Restructuring Practice Form (Figure 10.4)
- A newsprint easel
- A marker pen
- Audio- or videocassette recorder and tape
- This manual

TOPICS

- Assessment of fear of negative evaluation
- Review of Session 1 homework assignment
- Identification of thinking errors in automatic thoughts
- Disputing automatic thoughts and developing rational responses
- Homework assignment for Session 2: Cognitive restructuring practice
- Preparation for initiation of in-session exposures

Assessment of Fear of Negative Evaluation

At the beginning of the session, clients should complete the Brief Fear of Negative Evaluation Scale.

Review of Session 1 Homework Assignment

At the close of Session 1, group members were asked to monitor and record automatic thoughts related to the experience of anxiety that occurred to them during the week. This homework assignment and the cognitive restructuring exercises in the latter portion of Session 1 were intended to help group members recognize that they are capable of producing maladaptive and distorted thoughts and that an excellent clue to the presence of such thinking is the experience of anxiety or other unpleasant affect (Sank & Shaffer, 1984). It should also be possible to use the results of the clients' homework efforts to emphasize the degree to which their own thinking causes them pain. It is important to pay substantial attention to the effort clients put into these homework assignments, as the discussion of their work during the past week will set the tone for homework assignments to come. The ATs that clients recorded during the week will serve as the basis for a discussion of the categorization of the errors in logic that they contain.

Therapists should ask group members for examples of ATs that they experienced during the week, and these should be recorded by one of the therapists on the easel. A list of 12 to 15 ATs should be collected from group members by a combination of soliciting volunteers and specifically asking each group member to contribute. Therapists should make every effort to assure that at least one AT from each group member is recorded on the easel if at all possible.

As each AT is collected, the therapists should ask the group member for a brief sketch of the situation in which the thought occurred and what effect the thought appeared to have on his or her mood. Therapists should ask other group members if they also have experienced the thoughts volunteered by their peers. Any similarities among the thoughts offered by different group members might be highlighted at this point and may serve as a segue into the discussion of thinking errors that comes next. If therapists encounter difficulty in generating a sufficient sample of ATs, they may ask group members to recall their responses to the Session 1 exercise on ATs about being in group treatment or probe for reactions that group members may be having at the moment about presenting their ATs to the group.

Identification of Thinking Errors in Automatic Thoughts

When a sufficient list of ATs has been elicited from the group, therapists should hand out the List of Thinking Errors (see Figure 10.1). Thereafter, the therapists should ask group members to keep their own ATs in mind as they read through

List of Thinking Errors

All-or-Nothing Thinking (also called black-and-white, polarized, or dichotomous thinking): You view a situation in one of two categories instead of on a continuum.

Anticipating Negative Outcomes: You expect that something negative has happened or is going to happen. There are two types of thinking errors that fall into this category:

> *Fortune Telling*: You predict that something negative is going to happen in the future, as if you were gazing into a crystal ball.

> *Catastrophizing*: You tell yourself the *very worst* is happening or is going to happen, without considering other possibilities that may be more likely and/or less negative.

Disqualifying or Discounting the Positive: You unreasonably tell yourself that positive experiences, deeds, or qualities do not count.

Emotional Reasoning: You think something must be true because you "feel" (actually believe) it so strongly, ignoring or discounting evidence to the contrary.

Labeling: You put a fixed, global label on yourself or others without considering that the evidence might more reasonably lead to a less disastrous conclusion.

Mental Filter (also called selective abstraction): You pay undue attention to one negative detail instead of seeing the whole picture.

Mind Reading: You believe you know what others are thinking, failing to consider other, more likely, possibilities, and you make no effort to check it out.

Overgeneralization: You make a sweeping negative conclusion that goes far beyond the current situation.

"Should" and "Must" Statements (also called imperatives): You have a precise, fixed idea of how you or others should behave, and you overestimate how bad it is that these expectations are not met.

*   *   *

Maladaptive Thoughts: Problematic thoughts that do not contain logical thinking errors. These thoughts may be true. However, dwelling on these thoughts makes you feel more anxious and may interfere with your performance.

FIGURE 10.1. List of Thinking Errors. Adapted from *Cognitive Therapy: Basics and Beyond* (Figure 8.2, p. 119), by Judith S. Beck, 1995, New York: Guilford Press. Copyright 1995 by The Guilford Press. Adapted by permission.

the list and discuss the meaning of each type of logical error. Therapists should refrain from simply reading the text provided on the handout but rather should explain each thinking error in detail, weaving into their discussion examples from the group members' own ATs.

This portion of the session must be carefully handled for a variety of reasons. First, it is easy for the therapists to become too abstract or long-winded in this section, and group members' attention may wane. Second, therapists may provide examples that are ambiguous or incorrect, and clients may react with confusion or pessimistic assessment of their ability to grasp the concept. Third, group members may see each and every logical error in their own thinking, and they may take this as a numerical sign of the seriousness of their affliction. It is useful, therefore, for therapists to:

1. Have a list of examples readily available (a discussion of each thinking error is presented in the next section).
2. Point out that some clients will see several of the thinking errors as personally relevant, whereas others will see only a few categories as applicable to themselves, and that the number of personally relevant thinking errors is *not* an index of disturbance.
3. Note that most negative thoughts contain more than one distortion. This statement will help to relieve the pressure many clients feel in being put on the spot to come up with the "right" thinking error during group discussions. There is no perfect match between AT and thinking error. In fact, we usually encourage clients to identify two to three thinking errors per AT.

After the therapists describe the several thinking errors, they should ask the clients whether any of the ATs they recorded for homework or any of the ATs that were recorded on the easel seem to reflect a specific thinking error. Whenever a client volunteers that a thought is an example of a specific thinking error, therapists should follow up with a question, such as "What aspect of that automatic thought is [specific thinking error]?" Therapists should note which thinking errors come up frequently for the group as a whole and which ones are heavily utilized by specific group members, and these assessments should be shared with the group. The goal is to help each group member learn about his or her own cognitive style and how it may affect his or her emotional state. If time allows, therapists may ask the group members if they experienced other ATs during the week that they had not previously volunteered or may return to thoughts listed on the easel during the previous session and examine the thinking errors contained therein.

Thinking Errors

Thinking errors are simply ways of thinking that people use to understand their worlds but that do not work in their best interests. They are often described as "irrational," but because some clients find this a difficult pill to swallow, it is generally better to focus on the idea that they are based on faulty logic and, therefore, do not stand up to close scrutiny. Because these errors are so often associated with emotional distress, identifying them is an important step toward more effective coping. For clients, becoming familiar with the errors in logic to which they are most vulnerable will ultimately help them to recognize problematic thinking earlier in their stream of consciousness and to intervene with themselves before anxiety spikes.

To assist therapists in conducting the exercise on identifying logical errors in automatic thoughts, the following sections discuss the thinking errors listed in Figure 10.1 and provide a series of examples relevant to clients with social phobia. These discussions rely heavily on the previous work of A. T. Beck, Rush, Shaw, and Emery (1979), J. S. Beck (1995), and Persons (1989). Examples are drawn from our clinical files and supervision notes. The thinking errors described subsequently and in Figure 10.1 originally appeared in the literature in the context of cognitive therapy for depression. However, our experience in using similar lists for the past several years suggests that each thinking error is quite relevant to the cognitive experience of clients with social phobia. Keep in mind that these thinking errors are not mutually exclusive. Any single thought may have aspects of several logical errors within it or may be classified into different categories depending on the specific aspect of the thought that is emphasized.

ALL-OR-NOTHING THINKING

Also described as dichotomous or black-and-white thinking, this pattern is characterized by a view of reality consisting of only two discrete categories. Everything is viewed as either black or white, never in shades of gray. Persons (1989) suggests that statements that include terms such as "always," "never," "completely," "totally," or "perfectly" are likely to involve all-or-nothing thinking, whereas statements that contain such terms as "sometimes," "usually," "frequently," "partially," "generally," "often," "somewhat," "or "occasionally" are likely to represent more adaptive thinking.

All-or-nothing thinking typically involves a dual process. First, the client views himself or herself or the world in dichotomous terms, with one category having a positive valence and the other having a negative valence. Examples might include good–bad, success–failure, attractive–unattractive (or beautiful–ugly), and intelligent–unintelligent (or brilliant–stupid). Second, the two categories are of unequal size. That is, the positive category is very small, and the negative category is quite large. As a result of this dual process, it is much easier to attribute the negative pole than the positive pole to oneself; it is easier to see oneself as bad, failed, ugly, or stupid than it is to see oneself as good, successful, beautiful, or brilliant. Because neutral or unbiased judgments become impossible, all-or-nothing thinking can therefore have extremely deleterious effects on clients' affect and motivation. For example, a female client believed that she was unattractive and had little to offer men. Not surprisingly, she was quite anxious in any heterosocial interaction because she believed it could only turn out badly. In fact, she was engaging in all-or-nothing thinking. She evaluated herself as unattractive, but when asked what "attractive" meant, she described models and movie stars. In order to see herself as attractive, she had to be as attractive as these beautiful people. Average attractiveness or even "good looks" were just not good enough. Other examples of all-or-nothing thinking abound among clients with social phobia. A client with a fear of public speaking saw any presentation in which he stumbled over his words or in which his voice cracked as a total failure. Because total avoidance of these frequent human foibles is not possible, he also knew that all future presentations would be similarly doomed, and he decided that he had to leave his executive position or face repeated and inevitable failure.

Clients also frequently report that they have refrained from attempting new activities because they would not be able to do them perfectly. If an AT implies that only perfect is good enough, then it is probably an instance of all-or-nothing thinking.

Presenting these thinking errors in a manner that keeps clients engaged is one of the most challenging parts of the early sessions of CBGT. We have often found it useful to ask questions along the line of "OK, if we are going to divide the world into two categories, one intelligent and one stupid, or one beautiful and one hideous, would these two categories be equally easy to get into? Where would we put ourselves most of the time? What kind of problems does that pose for us?"

FORTUNE TELLING

Fortune telling, or "the fortune-teller error," is also referred to as predicting the future without sufficient evidence (A. T. Beck et al., 1979). When a person makes a fortune-teller error, he or she anticipates that some future event or effort will turn out badly and is certain that this prediction is accurate. Therefore, why should he or she try to do something difficult? It will only result in pain and suffering. Like all-or-nothing thinking, examples of fortune telling are numerous among our clients with social phobia. This distortion has been evident in the reported ATs of almost every client in most of our groups. A typical example is the case of a middle-aged gentleman with a fear of writing in front of other people. He was unable to sign checks, use credit cards, or engage in any sort of writing behavior when other people might be watching, although he was quite capable of doing these things when alone. In public writing situations, his hand would shake, and he would experience profuse sweating, heart palpitations, and a fear of passing out. He reported a number of ATs, including "My hand will shake," "I won't be able to write anything at all," "I'll look like a damned fool," and "I'll panic." Of course, the difficult issue for this client was that his past experience supported these predictions (see the discussion of prediction on the basis of pre-treatment experiences in the section titled "Overgeneralization"). However, it became clear during treatment that these dire predictions played a major role in producing the very symptoms he feared. For this client and for others, an important aspect of undermining fortune telling was to get him to question his thoughts: "Do I know my hands will shake?" "Has it ever turned out as badly as I predict?" "Even if my hand does shake and I do have trouble writing, does this have the terrible meaning that I attach to it?"

Another common example of fortune telling occurs among clients with social interaction fears. They quite commonly report thoughts such as, "I'll freeze," "I won't be able to think of anything to say," "I'll look foolish," "I won't be able to keep her interest," or "She won't want to go out with me again." A common theme for clients is that their anxiety will be visible to others and that this will have a negative impact on the outcomes of social interactions.

A helpful way to introduce the concept of fortune telling is to say something like "OK, who in here can really predict the future? Which of you has made a fortune on the stock market or playing the horses? Isn't it true that we act as if we can tell the future when it comes to social situations? How well does that usually work?"

CATASTROPHIZING

Like fortune telling, catastrophizing has to do with the unwarranted anticipation of negative outcomes. To catastrophize is to attribute extreme and horrific consequences to the outcomes of negative events. Being turned down for a date means that the person will never have another opportunity to date. Therefore, he or she will never have a meaningful relationship with a potential partner, never get married, never have children, never have grandchildren, and die all alone, unloved and unnoticed. Making a mistake on a job means being fired and publicly humiliated, never being able to find another job because people now know you are incompetent, and remaining unemployed for the rest of your life. A good example of catastrophizing is the case of a young, attractive female client who was very anxious at the prospect of engaging in conversations with men of her age whom she found to be physically attractive. She avoided contacts with young men and interacted with them only if they made the approach. She would then make an excuse to leave and cut the interaction short. At the beginning of treatment, she had a minimal dating history and suffered intense anxiety on a daily basis. In discussing her fears, she reported the AT, "He'll be able to tell that I'm nervous." Although her anxiety was, in fact, considerable, it is doubtful that any but the most astute observer would have noticed, as the client was not only quite attractive but also able to carry on very pleasant conversations despite her anxiety. The fortune telling and catastrophizing aspects of this thought are evident in the following passage:

THERAPIST (T): Why is it so important to you that the young man might be able to see that you're nervous?

CLIENT (C): He'll think there's something the matter with me.

T: What might he think was wrong?

C: Oh, just that something was wrong with me, like I was mentally ill or something.

T: You don't seem to like that idea. What would it mean to you if he did think you were mentally ill?

C: He wouldn't want to have anything to do with me. He'd just think of me as defective.

T: Defective?

C: Yes! Like I'm flawed. He wouldn't want to have anything to do with me because he'd think I'm defective!

T: That certainly seems important to you. What would it mean if he really did think you were defective?

C: He'd just be another one of many.

T: Many who think you're defective? (*Client nods and begins to cry.*) If many men do think of you as defective, what would that mean to you?

C: **NOBODY** would want to have anything to do with me. **I'D BE ALL ALONE FOR THE REST OF MY LIFE!**

One good way to dramatize the thinking error of catastrophizing is to read the preceding dialogue. However, the main goal is to show the clients that their reactions to specific events may be more than extreme. For example, "So let's say that you give a presentation during a meeting at work, drop your notes, and say only part of what you want to say because you get really anxious. Do you stop there or does your thinking take on a life of its own? Where do your thoughts go? Think about losing your job? What other bad thing might you think could happen next? Then what? Then what? And after that? Do we help ourselves with this type of thinking?"

DISQUALIFYING OR DISCOUNTING THE POSITIVE

This thinking error involves the rejection of positive experience. The client discounts positive experiences or outcomes by coming up with explanations that have nothing to do with his or her own ability or effort. With positive information invalidated, the client's negative belief system is supported and maintained. This distortion is among the most frequently encountered in our experience and represents a significant threat to therapeutic progress if left unaddressed. Three examples serve to illustrate how clients with social phobia disqualify the positive. First, several clients have explained away apparent successes in homework assignments or in naturally occurring events by saying, "It was easy to do. I don't know why. I just must have been having a good day." Thus they attribute their successes to the great unknown, the stars above, or anything other than themselves. Second, clients may similarly discount accomplishments by saying, "I don't know what I was so worked up about. It was easy," and attribute their success to misestimation of task demands rather than personal effort. Third, the person may attribute success to the kind hearts and support of others. This is the most common version of disqualifying the positive among clients with social phobia and is illustrated in the following example. A male client who sought treatment for heterosocial interaction fears took a significant risk and asked a woman for a date. She accepted, and at the next session, he reported that they had a marvelous time. When asked why this might have been the case, he reported that the successful evening occurred because she was so nice and easy to talk to. Although this statement included an honest and heartfelt compliment, it also implied that if it was not for her niceness, the evening would have been an abysmal failure. His willingness to take a risk, his appeal to others, and his improved social skills had nothing to do with it. He went on to say that she probably would not want to see him again and that he did not intend to call her just to be rejected. She was very nice, but niceness only goes so far. To quote Persons (1989, p. 114), "This logic can make a therapist's head hurt!" Thankfully, this is one of the easier errors for clients to identify, at least in the thoughts of their fellow group members, if not in their own thinking.

EMOTIONAL REASONING

In emotional reasoning, the client makes an inference about himself or herself or the world on the basis of a feeling state or emotional experience (Persons, 1989). As J. S. Beck (1995, p. 119) puts it, "You think something must be true because you 'feel' (actually, believe) it so strongly, ignoring or discounting evidence to the contrary." Again, emotional reasoning is a common thinking error among clients with social phobia. A typical statement is that of a client who became nervous when she had to eat or drink in front of other people: "I'm so nervous, other people *must be* thinking bad things about me." Another is the heterosocially anxious man who said, "I feel so foolish, I must really look foolish." Yet another is the client with public speaking fears who said, "I get so anxious, I know I must be coming across badly."

Clients who engage in emotional reasoning fail to realize that feelings do not equal reality (Hope & Heimberg, 1990). They make a fundamental error in assuming that the other person has access to the same information that they themselves have access to. However, this cannot be true, because only the client can truly know his or her internal subjective state or degree of physical arousal. Although arousal *can* be visible to others (e.g., blushing or profuse sweating), this is not always the case (e.g., rapid heartbeat), and even if it is visible, it rarely has the meaning to others that it has to the client.

Clients who engage in emotional reasoning may also make the rather common confusion between feelings and thoughts. Consider the young woman with a generalized fear of interacting with others who believed, "I feel so stupid, I must look stupid." "Stupid" is not an emotional state. Rather, this client felt distressed because she had experienced a number of negative *thoughts* about being stupid. Thus the approach to emotional reasoning with this client was to help her understand that she was engaging in thought–feeling confusion and to help her question the meaning, accuracy, and implications of labeling herself as stupid (see the next section).

LABELING

This thinking error involves summarizing one's feelings about oneself or others with a negative label. To do so is to fan the flames of negative feelings toward the labeled person. Although clients with social phobia may apply labels to other people, they do so most readily to themselves. They observe their behavior, judge it negatively, and apply summary labels to themselves. Clients frequently describe themselves as losers, jerks, stupid, foolish, boring, incompetent, or inadequate. The client whose dialogue was presented earlier (in the section on "Catastrophizing") labeled herself as defective.

An effect of this labeling process is to take an observation about one's *behavior* and turn it into an observation about one's *personality* or *character.* As a result, the client may feel hopeless about his or her ability to change and may believe that change efforts are futile. Labeling oneself in this way may inhibit problem-solving efforts because problems may be viewed as unsolvable (Persons, 1989).

Most of the time, when a person applies a label to another person, it is because of (often legitimate) anger over that person's misdeeds. Socially anxious persons sometimes apply negative labels to others because other people may put them in positions of anxious vulnerability. Consider the example of the college student who called his professor a "total jerk" and "incompetent" because the professor insisted that the student give a required classroom presentation (Hope et al., 2000). Of course, these labels were a reflection of the student's concerns about public embarrassment and had little to do with the character or qualifications of the professor. However, the student's focus on the professor's character was not helpful because it did not address the real cause of concern.

MENTAL FILTER

In mental filter (also called selective abstraction), the person becomes obsessively focused on a specific negative aspect of a situation and loses his or her ability to objectively view the situation in its entirety. The client with public-speaking phobia described previously was also engaging in mental filtering to the extent that he was unable to see that, despite stumbling over his words or having his voice crack, he made a coherent presentation, made a number of important points, and kept his audience's attention during his talk. His negative evaluation was based entirely on the negative details without consideration of the "big picture." Other examples include the college lecturer who became distressed when he saw a single student (in a class of 75) yawn during one of his lectures, the female client who gave a cocktail party for her husband's business associates and saw it as a terrible experience because she had spilled a drink, the young man who believed that his relationship with a woman was doomed to failure because they had had a single argument, and numerous clients who believed that their behavior in social interaction or performance situations was a failure because they became anxious.

MIND READING

In mind reading, the client arbitrarily concludes that someone is reacting negatively to him or her. However, rather than check this out with the other person, the client simply assumes the accuracy of this conclusion. Examples from our files are abundant:

> "He doesn't like me."
> "My boss and coworkers think I'm incompetent."
> "She must think I'm boring."
> "She's not interested in what I'm saying."
> "He (she/they) must think I'm unfriendly, weird, a nut case, mentally ill, defective, flawed, unacceptable."

Because these conclusions are based on clients' internal processing, they often are very far from the truth. However, they may be quite compelling to the client and reduce his or her willingness to approach others. Clients may be helped to cope with mind-reading errors by asking themselves to examine the evidence on which their conclusions are based. An example of mind reading and methods for coping with it are presented as part of the next exercise.

OVERGENERALIZATION

In overgeneralization, the person overinterprets the meaning of a negative outcome. The client draws unwarranted conclusions about the representativeness of the outcome for similar situations or events in the future. For example, a male client who wanted to increase his interaction with women was afraid to approach a woman and ask her to join him for an evening's activities. After much anxious anticipation, he worked himself up to it, only to have the woman refuse the invitation. He reported this outcome in the following group session and appeared quite down on himself: "She wouldn't go out with me. No one ever will!" He went on to describe his catastrophic belief that he would be alone for the rest of his life. Of course, as Persons (1989) points out in describing a similar client, all this proves is that he will not be going out with this woman at this time. It says nothing about his future dating prospects with other women or even with this same woman at a later time.

Another variation on overgeneralization that is common among clients with social phobia is to overgeneralize from past experiences to experiences in similar situations during treatment. One client, in discussing a potential homework assignment to enter a feared situation (attending a work-related social event) after several weeks in treatment, stated that he knew he would become overwhelmingly anxious and that he would rather not accept this assignment because it was doomed to failure. When questioned about his predictions of anxious doom, he stated, "I *always* get anxious!" (Note the all-or-nothing flavor to this statement as well: It always happens, and he describes becoming anxious as if it happens to the full extent or not at all.) However, this is an inappropriate generalization, as he had built up a number of success experiences in treatment and had learned a number of new coping skills.

"SHOULD" AND "MUST" STATEMENTS

"Should" statements capture the rules that persons have about the ways that they (and others) should live their lives. Although they may be helpful to persons who are not prone to anxiety or depression, clients' "should" statements are often extreme and perfectionistic. In the case of clients with social phobia, self-directed "should" statements may be summarized as, "I should always be perfect." Of course, these rules are strongly felt but impossible to live up to. Therefore, they may be a potent source of negative thoughts and feelings about the self.

Examples of self-directed "should" statements from clients with social phobia include, "I should be able to say the right thing," "I should always be in control," "I shouldn't show my anxiety in front of others," "I have to be perfect," and "I shouldn't be inappropriate; there are rules for how I should act." In each case, "should" statements encourage clients to become maladaptively focused on themselves, to be constantly checking out their behavior and the reactions of others, and to become distant observers rather than participants in social interaction.

"Should" statements may also be directed at others. Another person *should* act this way or that way. When "should" statements are directed in this manner, the result may be feelings of anger or hostility toward others. Our clinical and research experience suggests that these types of "should" statements do occur among persons with social phobia. Individuals with social phobia tend to believe, more than persons with panic disorder or without an anxiety disorder do, that the good things in life are controlled by powerful others (Cloitre et al., 1992b; Leung & Heimberg, 1996). They also tend to believe that these powerful others will overlook them or not take them into account. The college student who called the professor names when the professor required him to give a presentation in class was saying to himself something like, "He shouldn't make me do this. He knows I can't handle it."

MALADAPTIVE THOUGHTS

Persons (1989) includes an additional category that she labels "maladaptive thoughts." Maladaptive thoughts are not necessarily irrational or distorted. Nevertheless, it may be harmful to the individual to dwell on them. Examples include, "I've never done this before," "He's the president of the company," and "It's not fair that it's so hard for me to overcome my anxiety." Maladaptive thoughts are often self-critical and may have a ruminative flavor to them. They may distract the person from his or her purpose or decrease the chances of attempting new behaviors.

Persons (1989, p. 103) poses several questions that may help to determine whether a thought is maladaptive: Does the thought help my mood? Does the thought help me to think productively about my situation? Does the thought help me to behave appropriately? and Does the thought reinforce my irrational beliefs? It is useful to take this approach when thinking patterns are not clearly distorted.

Although Persons's questions suggest an excellent way of working with maladaptive thoughts, they may not readily determine whether a specific thought is best considered an example of maladaptive thinking, that is, a thought that is not distorted but is otherwise unhelpful. A thought should not be placed in this category until it is determined that none of the thinking errors described earlier can be appropriately applied to it. Clients are often quick to classify as maladaptive thinking such automatic thoughts as, "I'm going to be anxious" or "I'm not good at public speaking" (better classified as instances of fortune telling or all-or-none thinking). Beginning therapists will all too often find themselves agreeing when a client labels an AT as maladaptive thinking "because it is true." However, the thought may not be at all true, just very strongly held by the client. It is also the case that apparent maladaptive thoughts, when elicited, may hide distorted thoughts, and it is useful to probe these thoughts a bit before yielding. For example, "I've never done this before" might easily be a veiled expression of "I'm going to make a fool of myself."

Disputing Automatic Thoughts and Developing Rational Responses

The following exercise (adapted from Sank & Shaffer, 1984) introduces two of the remaining steps in the cognitive restructuring process, disputing automatic thoughts and developing rational responses. It also allows clients to see the cognitive restructuring process unfold in the context of a specific situation. The exercise (see Figure 10.2) begins as one of the therapists describes an anxiety-evoking situation. The therapists elicit from the group emotional, physiological, and behavioral consequences that might occur to the person in this situation. The group members generate potential ATs about the event that might serve to produce these emotional, physiological, and behavioral reactions. The group members are then asked what thinking errors they see in each AT. Then, using the List of Disputing Questions (see Figure 10.3), that is, a list of questions designed to dispute the content of automatic thoughts, the group members and therapists question each AT. Using the contrary information generated by this questioning procedure, group members and therapists collaborate on the development of more balanced rational responses to the situation. The group then reviews the situation and makes a judgment about the potential anxiety-reducing effect of viewing the situation in a rational manner and how the negative emotional, physiological, and behavioral reactions may also be reduced.

Referring to Figures 10.2 and 10.3, these steps should be followed in implementing this exercise:

1. T1 introduces problematic situation (activating event): "As you sit eating lunch with a friend in the employee cafeteria, the boss walks by and says to you in an irritated tone, 'Please see me in my office as soon as you are done eating.' "

2. T2 asks the group: "What would be your immediate reaction? How would you feel? What physical symptoms might you have? What would you do?" T2 lists these responses on the easel and adds any negative emotional, physiological, and behavioral reactions from Figure 10.2 to the list if they are relevant and were not mentioned by a group member.

3. T1 asks the group to generate a list of ATs that they would experience

Problematic Situation: As you sit eating lunch with a friend in the employee cafeteria, the boss walks by and says to you in an irritated tone, "Please see me in my office as soon as you are done eating."

Negative Emotional, Physiological, and Behavioral Reactions
- Your anxiety increases dramatically.
- You become physically tense.
- Your heart starts to pound.
- You lose your appetite for the rest of your lunch.
- You feel frozen in your chair.
- You find it difficult to concentrate on anything else.
- You ask your friend to tell you that it's OK but reject your friend's attempts to reassure you.

(Other consequences as generated by group)

Automatic Thoughts (ATs)
- "I must have really messed up."
- "Oh, no. Not again!"
- "The boss must think I'm so incompetent."
- "Everyone will find out. I'll be humiliated."
- "He's going to fire me."
- "I'll never find another job."

(Other ATs as generated by group)

Positive Consequences of Disputing ATs and Developing Rational Responses
- Less anxious
- Less physically tense
- Feel better about self
- Feel more confident in your skills and abilities
- Able to reflect on current circumstances and make a rational plan
- Able to get up and walk relatively calmly into boss's office

(Other positive consequences as generated by group)

FIGURE 10.2. Exercise in disputing automatic thoughts and developing rational responses. Based on an exercise in Sank and Shaffer (1984), pp. 233–234.

if they were to find themselves in this situation. T2 lists these ATs on the easel below the emotional–physiological–behavioral reactions already listed and adds any relevant ATs from Figure 10.2 that were not mentioned by a group member. T1 facilitates the group members' identification of thinking errors for each AT.

4. T2 passes out the List of Disputing Questions and describes it to the group: "This is a list of questions that you can use to dispute and argue with your ATs. They are presented in a general form so that you can apply them to a range of situations and so that you may adapt them in the way that works best for you. It is not an exhaustive list, and you may come up with other disputing questions that work even better for you. This is very similar to the ques-

---

List of Disputing Questions

Use these questions to challenge your automatic thoughts. Be sure to *answer* each question you pose to yourself. You will find each question helpful for many different thoughts. Several examples are also presented to help you get started.

1. Do I know for certain that _____?
   Example: Do I know for certain that I won't have anything to say?

2. Am I 100% sure that _____?
   Example: Am I 100% sure that my anxiety will show?

3. What evidence do I have that _____? What evidence do I have that the opposite is true?
   Examples: What evidence do I have that they DID NOT understand my speech?
                   What evidence do I have that they DID understand my speech?

4. What is the worst that could happen? How bad is that? How can I cope with that?

5. Do I have a crystal ball?

6. Is there another explanation for _____?
   Example: Is there another explanation for his refusal to have coffee with me?

7. Does _____ have to lead to or equal _____?
   Example: Does "being nervous" have to lead to or equal "looking stupid"?

8. Is there another point of view?

9. What does _____ mean? Does _____ really mean that I am a(n) _____?
   Example: What does "looking like an idiot" mean? Does the fact that I stumbled over my words really mean that I look like an idiot?

10. Is focusing on this helping me?

FIGURE 10.3. List of Disputing Questions. Adapted from *A Therapist's Manual for Cognitive Behavior Therapy in Groups* (p. 223), by L. I. Sank and C. S. Shaffer, 1984, New York: Plenum. Copyright 1984 by Kluwer Academic/Plenum Publishers. Adapted by permission.

tioning I asked you to help me with in the first session when I shared my ATs about giving that speech to the group of psychologists. Remember how we questioned each one of my ATs and found out that I was thinking myself into a lot of anxiety.

"Here's how it works. Let's say that I had the AT 'The boss must think I'm so incompetent' to the situation [cotherapist] presented. This is an example of mind reading. I could ask myself the following questions:

- "Do I know for sure that the boss thinks I'm so incompetent?"
- "What evidence do I have that the boss thinks I'm so incompetent?"

- "Could there be other explanations for his calling me into his office?"
- "What is the likelihood that he is so sure I'm incompetent that my job is really in trouble?"
- "What is truly the worst thing that could happen if he does think I'm so incompetent? How bad is that? How can I cope with that?"

5. T1 suggests to the group that they attempt to answer the questions just posed by T2 and emphasizes to the group that *it is the answers to the Disputing Questions that are really important*. Simply asking the questions is not good enough. Each question is repeated, and the group generates an answer to it.

A very important concept that needs to be communicated to the clients is that *effective disputing of automatic thoughts is an ongoing process in which an AT is examined by questioning it, answering the question, questioning the answer, and so forth* Additional useful disputation may be accomplished by starting the process over with a different question. Disputation involves microanalytic examination of closely held assumptions, not easy answers to clichéd questions. It is hard work, plain and simple.

---

6. The therapists record the answers to the questions on the easel. These are what we call *rational responses*, that is, responses based in logic and evidence that rebut the content of the AT (information about the nature of effective rational responses is provided in the next section).

7. T2 then selects an AT from the easel and the process is repeated, coaching the group members through the process of identifying the thinking error(s) in the AT, disputing it, and developing a rational response.

8. T1 and T2 alternate the rest of the way through the list of ATs, identifying the thinking error(s) in each AT, disputing it, and developing a rational response.

9. When the list of ATs is exhausted, or when it is clear that all group members have grasped the basic concepts, one of the therapists should pose the question to the group: "What would be the effect of disputing these ATs in this situation?" Each of the negative emotional, physiological, and behavioral reactions originally elicited from the group should be reviewed, and the group should be prompted to consider whether these consequences would be less likely to occur or, at least, to occur in lesser degree.

As time allows, the therapists and group members should return to the ATs that were generated as homework or as a part of the previous discussion of thinking errors and practice as much as possible the process of posing disputing questions and generating rational responses.

Effective Rational Responses

A rational response is a statement that summarizes the key points that a client "discovers" as he or she works through the process of disputing automatic thoughts. It is based on logic and evidence rather than on negative emotion, cognitive distortion, and pessimistic prediction. Engaging in the disputation process and deriving a workable rational response before entering a feared situation allows the anxious person to more easily strive against his or her ATs in the situation. It also provides a focus for cognitive debriefing after the situation has run its course, an important part of the cognitive-behavioral treatment of social phobia (see Chapter 12).

It is hard to give a more precise definition of a rational response, because it can take many forms. In a sense, if it helps the person function more adaptively in a situation, it is a more rational response than he or she had before. A rational response may be (among other things):

- A statement of the "final answer" to the disputation of a specific AT (e.g., "Blushing does not equal incompetence.").
- A summary of the answers to the disputations of several related ATs (e.g., "I have no reason to expect the worst"; "It is OK to be anxious").
- A reminder to stay focused on the task, to think rationally, and to cope with whatever transpires (e.g., "If there really is a problem, I'll just let my boss know that I will do my best to fix it.").
- A suggestion that certain behaviors are acceptable in the situation (e.g., "Remember that it is OK to talk about the weather and current events.").
- A statement of the person's goals in the situation (e.g., "My goal is to ask another person three questions and say three things about myself.").
- A reminder that the client should be on the lookout for certain types of ATs to which he or she may be vulnerable (e.g., "When I think 'I can't cope with this,' remember that is just my anxiety talking.").

In addition to its content, it is also important to focus on the form of a rational response. If a person is to use it effectively in a feared situation, a rational response should be brief enough to be easily remembered and repeated without itself becoming a distraction. It should be specifically related to the situation of concern rather than stating some broad generality ("I'm a nice guy and people like me!"). It should also be realistic, suggesting that positive or neutral outcomes are possible, but not naively so. Regarding the latter, consider the fellow who wanted to ask a woman out on a date. He had the AT that "She would never go out with someone like me." Clearly, this thought was unlikely to help him put his best foot forward. However, it would be just as inaccurate to substitute the thought, "She certainly will accept my invitation." A truly rational response here might suggest that he has no way of knowing whether she will accept or not but that he can give it a good effort and it *may* work out to his satisfaction. However, if he does not ask, she will surely not accept! A good rational response here might be very simple: "Nothing ventured, nothing gained." As we have said in other writings (Hope & Heimberg, 1990), this may sound like a cliché to us, but it may be a major revelation to the person struggling with social anxiety.

The client does not have to believe the rational response (especially early in treatment), but he or she must be willing to entertain the logical possibility that it is accurate. It would be naive for therapists to assume that, on the basis of simple questioning and disputation of an AT, a client would toss aside years of negativity. However, if the client can endorse the notion that there is a small possibility that the rational response is accurate, it becomes possible to reexamine the rational response and AT after the feared event has transpired and to make a judgment about the relative utility of each. In most cases, this effort should increase the client's belief in the rational response.

It is often useful to ask the client to give 0–100 ratings of his or her belief in the AT and the rational response before and after in-session exposures or homework assignments. The use of belief ratings is further discussed in Chapter 12.

The rational response can have other benefits, as well, simply as a side effect of the client's attention to it in feared situations. Attention to the rational response should disrupt the sometimes intense focus on automatic thoughts and interrupt the common phenomenon of cycling from one negative thought to another. Its introduction of an alternative viewpoint should make it more difficult for the client to simply accept the reality of his or her automatic thoughts. Finally, repetition of the rational response in the feared situation should cue the client to adopt a coping posture rather than to play the role of the victim.

Over the years, we have seen a number of rational responses usefully applied by persons with social phobia (some of these are described in more detail by Hope et al., 2000). These include the "nonequation," a rational response that is very useful when a client overgeneralizes the meaning of a behavior or outcome. For example:

- "Looking nervous does not equal [≠] looking foolish."
- "Being rejected ≠ Being alone forever."
- "Not getting this job ≠ Never getting a job."
- "Blushing ≠ Looking stupid."
- "Feeling anxious ≠ Looking anxious."

Another approach to rational responses is to focus on the worst possible outcome. When a client states that some outcome would be "awful" or that he or she "could not stand it," it is worthwhile to consider rational responses such as, "The worst that could happen is that she might refuse my invitation *and I can live with that.*" Depending on the realistic aversiveness of a negative outcome, an alternative might be, "The worst that could happen is that I might get fired *and that is unlikely.*"

Other examples of rational responses culled from our files include:

- "It's OK to take a pause in the middle of a conversation."
- "If I lose my place, I can take a second to collect my thoughts."
- "I can carry on a pleasant conversation even if I am anxious."
- "I don't have to be perfect to be hired."
- "Making mistakes makes you more human to others."
- "I'm only responsible for 50% of this conversation."
- "Conversation is a two-way street."
- "Speak slowly and remember to breathe."
- "I don't have to know the answer to every question."
- "The important things in life are sometimes difficult."

These rational responses are not simple affirmations. They are summaries of important information or self-instructions that keep the client on a path toward successful goal attainment. Just as positive reinforcement is defined by the increase in the frequency of the behavior it follows, rational responses are ultimately defined by their utility to the person and whether they serve to help the person manage anxiety and facilitate action that might otherwise have faltered.

Homework Assignment for Session 2: Cognitive Restructuring Practice

Our experience with CBGT suggests that these exercises will fill the time available for Session 2. However, two tasks remain before the session may be adjourned. The first task is the assignment of homework for the week between Session 2 and Session 3. Group members are asked to monitor ATs as in the previous week, but this time they are to use the List of Thinking Errors and List of Disputing Questions to assist them in the completion of a more complex self-monitoring and cognitive restructuring task. Group members should be instructed to list ATs that occur over the week and to use the Cognitive Restructuring Practice Form (Figure 10.4)[1] to:

1. Briefly describe the situation.
2. Record their ATs.
3. Identify and record the thinking error(s) in each AT.
4. Identify and record the emotions that are associated with the ATs.
5. Select the AT that seems most important to their anxiety and challenge it

Cognitive Restructuring Practice Form

1. **Situation**	
2. **Automatic Thoughts**	3. **Thinking Errors**
	THINKING ERRORS: All-or-Nothing Thinking, Overgeneralization, Mental Filter, Disqualifying the Positive, Mind Reading, Fortune Telling, Catastrophizing, Emotional Reasoning, "Should" Statements, Labeling, Maladaptive Thoughts

4. Emotions *(Check all that apply.)*

❏ Anxious/nervous   ❏ Frustrated   ❏ Irritated   ❏ Ashamed

❏ Angry   ❏ Sad   ❏ Embarrassed   ❏ Hateful

Other: _____

5. **Challenges** *(Use the Disputing Questions below or others you prefer. Challenge the most important AT(s) you listed above. Be sure to answer the question raised by the Disputing Question.)*

DISPUTING QUESTIONS: Do I know for certain that _____? Am I 100% sure that _____? What evidence do I have that _____? What is the worst that could happen? How bad is that? Do I have a crystal ball? Is there another explanation for _____? Does _____ have to lead to or equal _____? Is there another point of view? What does _____ mean? Does _____ really mean that I am a(n) _____?

6. **Rational response(s)**

FIGURE 10.4. Cognitive Restructuring Practice Form. Adapted from *Managing Social Anxiety: A Cognitive-Behavioral Therapy Approach* (Client Workbook) (Figure 6.4, p. 105), by D. A. Hope, R. G. Heimberg, H. R. Juster, and C. L. Turk, 2000. Copyright 2000 by Graywind Publications. Adapted by permission.

with Disputing Questions. Remember that disputing an AT is not usually accomplished with a single answer to a single question but by asking a question, answering it, questioning the answer, asking a new question that examines the AT from a different perspective, and so forth.

6. Develop and write out a rational response to the target AT.

This procedure is arduous but extremely helpful. It is also complicated and should not be given to group members unless it is thoroughly explained to them and discussion about recording a hypothetical situation has taken place in the group. Group members should be encouraged to complete forms for two or three situations that arise during the week, including an analysis of any anxiety they may feel in anticipation of Session 3 (see the next section). Several copies of the Cognitive Restructuring Practice Form should be distributed to group members for this purpose. Group members should also have copies of the List of Thinking Errors (Figure 10.1) and List of Disputing Questions (Figure 10.3).

Occasionally, our clients have produced miniaturized versions of the List of Thinking Errors and the List of Disputing Questions so that they can have these cognitive restructuring aids easily available. We encourage therapists to produce these forms in miniature for clients. Single-spaced, photo-reduced, two-sided copies of these forms can easily be reduced to the size of an index card and laminated.

Clients may also be instructed to read and study Chapter 6 in the Client Workbook, which should serve to reinforce the major content covered in this session.

Preparation for Initiation of In-Session Exposures

The final task in Session 2 is to prepare group members for Session 3. The clients will be aware that in-session exposures will start at the beginning of Session 3. For many, this represents an intensely anxiety-evoking situation, and the degree of anticipatory anxiety and negative thinking they experience may be extreme. It is a common experience for clients to entertain the possibility of avoiding coming to Session 3. It is very likely that group members will think of little else during the coming week and may be significantly distressed. We recall the young woman who arrived for Session 3 in an angry frame of mind, proclaiming to one of us that, "You ruined my week!" The temptation to take tranquilizing medication or a couple of drinks before the session may be great.

Because of this experience, it is best to confront the feelings of group members in a direct yet supportive manner. Therapists should inform group members that:

1. In-session exposures begin in Session 3.
2. Group members are likely to experience significant anticipatory anxiety during the week.
3. Group members may have a desire to avoid coming to the session or to self-medicate, but they should resist these temptations.
4. Group members' anticipatory anxiety is a function of ATs, and they can dispute their ATs (in fact, they might do so as part of their homework assignment if this is an issue).
5. Exposure is graduated. Group members will be exposed to less difficult situations first.
6. Group members will be given the opportunity to discuss the situations to which they will be exposed.
7. They will be learning new coping skills as they participate in exposures.

Note

1. The Cognitive Restructuring Practice Form presented here is a simplified version of the one that appears in the Hope et al. (2000) Client Workbook, redesigned to maximize consistency with other CBGT procedures. However, if the Client Workbook is used as an adjunct to treatment with CBGT, these differences may be confusing to clients and should be brought to their attention.

11

In-Session Exposures

In this chapter, we begin to describe the treatment techniques that will be the primary focus for the remaining sessions of CBGT: in-session exposures, cognitive restructuring, and homework assignments. These techniques are delivered in an integrated manner throughout CBGT. However, the integration of treatment components, especially of in-session exposures and cognitive restructuring, is difficult to grasp without a fully developed knowledge of each. We devote this chapter to the description of in-session exposures. The remaining techniques and technique integration are described in Chapters 12 and 13. The structure of Session 3 and beyond is described in Chapter 14.

Rationale for In-Session Exposures

In vivo exposure, that is, exposing oneself to feared situations in real life, is a key component of most cognitive-behavioral treatments for the anxiety disorders. However, *in vivo* exposure treatments for social phobia are often difficult to design and implement. First, *in vivo* exposures for clients with social phobia are inherently more complex than exposures for other anxious clients. Exposure for clients with other anxiety disorders requires only that they enter situations or confront objects that they fear. Exposure for clients with social phobia involves entrance into feared situations *but also requires that they execute complicated chains of interpersonal behavior while in the feared situations*. It is the fear of performing these behaviors (or of not being able to perform them) while under the scrutiny of others and the resultant fears of humiliation and embarrassment that define social phobia. As a result, *in vivo* exposures may be extremely anxiety provoking for clients with social phobia, as they also involve the reactions of others and a variety of feared interpersonal consequences.

Second, *in vivo* exposure for other anxious clients may be more or less easily available, but this is not always the case for the client with social phobia. Clients with panic disorder and agoraphobia may take a walk or drive away from home or visit a shopping mall at almost any time, and they may engage in interoceptive exposure (i.e., exposing themselves to feared sensations) in the privacy of their homes. However, the person with social phobia who fears speaking up in a weekly staff meeting may find his or her opportunities a great deal more limited. Consider also the following case examples. A male client with generalized social fears of many years' duration had, because of his fears, obtained employment as a night watchman at an industrial warehouse. He worked alone during late-night hours and rarely had interpersonal contact with anyone beyond cashiers and sales personnel when he had to buy food or other necessities. He had made so many isolationist choices over so many years that few *in vivo* exposure situations were available to him. We started his treatment by having him make eye contact and then say hello to passers-by on the street, but when it came to making conversations, few alternatives were available, and most of these were too anxiety-provoking for him to attempt. Similar concerns have arisen in the treatment of heterosocially anxious men who must engage in conversations with women but who have designed their lives to facilitate social avoidance and who are initially too fearful to join clubs, interest groups, or singles organizations. Also consider the case of the male client who had dropped out of doctoral study on two previous occasions because of fears about giving presentations. At first contact with this client, he worked in a gas station and had little opportunity to make presentations to others.

Butler (1985, 1989) has described additional difficulties in the conduct of *in vivo* exposure with clients with social phobia:

1. Social situations are, by their very nature, variable and unpredictable. It is often difficult to schedule exposure to social situations in advance of their occurrence, to repeat an exposure to the same situation, or to expose clients to easier situations before exposing them to more difficult ones.

2. Several situations involve only a brief exchange, thus defying traditional wisdom that exposures should be of prolonged duration. In these situations, clients who experience an initial surge of anxiety may be unable to see their anxiety stabilize or decrease over time. Clients who fear saying hello, interjecting a brief comment into an ongoing conversation, or responding to a question posed by a teacher or professor may find that the situation comes to an end while their anxiety is still at its peak.

3. Many clients do not avoid social situations but simply endure them at great personal cost. In these naturally occurring situations or during assigned exposures, some clients may withdraw into themselves and fail to attend fully

to situational cues. As a result, their anxiety may not have been fully elicited, and it is unlikely that they will be able to engage in meaningful emotional processing of the experience (Foa & Kozak, 1986).

4. Persons with social phobia are, by definition, preoccupied with the way they will be evaluated by others. However, how they are being evaluated may not be easily discerned in many social situations, and exposures may not provide information that will help them put this fear aside. Exposure alone has not always had a substantial impact on fear of negative evaluation in controlled studies, an important point because change in fear of negative evaluation has a strong relationship to treatment outcome (Mattick & Peters, 1988; Mattick, Peters, & Clarke, 1989). Given the frequency of thinking errors among persons with social phobia, we are not surprised. We frequently see clients who have completed an *in vivo* exposure in objectively successful fashion, only to turn it into a terrible failure experience by assuming the negative response of others (the mind-reading error).

For these reasons, we have deemphasized *in vivo* exposure as the primary means of exposing clients to their feared situations, especially early in treatment. (It is still utilized extensively in CBGT, and its use is described in detail in Chapter 13.) Instead, we have utilized the treatment group as a forum to create *simulations* of client's feared situations to which they may be exposed. In-session exposures have a variety of characteristics that make them attractive for the treatment of clients with social phobia:

1. In-session exposures are always *available*.

2. In-session exposures are *schedulable*. That is, we can expose a client to his or her feared situation at the appropriate time. It is a simple matter to determine a graduated exposure schedule, so that the client may first be exposed to a relatively mild situation and then to more difficult ones.

3. In-session exposures are *controllable*. By appropriate definition of the situation and coaching of the therapists and other group members who may take part in an in-session exposure, it is possible to include the necessary aspects of a situation and to make sure that hurtful aspects are omitted. In this way, the chances that a client may "get in too deep" are minimized.

4. In-session exposures are *moldable to the needs of the individual client*. Situations can be constructed that will evoke the "right" amount of anxiety and that will include the specific, often idiosyncratic, events or reactions that a client fears.

5. In-session exposures *occur under the observation of the therapists*. As a result, therapists are more able to know "what is really going on," may be less dependent on client report (which may often be negatively biased), and are better able to design interventions that will maximize the utility of the experience for the client.

6. In-session exposures are *easily integrated with cognitive restructuring activities*, thus increasing the chances that clients will practice these important skills and learn to utilize them outside of group sessions. The integration of exposure and cognitive restructuring is described in Chapter 12.

7. In-session exposures are *less easily avoided by clients* than homework assignments and less easily disrupted by extraneous events in the client's life.

8. In-session exposures may *facilitate compliance with homework assignments for in vivo exposure* by providing clients with a success experience prior to the demand to try something in real life.

Preparation for an In-Session Exposure

Selecting a Situation for Attention

Preparation for an in-session exposure begins by selecting a situation of relevance for the targeted client. The situation may be suggested by the client and may represent something that he or she wishes to work on in general or an upcoming situation with which the client is concerned. However, exclusive reliance on the client in selecting situations may be risky. Clients may avoid suggesting situations because they are afraid to attempt them or because they believe they will fail. They may simply not think of a particular situation that might be beneficial to confront. Also, they may become preoccupied with upcoming situations, but these situations may be very different in content from their stated goals (see Chapter 8) or too difficult to confront at a particular time in treatment. Situation selection is a negotiated process, often beginning with the therapists suggesting a situation for attention.

Therapists should develop a list of potential exposure situations for each client in advance of group sessions, based on the client's goals as stated in the treatment orientation interview, his or her fear and avoidance hierarchy, and the events that have transpired in earlier group sessions and homework assignments. With this list in hand, therapists will minimize the need to create a suitable situation "on the fly." Furthermore, because some in-session exposures may require that additional people or materials be available (discussed later), advance planning allows for the recruitment of these resources.

Selected situations must reflect the client's goals. Because treatment is time-limited, all situations that may engender anxiety will *not* be confronted in the group, and shifting back and forth between very different types of situations (e.g., dating and public speaking) may rob the client of a sense of continuity and limit progress in each area. Once a determination is made that a situation is consistent with the client's goals, the next step is to review the client's hierarchy. For a client's first in-session exposure, a situation that was rated about 50 on the 0–100 SUDS scale (or a situation that is similar to it) is selected. This situation should be one that is within the client's ability as determined by the therapists and that does not require extremely complex and difficult behavior on the part of the client (first exposures are discussed more thoroughly later). Thereafter, the client should progress up the hierarchy a step at a time so that his or her most feared situation (related to the specific goal) may be confronted before the end of treatment.

Designing the In-Session Exposure

No matter whether a situation is suggested by the client or by the therapists, the specific nature of the situation must be discussed. If the situation selected is a presentation of a committee report at a staff meeting, for example, the room in which the meeting will take place and the arrangement of the furniture should be discussed, and either the in-session exposure should occur in a convenient similar setting or (more commonly) the furnishings of the group therapy room should be arranged within reason to approximate the real-life setting. The specific behavior required of the client should also be established. Will he or she sit at a conference table, stand by the seat, or move to a lectern? Will he or she be required to use handouts or additional materials? Would the client be likely to speak spontaneously or from prepared notes? How controversial or technical is the subject matter he or she would be discussing? It is also important to determine what other people will be present and what their roles are in relation to the client (e.g., supervisor, peers, subordinates, strangers, customers, etc.).

To take another example, consider a client with a fear of dating. If the target situation is to initiate a first conversation with a potential dating partner, it is important to know the setting in which this would occur. Will it be a health club, a classroom, a church group, a business meeting of a charitable organization, a mixer for a singles' club, or a party at a friend's house? Within the target setting, what is the very specific situation in which the conversation would be initiated? Will it be initiated by turning to talk to the person sitting beside the client? Will it occur at a refreshment stand? Will there be other people in close proximity when the approach is made? Is the other person someone the client has some acquaintance with, will they meet through a mutual friend, or in some other way?

A particularly important aspect of this discussion is the determination of the behavior of the other people to be involved in the in-session exposure. Therapists and other group members will assume these roles and must be informed how to behave. For instance, in the dating example, the person to be approached could be either receptive to conversation and interested in getting to know the client, uninterested, involved in a committed relationship, or shy and introverted. In the staff meeting example, the "audience" would be composed of group members who assume the roles of people who have specific behavioral styles and relationships to the client. The client may expect them to behave in certain ways, and this may be a source of considerable anxiety.

When the client reports on situations of concern, these situations will be populated with real people rather than social roles. That is, the client will typically report anxiety talking to "Jane" or "Robert," not anxiety about the prospect of talking to "dating partners." Although in-session exposures should be realistic, it is often a mistake for role players to be instructed to take on the roles of the specific people of concern, the Janes and the Roberts. It leaves the door wide open for the client to discount the experience if the behavior or appearance of the role player differs from those that the client would expect from the specific person in the real situation. In most situations, it is preferable to construct the in-session exposure to involve other people in similar roles. In dating contexts, *it is also important that therapists not communicate to the client that it is critical to his or her success in therapy or in life that he or she pursue a specific romantic interest.*

Use of Additional Personnel from Outside the Group

Most in-session exposures are conducted with the therapists and group members playing the required roles, and it is possible to conduct groups in which no one else is involved. However, several situations may arise in which it would be useful to recruit other available individuals to assist in the conduct of in-session exposures. For instance, it may be that a male client has a fear of dating or making conversation with women but the specific group includes no female clients of the right age. In the later stages of the group, a client may have interacted repeatedly with all the age-appropriate members of the group, and they may no longer be maximally useful for in-session exposures on the topic of interaction with strangers. Earlier in the group, appropriate group members may be available, but they may themselves be too anxious about similar situations to adequately fill the necessary role(s). A client with public-speaking phobia may become anxious only with audiences of unfamiliar people or of larger size than the group itself can provide. In situations like these, other individuals may be brought in to assist. At the Adult Anxiety Clinic of Temple University, we typically make use of undergraduate research assistants, doctoral students, and support staff to fill these roles, but any person who has adequate social skills and the right characteristics for the specific in-session exposure may be recruited. When recruiting outside persons, we typically ask the permission of group members and take care to instruct the recruit on issues of confidentiality. They are also carefully instructed about the role they will be asked to play. The use of outside persons requires that therapists formulate topics for in-session exposures at least one session in advance so that there is adequate time for recruitment.

Therapists who work in nonuniversity settings often remark that there is no one else that they can bring into their social phobia groups. They may work in independent practice or with colleagues who are conducting their own sessions during the time of the group. It is important to emphasize that the use of additional personnel is not required for the successful conduct of CBGT; it only makes it easier to create situations in which novelty or group size are maximized. However, clinicians may easily overlook potential role players who are available in their settings. Our experience suggests that support staff are often willing to participate for the few minutes at a time that are required and that they may enjoy a sense of contribution to the overall effort by their participation. Professional colleagues may also be asked to participate when they are available or when advance notice can be given.

Advance Preparation and the Use of Props

Some in-session exposures may require special preparation on the part of the target client. A frequent example is the client with public-speaking phobia who fears making presentations on specific (often technical) topics that require advance preparation, such as the development of notes, handouts, or charts. Although many of these clients' fears may be confronted in the context of extemporaneous talks on any topic, they must eventually talk on the feared topics. Assigning as homework the development of notes and materials gives the target client the opportunity to work on these situations. Furthermore, many of these clients experience substantial anticipatory anxiety that inhibits their preparation, reinforces procrastination, and creates a situation in which they may in reality be poorly prepared. An assignment to prepare presentation notes or other materials provides the opportunity for the client to work on anticipatory anxiety and procrastination using cognitive coping skills (see Chapter 12).

Other situations may also arise that require the use of props. These situations frequently involve clients with specific fears of eating, drinking, writing, or working in front of others. Obviously, in-session exposures for clients with eating or drinking fears will require that food or drink be obtained in advance and brought to the group. Most typically, these will be salads (with dressings), soups, or other "messy" foods and appropriate utensils or drinks, glasses, and pitchers. It is important to carefully determine the types of food that are anxiety-evoking, but water will typically suffice for drinking phobics. Other in-session exposures may be more idiosyncratic and require the therapists to obtain props appropriate to the situation. For instance, one female client who worked as a secretary became quite anxious whenever her boss would hover over her typewriter. A typewriter was necessary for conduct of exposures pertaining to working under observation and to asserting her wishes to her boss that he not hover over her. A hair stylist who became anxious when making conversation with the person whose hair she was cutting never looked at the person directly but kept eye contact through the mirror she was facing. To do this exposure, a mirror was necessary. A nursing student became quite anxious at the prospect of measuring blood pressure or giving injections while being observed by her supervisor, and a blood pressure cuff and syringe became necessary props for her in-session exposure. A male client with a fear of writing in public was specifically concerned about signing credit card forms and rebate certificates, and these had to be obtained in quantity. Furthermore, this client's anxiety increased as the size of the signature space decreased, and we prepared a series of mocked-up rebate forms that required increasingly smaller signatures. As with the use of other props or personnel, these in-session exposures had to be planned at least one session in advance.

Incorporating Feared Outcomes

Before an in-session exposure, the target client is asked about the specific aspects of the situation that he or she fears. In most cases, the primary fear is that the client will not be able to perform in the desired manner and that other people will have a negative reaction to this state of affairs. If this is so, the client's fear will be addressed in cognitive restructuring activities prior to the in-session exposure. However, two other types of fears deserve attention and may influence the shape of the in-session exposure. In one situation, the client fears that a specific symptom of anxiety will be present, for example, that he or she will blush or sweat profusely and that this will be visible to others. If this symptom does not occur, the client may experience some anticipatory anxiety but may soon realize that the situation is well in hand, and anxiety may subside. Although this sounds like a successful outcome, it is not. Rather, the client may trivialize the experience, saying to himself or herself, "I did all right, but I didn't sweat. If I did sweat, it would have been terrible." In this particular case, we have found it useful to elicit the specific symptom of anxiety feared by the client (e.g., have the client wear a wool sweater, drink hot tea, or engage in a brief period of exercise) immediately before the in-session exposure.

In the second case, the client is afraid that another person will have a specific reaction or that there will be some event that will complicate the situation; if this does not happen, we again run the risk that the client will trivialize the experience. One public-speaking phobic believed that he could perform adequately if he was allowed to make his presentation from start to finish without interruption but that he would "fall apart" if interrupted with questions. He feared that he would lose his place and not be able to get back to it, and, as a result, he would stand silent at the podium while everyone stared at him. As this was not apparent to the therapists at the start of treatment, his first in-session exposure was designed for him to give his talk to a receptive *but quiet* audience. He experienced no anxiety and saw no benefit because the situation he feared had not occurred. In our next attempt, we instructed the group members to ask frequent questions, and the results were dramatically different. He became very anxious, but he found that he was able to respond to the questions and continue with his talk, and his anxiety spiraled downward. Another client who experienced intense anxiety around public-speaking situations on his job viewed these situations as opportunities for his supervisors and others to disparage his poor job performance. He believed that he would be publicly humiliated, would not be able to respond, and would lose his job. Although all of these aspects could not be incorporated into an in-session exposure, group members who took on the role of his supervisor and coworkers were instructed to interrupt the client and make negative comments about his presentation, his job performance, and so forth. Thus he was able to place himself in a version of the feared situation and, with time, to adjust his prediction of how likely this feared outcome might be.

An interesting question arises from the preceding examples. Is it most important to design the in-session exposure to match objective reality or the client's sometimes distorted view of it? Of course, the answer is "both." The exposure situation must incorporate those aspects feared by the client. If an objective aspect of the situation is feared (e.g., people might ask questions), it should be included. Likewise, if the client fears an unlikely circumstance and focuses on it as the key to his or her anxiety, the in-session exposure will be of little value if this aspect is not included. Keep in mind that the goals of engaging clients in in-session exposures include:

- Exposing the client to a realistic dose of his or her anxiety experience.
- Helping the client to remain in the situation and continue performing despite his or her anxiety.
- Eliciting relevant cognitions for use during cognitive restructuring periods.
- Giving the client an opportunity to practice cognitive coping skills while in a state of arousal.

Obviously, to meet these goals, the in-session exposure must be realistic, but the "reality" it must match is that of the client. One additional example may further illuminate this issue. A client wanted to work on his anxiety about giving committee reports in staff meetings at his job. Like the client described previously, he was afraid that he would lose his place and not be able to complete the task without humiliation and embarrassment. Early in treatment he gave a mock committee report for his in-session exposure. He did very well and experienced very little anxiety. He also saw it as a trivial result because the situation that he feared had not occurred. He feared the unlikely event that a burst of air from a nearby air-conditioning vent would blow his notes off the podium and that he would be left standing there with no notes, nothing to do, and nowhere to hide. When we brought an electric fan to the next session and placed it where the air-conditioning vent was in his conference room, he became very anxious but then began to cope with (and benefit from) the experience.

SUDS Recording

Clients should be asked to provide an ongoing record of their anxiety during in-session exposures. They have been trained in the use SUDS ratings during the treatment orientation interview, and individualized anchor points have been derived for each client (see Figure 8.2). During the in-session exposure, the target client is prompted every 60 seconds or so to give a SUDS rating. This prompt is delivered by a therapist who is not participating in the in-session exposure or by another group member. It is most helpful and least intrusive if the person simply says "SUDS?" The client responds with a number between 0 and 100 and may also be asked to engage in some cognitive coping activities. SUDS ratings are recorded on the In-Session Exposure Recording Form (Figure 11.1).

The record of SUDS ratings delivered by the target client is extremely useful during the cognitive restructuring period that follows the in-session exposure (see Chapter 12). However, the incorporation of this assessment into the in-session exposure is not without consequence. The probe presents an unnatural break in the flow of the in-session exposure. Nothing like this ever happens in real life! Therefore, the client may lose track of his or her thoughts momentarily, and it is incumbent on the role players or nonparticipating therapist to help the client out.

FINAL PREPARATIONS

At this point, therapists will engage the target client in a period of cognitive restructuring activity to help him or her develop adaptive responses to anxious thoughts that will occur during the in-session exposure and behavioral goals for the exposure (see Chapter 12). Thereafter, the last pieces of preparation for the in-session exposure should be completed:

1. Arrange furniture in the group room as necessary or move to an alternate site (e.g., reception area, conference room, coffee area, etc.).
2. Choose specific persons to play required roles and make sure that they understand what to do.
3. Assign a therapist or group member who will not participate in the in-

In-Session Exposure Recording Form

Client _____

Date _____ Session # _____ Client's exposure # _____

Description of exposure situation: _____

_____

_____

Others involved: _____

_____

Client's goal(s) in exposure:

Rational response(s) used in exposure:

SUDS Record:
_____

Time	Rating	Time	Rating
Initial	_____		
1 minute	_____	6 minutes	_____
2 minutes	_____	7 minutes	_____
3 minutes	_____	8 minutes	_____
4 minutes	_____	9 minutes	_____
5 minutes	_____	10 minutes	_____

FIGURE 11.1. In-Session Exposure Recording Form.

session exposure to probe for SUDS ratings and record them on the In-Session Exposure Recording Form (Figure 11.1).

4. Negotiate with the target client a goal for the in-session exposure (see Chapter 12).

First Exposures

With the beginning of in-session exposures in Session 3, a new phase of treatment begins. Clients will be expected to participate in anxiety-evoking events on a regular basis, unlike their experience in the first few sessions. As noted in Chapter 10, they may approach Session 3 with trepidation, hoping against hope that they will not be chosen for the very first in-session exposure. Even if they are "lucky" enough to avoid this particular anxiety-evoking event, they will watch the initial in-session exposure with rapt attention, attempting in their own minds to make a determination of what they may be asked to do and whether or not they will be able to do it when their turn comes. Because clients may be extremely anxious and self-focused at the beginning of Session 3, the success of the very first in-session exposure may have a significant impact on the future history of the group and on its ultimate effectiveness in reducing the anxiety of the group members. Therefore, we encourage therapists to carefully consider which group member will be selected and to what situation he or she will be exposed.

The selected client should be one whom the therapists believe will be able to handle the in-session exposure successfully. Also, it is probably good to pick someone who is a good "coping model." Picking the least impaired member of the group may set the bar too high for the ones to follow. A moderately impaired member who is anxious but who can have a success experience is probably the best.

The target situation should be one that the remaining clients will not see as beyond their own abilities. Also, because of the anxiety inherent in this situation, the therapists should select a situation that does not require elaborate set-up or the utilization of additional personnel or props. Nor should they select a situation that requires multiple or complex roles that must be played by group members. Group members may simply be too anxious to execute these behaviors well and may become additionally preoccupied with the notion that they might become responsible for "ruining" someone else's in-session exposure. Of course, they may also have a phobic reaction to playing the role of an attractive dating partner, authority figure, and so forth. As a result, therapists will find that the best situations for initial exposures will often be conversations with a single other person (e.g., a potential romantic interest) whose role may be assumed by one of the therapists or a presentation to a passive, receptive audience.

One other caveat about first exposures is in order. Because the target client's anxiety may be higher than will be the case for subsequent exposures, it is important for the therapists to keep the preparatory activities simple. The client may be less able to retain information or respond to questions and may be more distractible. The therapists should avoid becoming bogged down in details of exposure set-up and cognitive restructuring. Do only what is necessary and get on with it!

Choosing Role Players and Combined Exposures

An important issue in the conduct of in-session exposures is the selection of the persons to play the various roles. Early on, it is necessary to rely mostly on therapists or recruited personnel to play complex roles. However, as treatment proceeds, these tasks should be increasingly handed over to other clients. In selecting a client to play a specific role in the in-session exposure of another client, it is necessary to consider the following two points. First, it is preferable to select a client who does not have a complementary fear whenever possible. For example, a woman with fears about being approached by men may not be a wise choice for an in-session exposure for a man with a fear of asking women for dates. Second, the therapists should carefully assess whether or not the potential role player has the capacity to play the role well. Can he carry his weight in a conversation? Will she go silent or attempt to dominate the conversation? Will he or she attempt to "rescue" the target client? If she will be required to give feedback to the client after the in-session exposure, will she do so straightforwardly? Will he pick out a number of trivial negatives? Will he, on the other hand, ignore any negatives and give unrealistically positive feedback? These judgments may be highly subjective ones, but they may be quite important to the success of the in-session exposure.

Alternatively, it is possible to pick multiple clients with similar fears to go through an in-session exposure together, especially in the case of in-session exposures such as the cocktail party or wine-tasting situations described later in this chapter. Similarly, therapists may purposely select clients with complementary fears (e.g., men and women with heterosocial fears) to participate in the same in-session exposure, especially if the clients appear to possess reasonable behavioral skills. In this case, it is necessary to devote cognitive restructuring time to each of the participants before and after the in-session exposure. However, it is often a useful strategy for demonstrating to clients that the second person in an interaction may be focused on his or her own personal concerns and not on the first person's inadequacies. If this strategy is selected, care must be taken not to devote so much time to preliminary activities that the in-session exposure drags to a conclusion.

In-Session Exposures versus Social Skills Training

In-session exposures are not primarily intended to teach specific behavioral skills, as in social skills training. Although there is undoubtedly some benefit that arises for clients in terms of behavioral skill acquisition, in-session exposures do not provide the brief repeated rehearsals that are the hallmark of social skills training, nor is there a systematic effort to provide specific feedback about the microlevel behaviors that are the focus of social skills training. Throughout the in-session exposure and its associated activities, the focus is on the physiological and subjective components of the anxiety response, and the in-session exposure is used primarily as a tool for providing affectively compelling information to the client that may result in cognitive, affective, and behavioral change. It has been our experience that many persons with social phobia possess adequate behavioral skills but are inhibited by their maladaptive belief systems and that therefore a social skills training approach is unnecessary. However, some clients may have meaningful social skills deficits. In these cases, social skills feedback *may be* incorporated into the standard procedure for in-session exposures, which may be shortened to give more opportunities for specific behavioral feedback. For example, a client who carries on a delightful conversation with a role player but never once makes eye contact might benefit from feedback about this. This feedback can then be integrated into future exposures, when an additional goal might be to maintain eye contact over the course of the conversation.

Do In-Session Exposures Make Clients Anxious?

Not surprisingly, we have been asked on several occasions whether the simulated nature of these exposure exercises reduces the client's involvement or the magnitude of their anxiety response, and the reader may have entertained similar questions while reading this chapter. In fact, it is possible for a client to focus on the artificial nature of the in-session exposure as a means of cognitive avoidance, and clients who do so may keep their anxiety at a minimum. Clients who focus on the artificial nature of in-session exposures as a means of controlling their anxiety are confronted about this issue early in therapy. Talking about the need to let go of this avoidance strategy and to work on making the in-session exposures as real as possible in order to fully benefit from treatment is usually sufficient. Of course, if clients do not let go of this coping strategy, the potential for positive treatment response may be compromised. Although this does occur for a small percentage of clients, it has not been a problem for the large majority.

In fact, many clients do not *expect* to feel anxiety during in-session exposures but end up feeling it quite strongly! In our clinic, clients come into treatment aware of this fact because they typically experienced substantial anxiety during our behavioral assessments. In other settings, it is useful to encourage clients to try as hard as they can to really throw themselves into the situation and to judge the efficacy of in-session exposures once they have actually participated in one.

Typically, clients are quite anxious during in-session exposures, their anxiety arising from several sources. First, there is typically a similarity between the simulated situation and the client's cognitive representation of the real one. Although the in-session exposure will not contain all the imagined consequences feared by the client (he or she cannot really lose his or her job or will not really be rejected by the other person), he or she can do badly in his or her own eyes and provide evidence for his or her inadequacies. Second, the clients are aware that they are being observed and evaluated by a "panel of experts" (the therapists) and by a group of their peers (the other group members). These two factors are legitimate anxiety-elicitors for clients with social phobia. Anecdotal reports are that anxiety is initially high during in-session exposures, as clients fear looking bad in front of strangers. As they become more familiar with other group members, however, their fears of disappointing significant others may come into play and keep their anxiety high. Thus the CBGT group provides a mix of "simulated" and "real" anxiety experiences with which the clients must learn to cope.

Examples of Common In-Session Exposures

The content of in-session exposures is as varied as the circumstances of the individual group members and will always be highly individualized. However, several situations have occurred repeatedly in our experience. In this section, we describe the themes of several of the more frequent in-session exposures and the variations on these themes.

Initiating Conversations with a Person of Potentially Romantic Interest

This is one of the most common topics for an in-session exposure. It is also a situation that can vary on a large number of important characteristics. These include the setting, the amount of familiarity the client has with the person, the behavior of the person, and the goal of the interaction.

SETTING

As noted in an earlier section, these interactions can occur almost anywhere—in a college class, a church group, a singles club mixer, a health club, or a party hosted by a mutual friend, to name just a few. Examination of the setting is extremely important because it may dictate the physical proximity of the interactants, as well as the appropriate topics of conversation. For instance, a health club setting pulls for talk about exercise routines or how to use a specific exercise machine, whereas a party at a friend's house may lead to conversation about the host or hostess.

FAMILIARITY

Has the client met, talked to, or been in the same place as the other person on previous occasions? Do they have common experiences to talk about? Has a previous interaction gone badly? Has conversation with the same person been the topic of a previous in-session exposure?

BEHAVIOR OF THE OTHER PERSON

Is the other person receptive or uninterested? Warm or aloof? Outgoing or shy? Will he or she carry the weight of the conversation or will he or she take leads from the client? Most important, will the other person notice the client's anxiety and say something about it?

Asking for a Date

Most of the issues raised herein about conversations with a potential romantic interest apply here as well. In fact, they define the general form of the in-session exposure, as asking for a date may actually take only a few seconds. A client may actually reduce his or her anxiety rather considerably by asking for a date almost immediately, but it is unlikely that a real-life situation would take that shape. As a result, we typically require that the client engage the other person in a period of conversation before making the request and allow him or her to ask for a date only after a prearranged period of time has elapsed and a signal is given by a therapist.

SETTING

The major question here may be whether the client will ask for a date in person or over the telephone. Telephone in-session exposures may be easily arranged by using local extensions or simply by having the players sit facing away from each other.

FAMILIARITY

This exposure topic assumes a degree of familiarity with the other person in most instances. In these cases, it may be helpful if the in-session exposure follows other in-session exposures in which the client has initiated conversations with the other person. Some exceptions are the blind date, a contact engineered by mutual friends, or a contact that results from use of a dating service.

BEHAVIOR OF THE OTHER PERSON

In addition to the concerns noted, therapists must determine whether or not the other person will accept the invitation, suggest an alternative arrangement (e.g., "I can't go out with you this Friday, but how about Saturday?" or "I really don't like to go to baseball games, but have you seen the latest movie with Tom Hanks? I hear its really good!"), reject the invitation, or give an ambiguous reply. In order to set up this in-session exposure effectively, it may be necessary to ask the target client to briefly step out of the room.

Other Conversations

The number of potential conversational topics for in-session exposures is truly infinite. Here we list for you a sample of the large number of different situations that have been targeted in our groups:

- Participating in conversations involving more than two people, as might happen at a party.
- Running into a friend at a store and making small talk.
- Running into a friend at a store when the friend is with another person who is unfamiliar to you.
- Working in your yard and talking to your neighbor.
- Talking to a classmate before or after a class.
- Talking to the parents of your child's friends.
- Making small talk with fellow employees during a coffee break or in the company cafeteria.
- Introducing yourself to someone.
- Joining in an ongoing conversation.
- Making small talk with strangers in a grocery store, movie line, or doctor's office.
- Starting a new job and meeting the people who work there.
- Getting to know friends or colleagues of your spouse or significant other.
- Conversing with someone on a date.
- Asking or answering personal questions.
- Making a telephone call to someone you like.

Public Speaking

Public speaking includes giving formal speeches to professional or political organizations, but it also includes a great deal more. Although we have encountered clients who fear speaking only in such lofty settings as international conferences or political events, the typical client with public-speaking fears is concerned with more mundane events, from giving class lectures or presentations to giving a toast at a wedding to expressing an opinion at a meeting of the PTA or the local Cub Scout pack. Public-speaking fears, as defined in this way, are extremely common and distressing to large numbers of people.

SETTING

Where will the client be required to speak, and what are the formal characteristics of the setting? Will he or she stand at a podium or lectern in front of an audience? Or will he or she be seated with the audience around a table? Will he or she write on the easel or use other visual materials? Will the speaking task be less formal or structured, as, for example, telling a story to a group of people at a party?

BEHAVIOR REQUIRED OF THE SPEAKER

Several issues need to be considered here. First, is the client to speak from notes or extemporaneously? If from notes, do they need to be prepared in advance, or can the client jot down a few notes before the in-session exposure begins?

Second, is the topic itself truly relevant to the client's fear, or, as is often the case, is it simply a fear of talking in front of people and being the center of their attention? If the latter, then it may be possible to have the client speak on any of a number of topics—for example, a hobby, a job, a recent vacation trip, or some aspect of personal history. These topics are typically easier to arrange as they are available to everyone and easily understood by the audience.

Third, will the speaker speak without interruption, or will he or she entertain questions from the audience? This decision is an important one because clients show a great deal of variability in their response to audience questions. Some find questions to be extremely anxiety-provoking, representing an opportunity for them to show their lack of knowledge or competence. Others find questions to be anxiety-reducing, as they find the interactive aspects of question-and-answer to be less artificial than lecturing to an unresponsive audience.

Fourth, will the speaker be asked to present purely factual or historical data, or will he or she be required to render an opinion on the topic? If relevant to an individual's concerns, expressing opinions may produce a substantial increase in anxiety, as one's opinions may be ridiculed or require defense.

Fifth, does the speaker fear the occurrence of a problem with his or her performance or behavior (instead of, or in addition to, the reactions of the audience)? For instance, does he or she fear stumbling over his or her words or mispronouncing words? If so, therapists must act to increase the probability that this will happen or that the speaker cannot discount the experience if it does not. Clients may avoid certain words or phrases they find difficult and then discount successful performances precisely because they did so. In this situation, asking the client to use the feared phrase a certain number of times or to read aloud a selection that contains several unfamiliar, foreign, or technical words may be necessary.

Sixth, the client may fear a physical symptom that may occur in the context of public speaking, such as blushing or profuse sweating. Failure of the symptom to occur may lead to discounting of success experiences. Consider the case of a professional man who had to do a fair amount of public speaking in his job as staff training director at a local facility. He was concerned that his profuse sweating would be visible to others and serve as an indication of his incompetence and unsuitability for the job. On days on which he had to speak in front of others, he would jog several miles before work, for the purpose of "sweating himself dry." He would then select one of a limited number of shirts that he believed hid his sweat reactions. In early in-session exposures, the sweat response did not occur, and little progress was made. The client did not start to make meaningful movement until we changed our approach. In later in-session exposures, he was requested to go to another room and engage in a period of intense exercise or drink a cup of hot tea before speaking. He was also asked to wear shirts that he had previously avoided wearing in these situations or to douse himself with water from a spray bottle before entering the room in which the speech was to take place.

BEHAVIOR REQUIRED OF THE AUDIENCE

Group members, therapists, or recruited persons who serve in the roles of audience members may be asked to behave in a number of different ways. Most simply, they may be asked to look attentive and say nothing. Alternatively, they may be asked to behave in a manner feared by the speaker. These behaviors may include asking questions, disagreeing with the speaker, looking bored and uninterested, or making disparaging remarks. When asked to engage in these behaviors, they should be coached by the target client and therapist in advance of the in-session exposure. In most situations early in treatment, therapists or recruits may need to assume active roles, but group members are often able to assume these roles quickly. Group members may be hesitant, however, if the topic of the speech is specialized or technical. In these cases, it may be useful to provide a specific question or comment to each group member so that they may participate more easily.

EXAMPLES OF PUBLIC SPEAKING IN-SESSION EXPOSURES

Examples of public speaking in-session exposures from our groups include:

- Giving a book report to an undergraduate literature class.
- Making a presentation as a graduate student in a seminar.
- Presenting a paper at a scientific meeting.
- Giving a toast at the wedding of a friend or at one's parents' anniversary party.
- Offering a eulogy at a friend's funeral.
- Presenting a treatment plan at a medical, mental health, or educational staff meeting.
- Offering an opinion on a controversial topic at a discussion group.
- Answering questions in a class or seminar.
- Presenting a committee report at a business meeting.
- Reading from a magazine, newspaper, or religious text.
- Introducing oneself and disclosing personal information at a meeting of Alcoholics Anonymous or other self-help group.
- Chairing a meeting of a self-help group.
- Training others in technical procedures.
- Giving workshops in one's area of expertise.
- Telling a story to a group of people at a party.

Writing in Front of Others

Typically, writing behavior is unimpaired and evokes little anxiety when a person is alone. The person who fears writing in public, however, actually fears that his or her anxiety will be visible to others, often in the form of a tremor of the writing hand or implement. For most clients, this concern is generalized to any situation in which others may view their writing behavior. Other clients may experience anxiety only in a limited subset of writing situations, and the specific cues that elicit their reactions should be incorporated into in-session exposures. Consider the case of the client who became anxious whenever he had to sign a credit card voucher in at an upscale men's clothing store but was relaxed and calm signing at K-Mart! Other clients may become more anxious when writing with pen rather than pencil because mistakes are harder to conceal and ink may be easily smudged. For others, a small space for a signature may signal anxiety. We have used the following situations in the treatment of writing-phobic clients:

- Taking notes during treatment sessions and showing them to the therapists and group members.
- Completing various forms, such as credit card blanks, rebate applications, counter checks, or rental agreements while group members and therapists crowd around, observe, and make comments.
- Writing on the easel the automatic thoughts reported by another group member in preparation for an in-session exposure.
- Registering at a motel and signing the many required forms.
- Completing an insurance application while sitting with the broker.
- Signing the many forms required at a real estate closing.
- Completing a detailed medical history form.
- Waiting in line at a bank to conduct business that will require writing in front of the teller; dealing with anticipatory anxiety while making conversation with other people in line.

Most episodes of writing in public involve small writing samples, often only a signature. In our experience, it is not helpful to the client if an in-session exposure involves only a single writing sample. Rather, if a small sample of writing behavior is targeted, it should be repeated many times during an in-session exposure. Also, if the client's anxiety increases as the signature space gets smaller and smaller, it is a good idea to take this to the extreme and have the client sign smaller and smaller and smaller and smaller forms until the process becomes absurd. The fact that it may never happen precisely that way outside the group is of little consequence.

Eating or Drinking in Front of Others

Persons with fears of eating or drinking in front of others appear to have the same general concerns as those expressed by persons with writing fears.

However, eating and drinking with others is less easily avoided than writing in public without extreme effects on one's life. Eating or drinking phobics often find that they are almost totally unable to socialize with other people, because socializing and food and drink are so intimately tied together in modern society.

Given this state of affairs, it is not difficult to come up with in-session exposures for eating and drinking phobics. Almost any conversational or social situation can be modified to include food or drink. However, formal situations, such as banquets, dinner parties, or cocktail parties, especially if important persons are present, may be extremely difficult for these clients.

Clients differ among themselves in the situations that are most difficult for them, and they also differ in the types of food they find most difficult or anxiety provoking. Finger foods are typically nonthreatening and may be preferred by clients as a subtle form of avoidance. (However, we recently encountered a client who feared eating french-fried potatoes that she held in her hands. She feared that the French fry would exaggerate the shaking of her hands so that it would be more visible to others, and this was especially the case if the French fry was "limp"!) "Utensil foods" are more difficult, and the level of difficulty appears to increase as the "messiness" of the food increases. This is presumably because the messier foods have greater potential for social embarrassment when there is a spill or food falls from a utensil onto one's lap (or the lap of someone with the client!). Salads with dressing, soups, pasta dishes, any dishes with cream or cheese sauces, soft or partially melted ice cream, and other desserts may be avoided when other people are present. Serving food to others may also be difficult as they will be watching rather closely.

The central task in an in-session exposure for an eating phobic is to eat. If the client simply plays with his or her food or moves it around the plate without eating it, the in-session exposure has become just one more episode of avoidance. Even if a difficult situation is handled well by the client in every other way (e.g., a woman with a fear of eating in public simulates a dinner date with an attractive man; the conversation goes well and he is responsive) but the client does not eat, this success will be discounted, trivialized, and quickly forgotten. Thus goal setting (see Chapter 12) becomes a very important activity for in-session exposures with eating phobics. The client will typically agree to take a predetermined number of bites of food but may need to be prompted repeatedly by the therapists lest he or she "forget."

Drinking phobics are similar in most respects to eating phobics. There is somewhat less variability introduced by the specific beverage, although beverages that may stain (e.g., red wines) are generally more anxiety provoking. One situation that we have utilized with clients with fears of drinking in public is the "wine-tasting party." The target client and two to three other clients "attend" a party in which the activity is taste testing several varieties of "wine" (actually any beverage will do). Another person plays the role of the expert who presents the wines. The situation requires repeated drinking behavior and can easily be modified so that clients purposefully spill drinks or fill their glasses to the brim to increase the chances of spilling. Many times, this exposure has been extremely powerful to the target client and highly involving for the other group members.

Serving drinks to others is a major source of distress for many of these clients, especially if the client pours from a pitcher into a glass held by the other person. A female client who was married to a business executive had for many years avoided having cocktail parties for her husband's business associates, despite rather considerable pressure from her husband to do so. She was extremely afraid that her hand would shake whenever she served drinks and that this clear demonstration of incompetence would reflect badly on her husband and his career. An in-session exposure was designed in which she was to host a cocktail party and move around the room, repeatedly pouring drinks (of water) to each of the seven guests (two therapists, five other group members). As a way of showing the intensity of her fear and how the best-laid plans of cognitive-behavioral therapists can go awry, the outcome of the in-session exposure is worth considering. The client poured a large number of drinks without incident. There were no major spills. In fact, there were few minor spills, save a single drop that went astray on a single occasion. During the postprocessing of the in-session exposure, the client reported that she was pleased with her performance. That evening she attempted to kill herself! She later reported that the "spill" confirmed her belief that she was incompetent. Although the attempt was not successful, it clearly taught us to consider the importance of every last drop! It also taught us the importance of cognitive restructuring *after* the in-session exposure (see Chapter 12).

Working/Playing While Being Observed

Fears of working or playing while being observed by others are extremely common. Earlier, we described the examples of the secretary whose boss watched her type and the student nurse who became anxious and froze when her supervisor was watching. Consider also the cashier who becomes anxious and cannot make change correctly while the customer is standing and waiting. We have also seen several clients who reported that they became anxious playing tennis, bowling, or shooting pool, simply from the knowledge that someone may be walking by and *may be* watching. Playing team sports may also be quite anxiety provoking, and the social costs of fielding errors, turnovers, or missed shots perceived to be very high.

These situations are not always easy to turn into in-session exposures. At the least, they require additional props. Paradoxically, some may be easier to arrange as *in vivo* exposures. However, if the key theme is being the center of attention, as it so often is, any activity that is performed under the close observation of others may serve as a reasonable substitute.

Assertion and Interaction with Authority Figures

Assertion and authority situations are frequent foci of in-session exposures. Frequent topics of in-session exposures from recent groups include:.

- Having a casual conversation with a boss or supervisor.
- Asking for and justifying a raise in salary.
- Asking others for favors or assistance.
- Refusing unreasonable requests.
- Turning down unwanted sexual advances.
- Making a mistake and having to talk to the boss about it.
- Receiving an annual evaluation from a boss or supervisor.
- Responding to unfair criticism from a boss or supervisor.
- Giving constructive criticism to others.
- Offering an opinion that is contrary to that held by a superior.

Job Interviews

Job interviews are difficult for many people. However, they are frequent events for clients with social phobia, as their anxiety may have led to disrupted employment. Almost every CBGT group will include at least one client who has concerns about interview performance. Job interviews put us in a position to prove our competence to others, a difficult position if you doubt your own competence, feel ashamed about your spotty employment history, or are concerned that your anxiety will show and leave a terminally bad impression.

In-Session Exposures for Specific Brief Behaviors

The in-session exposures described here were designed with the goal of putting the client in (an approximation of) the situation he or she fears. However, there are instances in which a relatively true approximation of the target situation may not contain the necessary therapeutic ingredients (or, at least, the right ingredients in the right doses). This is most often the case for situations that transpire quickly. Greetings, responses to questions, and check signings may take very little time. The client's anxiety may have gone up, but it would almost certainly have failed to come down before the situation ended. In these and similar cases, it is not in the client's best interest to replicate the situation closely. Rather, it is preferable to sacrifice a bit of the representativeness of the in-session exposure and require the client to perform the feared response repeatedly. This has been our standard practice with clients who fear writing in public. Rather than simulate a situation in which a single signature is required, the client is typically asked to perform a simple task repeatedly (e.g., sign 25 checks) or engage in a complex writing task (e.g., complete a long and detailed medical history or insurance application) while being observed by others.

A similar approach may be taken when a client fears specific interactional behaviors. If a specific, time-limited behavior or event is feared by the client, it may be performed repeatedly. Unlike public writing, however, the arrangements for these in-session exposures may sometimes be complex. In the remainder of this section, we describe examples of in-session exposures we have utilized to help clients overcome their fears of these specific behaviors.

Joining Ongoing Conversations

Many clients with social phobia fear breaking into ongoing conversations. They may fear that they will be viewed as intruders, that they won't be able to think of anything to say in the first few awkward seconds, or that they will somehow look stupid to the other people. However, many of these same clients do not fear continuing the conversation once it has begun (at least not to the same degree). For these clients, an in-session exposure that involves breaking into a conversation and then continuing to talk for several minutes might lose its anxiety-evoking potential after a very brief time, and the remainder of the exposure might be less relevant to the client's concerns. The task at hand is to design an in-session exposure that keeps the client focused on the act of joining ongoing conversations. Our solution has been to simulate a party setting. One therapist, the other group members, and additional persons recruited from outside the group (if possible) divide into dyads and stand around the room talking to each other. The target client is instructed to approach the nearest dyad and join in their conversation. One minute later, the second therapist prompts the client to leave that dyad and approach the next one. After another minute, he or she goes onto the next dyad, and so forth. In this manner, the target client is exposed to the feared action of joining an ongoing conversation 10 times in a 10-minute period, not just once. This exercise can easily be adapted to fear of serving drinks to others, as noted in the previous example.

Giving and Receiving Compliments

Compliments are another class of feared events that happen quickly. Clients with social phobia often have great difficulty giving compliments to themselves or others and may feel extremely uncomfortable receiving compliments from others. However, it seems stilted and artificial to require the client to engage a person in conversation and then hit them with (or be hit with) a barrage of compliments and praise. Thankfully, it is not necessary to do so, as the following procedure may work quite effectively. The therapists and other group members are seated around the room. The target client stands in front of one of the others and gives himself or herself a compliment. The other person agrees with the compliment and then expands on it ("Yes, you do have good taste in clothes. I very much like your blouse"). The target client then moves to the next person, and the procedure is repeated with each person in the room.

A few additional points should be made about this exercise. First, it is our clinical impression that the difficulty in receiving compliments is a consequence of the person's inability to see positive characteristics in himself or herself. Thus self-praise and receiving compliments may be logically linked together in the same exercise. Second, it is typically necessary to instruct the target client not to give himself or herself a compliment and then disqualify it (e.g., "I'm a good housekeeper, but then my house is so small anyone could keep up with it"). Our standard practice is to prohibit the client from (1) using the word *but* during this exercise and (2) saying anything other than "thank you" in response to the compliment from the other person. This exercise may be easily modified to focus on giving compliments to others. As the client approaches each person, he or she simply makes a complimentary statement about him or her, the other person thanks the client, and the client moves on. In both variations, the client is exposed to a high frequency of feared events in a brief period of time.

Making Mistakes in Front of Others

Most clients fear that they will appear awkward, incompetent, and imperfect in front of others. Thus they may require exposure to situations in which mistakes or obviously imperfect performances are likely. However, in our experience, some clients resist suggestions to make intentional mistakes during in-session exposures and homework assignments and have difficulty accepting the notion that making mistakes might not lead to catastrophic consequences. Others discount mistakes made in in-session exposures as trivial but remain afraid to do the same thing in real life. One solution is to create a situation in which mistakes are so likely to be made that the humor and futility of the situation become apparent. We have used the Stroop (1935) color-naming task as the stimulus for this situation. As we described in Chapter 4, the Stroop task requires the person to view words (color names) and, rather than reading the words, to report the colors in which they are printed (in this case, on poster board). The interference between the highly overlearned (but incorrect) response of reading the color name and the unusual (but correct) response of reporting the ink color virtually assures that a high frequency of mistakes will be made, and the client will easily be confronted with thoughts about looking foolish or incompetent in front of others. When the target client is asked to perform this task in front of the rest of the group, he or she will stammer, stumble over his or her words, and make a number of incorrect responses that are not being made intentionally. This exercise often has great emotional impact.

Revealing Personal Information

Not surprisingly, clients with social phobia are unlikely to feel comfortable talking about themselves, a task that puts them at the center of others' attention. This discomfort may rise exponentially when the person is called on to reveal private aspects of himself or herself and may increase further if the information disclosed is perceived as negative. Thus treatment of fears relating to disclosure of personal information requires a graduated approach, in which the client first reveals basic factual (e.g., demographic) information, then speaks about increasingly more personal topics over the course of time. This approach may be carried over the course of several successive in-session exposures, with each exposure involving a conversation with another person about increasingly personal topics. However, it is also possible to work with these issues in the context of a single in-session exposure. In one of our groups, we created a multistage in-session exposure that was designed to elicit increasing levels of self-disclosure from a male client who believed that no one would like him if they discovered what he was "really" like. As a result of this fear, the client avoided talking about any substantive personal topics. An in-session exposure was designed in which the client was asked to address the group for 3 minutes about his superficial characteristics (age, gender, physical appearance). In the next 3 minutes, he was instructed to talk about his typical daily activities. He then spent 3 minutes talking about his personal goals and dreams, including his own negative characteristics that he would like to work on changing. In other variations, clients could be asked to talk for specified times about positive characteristics, negative characteristics, or secrets they feel ashamed about. Cognitive restructuring efforts that were a part of this in-session exposure are described in Chapter 12.

Expressing Opinions

Clients with social phobia almost universally hesitate to offer opinions that might be perceived as contrary to the norm or to those of persons they perceive as important. In-session exposures on this topic may take several forms, including conversations about a specific topic in which the client is given the assignment to voice an opinion. A second person may be instructed to either agree with the client, disagree cordially, or disagree in a manner critical of the client. In addition, we have found it useful to engage the client in a public-speaking situation in which he or she is asked to present his or her opinion on a controversial issue and the reasoning behind that opinion. Topics have been selected from the important issues of the day and have included abortion, the death penalty, gun control, religious freedom, and environmental conservation. These in-session exposures require the client to express a potentially unpopular point of view in front of others and to do so much more strongly than he or she might in conversational settings. The client's presentation may be followed by a question and answer period in which the client is required to defend his or her point of view. Clients are deprived of the avoidance strategy of soft-pedaling their opinions, and, as a result, the anxiety-evoking potential of the in-session exposure is increased. The anxiety-evoking potential can be further increased by asking the target client to endorse the point of view *opposite* to his or her actual opinion (an interesting application of this concept is to ask a client who does not appear to embrace the logic of CBGT to give a presentation about how it works and why). We have also modified this in-session exposure to take the form of a formal debate between two clients with fears of expressing their opinions.

Fears of Being Trapped in a Social Situation

Some clients experience increasing fear when in a formal situation such as a meeting or dinner party. They have expressed the fear that they may need to leave the room (because their anxiety will become intolerable or simply because they need to use the facilities) and that they will become the center of others' attention if they get up to leave. Thoughts related to this theme come to occupy their attention and may contribute to a steady rise in anxiety. These clients require repeated exposure to the sequence of getting up, leaving, and returning to the setting.

The client with the fear of leaving or returning is first taken through the steps of preparation for his or her in-session exposure and the necessary cognitive restructuring activities (see Chapter 12). He or she is then assigned the task of getting up and leaving the room at 2- to 3-minute intervals and returning after an absence of 30 seconds. The client will repeat this sequence several times while the next client prepares for and goes through his or her own in-session exposure. On each return, the first client may take a seat next to one of the therapists (the one least involved in the next in-session exposure) and quietly provide a SUDS rating to that therapist. After the next client has finished processing his or her own effort, the client may stop leaving and returning and process his or her own experience.

Fears of Being in the Group

Several clients have reported that they become anxious simply being in group situations, even when they know there will be no demand made on them to perform or interact with anyone. These fears usually revolve around an inaccurate prediction that they will be the center of others' attention. In-session exposures for this fear have taken two forms. First, when another client is doing an in-session exposure for a public-speaking fear, this client may be seated facing the speaker but in front of the other members of the audience. He or she may be given writing materials and may record his or her own SUDS rating when the speaker is prompted to do so (SUDS ratings during exposures were described earlier).

Second, a client may report that the experience of sitting in the therapy

group is in itself a focus of extreme anxiety. If this is the case, it may be necessary to confront this anxiety before other anxieties can be effectively dealt with.
Most clients will be sufficiently desensitized during the structured exercises conducted in the first two sessions. For others, however, this fear becomes the focus
of their first in-session exposure. This client is guided through all the necessary
preliminary activities, but the in-session exposure simply involves sitting in the
room while the group shifts its attention to another client. As described for the
client with fears of leaving the room, the client processes his or her attempts to
use cognitive coping skills to control anxiety about sitting in the room after the
next client has finished.

12

Integrating Cognitive Restructuring Procedures with In-Session Exposures

In the two decades since we started to treat clients with social phobia, the cognitive restructuring procedures have undergone continuous revision, more so than any other component of CBGT. In their current form, cognitive restructuring procedures follow a specific sequence, but there is a great deal of latitude for therapists to design specific interventions for individual clients.

Cognitive restructuring activities take place before and after each in-session exposure, and the target client is required to use cognitive skills during exposures as well. The specific procedures are described in detail in the next several sections.

Before an In-Session Exposure

The goals of cognitive restructuring activities prior to in-session exposures in CBGT are for the client to question his or her thoughts, to develop alternative ways of viewing the situation, and to develop an approach to coping with negative thinking in the in-session exposure. Cognitive restructuring prior to an in-session exposure follows a series of steps, which are outlined in the upper portion of Figure 12.1. These steps are elaborated in the sections to follow.

Identification of Automatic Thoughts in a Selected Situation

After a situation has been selected to be the focus of an in-session exposure and its specific characteristics have been agreed on, the target client is asked to imag-

---

Before the In-Session Exposure Begins

1. Review target situation.
2. Identify automatic thoughts.
3. Identify thinking errors in automatic thoughts.
4. Question and dispute thinking errors in automatic thoughts.
5. Develop rational response(s) to selected automatic thought(s).
6. Obtain ratings of the degree of belief in automatic thought(s) and rational response(s).
7. Set appropriate goal(s) for performance in the in-session exposure.

During the In-Session Exposure

1 Repeat rational response(s) and provide SUDS ratings at 1-minute intervals.
2. Use disputing questions and rational responses as automatic thoughts occur.
3. Maintain focus on agreed-on goals for in-session exposure.

After the In-Session Exposure Concludes

1. Review goal(s) and determine goal attainment.
2. Review occurrence of targeted automatic thought(s).
3. Review use of rational responses and other cognitive coping attempts.
4. Review evidence in support of automatic thoughts versus rational responses.
5. Query occurrence of other automatic thoughts and client's attempts to cope with them.
6. Examine SUDS ratings and their relationship to automatic thoughts and rational responses.
7. Obtain postexposure ratings of the degree of belief in automatic thought(s) and rational response(s).
8. Ask client to summarize the main points he or she has drawn from the in-session exposure and cognitive restructuring activities.

FIGURE 12.1. Cognitive restructuring activities before, during, and after in-session exposures.

ine himself or herself in the situation (or in anticipation of it). He or she may be asked to visualize the situation in all of its detail and to report to the therapists and group members the thoughts that occur to him or her. The client is encouraged to give a complete reporting of experienced thoughts and to do so without any attempt to edit their content. Therapists may facilitate thought recall by prompting the clients with such questions as:

- "What went through your mind when . . . ?"
- "And what thoughts occurred to you next?"
- "Did you have any more thoughts about . . . ?"
- "What was your cognitive reaction to . . . ?"
- "Did you have any images about . . . ?"

Therapists should not assume that clients will provide a complete listing of ATs or even that they will spontaneously offer the thoughts that represent their greatest concerns. Clients may not be completely aware of their automatic thoughts, may not have fully articulated them, or may have experienced them as images rather than words. They may consider their automatic thoughts to be sources of embarrassment. They may be hesitant to report automatic thoughts because, "They'll really think there is something wrong with me if they know I think. . . . "

Because any negative reaction may inhibit clients' attempts to disclose ATs that they view as stupid, silly, or shameful, therapists must strike a nonjudgmental pose about the content of ATs.

As one therapist sits with the group and facilitates the client's recall of automatic thoughts, the other therapist stands by the easel and records them for all to see. However, especially in the early sessions, the client is unlikely to report thoughts in a manner that will be most productive for work. Thoughts may be reported as questions rather than statements, two or more thoughts may be run together, or the client's statement may simply be unclear.

The recorder should edit the client's reported thoughts and (nonjudgmentally) record them in a manner that is true to the client's meaning, but clear, concise, and to the point. "Maybe I was thinking that they might not think much of me" may be best summarized as "They won't like me." "What if I can't do it?" may be edited to "I won't be able to do it." Edits are intended to bring out the emotional impact of the AT and to facilitate working with it, but any changes should always be agreed on with the client.

Although the client should be encouraged to give as complete a listing of ATs as possible, it is not necessary to press too hard for this. **Two or three automatic thoughts that have relevance to the client will provide more than enough data for productive work.** However, it is important that automatic thoughts be reported in sufficient detail. Automatic thoughts result in anxiety because the client assumes that they are true and that certain negative consequences inevitably follow from them. However, the connection between the thought and the consequence may be so self-evident to the client that he or she may not spontaneously report it. Therefore, **after a list of ATs has been collected, therapists should question the client about the meaning of these thoughts**. The importance of this strategy is evident in the case of the woman described in Chapter 10 who reported extreme anxiety when interacting with men she found attractive and who avoided these situations whenever she could (see section on "Ca-tastrophizing"). She reported, "He'll be able to tell I'm nervous" as her first and foremost automatic thought and shared it with the group with considerable distress. *But why was that thought so distressing? It was distressing because it had a variety of very negative meanings to the client.* First, she would be nervous. Second, the man would detect her nervousness. These meanings are obvious in the way she reported her AT. The beginning therapist will often stop there, but it is important to ask why it matters if she is nervous and he knows it. The answer is that his knowledge of her nervousness will lead to further negative consequences:

She will be nervous →
    he will know →
        he will think badly of her →
            he will not want to be around her →
                neither will anyone else →
                    she will always be alone.

Gentle but persistent questioning of the content of ATs helps the therapists understand why the client is so mortally afraid of everyday situations and to be better prepared for later efforts to dispute their meaning. After the list of ATs is judged to be sufficiently complete, it may be useful for the therapists to review them, doing so in a logical order that ties the various ATs into an integrated whole (as much as possible) and suggesting thoughts that may have been omitted by the client. Early in treatment, it may also be useful to comment, "Who wouldn't be anxious with these thoughts running through their head?"

Identification of Thinking Errors in Recalled Thoughts

The List of Thinking Errors (Figure 10.1) should be presented to the target client, and he or she should be asked to identify the thinking errors present in each one of his or her automatic thoughts as recorded on the easel. To increase the depth of the client's understanding of thinking errors, *he or she should be encouraged to go beyond simply naming the thinking error in each automatic thought and to provide the specific reason why the thought is problematic.* Because any AT may contain several thinking errors, it is not necessary for the client to provide a comprehensive list, just a sampling that will help him or her develop an understanding of his or her own cognitive habits. It is also important for the therapists to avoid forcing the client to adopt their specific interpretation of an AT.

Why is it important for the client to identify the distortions in his or her ATs? Identification of thinking errors (or of the maladaptiveness of specific thoughts) helps the client to move away from the amorphous experience of negative affect and streams of ATs toward the task of questioning specific thoughts and developing rational coping responses. It does so by providing a structure within which the client can effectively operate. The many automatic thoughts are reduced to a few thinking errors, and the client can develop questioning routines that are specific to his or her own "preferred" errors.

The Process of Disputation of Automatic Thoughts and Development of Rational Responses

After identifying thinking errors, the client attempts to develop rational responses to specific automatic thoughts, using the List of Disputing Questions (Figure 10.3) and additional questioning by therapists and group members. In this section, we present some common automatic thoughts and dialogues between therapist(s) and client(s) that demonstrate tactics for disputing these thoughts and developing rational responses clients may use to cope with them.

The examples that follow demonstrate the primary tasks involved in disputation of automatic thoughts. An important point, especially for the beginning cognitive-behavioral therapist, is that the process of disputing automatic thoughts and developing rational responses is exactly that—a process. It is the rare case in which the therapist can pose a single question like those listed in Figure 10.3 and watch the client quickly produce a useful rational response. **The process of disputation is a continuous interchange in which the therapist(s) gradually leads the client in the direction of a useful rational response.** The therapist's goal is to continuously question the client's statements and gently suggest alternatives to automatic thoughts and thus to bring him or her around to consideration of a more adaptive viewpoint. The specific strategies that may be used are unlimited, although any strategy should allow the client to struggle with the issues and come up with alternatives himself or herself.

The rational responses that are generated at the end of these dialogues are intended to serve as personally meaningful self-instructions for clients to use during in-session exposures. The process of generating rational responses is demonstrated in these dialogues and was described in Chapter 10. Although the rational responses may sound a bit like slogans, they can be extremely meaningful to clients and may serve multiple functions during times of anxiety. To reprise some of the major points from Chapter 10, rational responses:

- Focus the client on a positive, coping message.
- Alert the client that he or she should engage in active cognitive coping.
- Alert the client that he or she is engaged in a negative internal dialogue that he or she should stop.

- Distract the client from negative thinking or physiological arousal and thus serve to break into an escalating pattern of focusing on the negative.

An effective rational response should have several characteristics:

- Its content is specifically relevant to the situation at hand.
- It is realistic.
- It has some degree of plausibility to the client.
- It is stated in the client's own words.
- It is brief, easy to remember, and efficient to use.

It is not important that the client accept the rational response as totally true and reject the automatic thought as totally false, only that the client endorse the possibility that the rational response might be accurate and helpful.

Before we present examples, consider the context. The client has generated a number of automatic thoughts about the situation that will soon be the focus of an in-session exposure and has attempted, with the group's help, to identify thinking errors that characterize these thoughts. The client knows that he or she will soon be expected to "perform" and may be quite anxious. If so, his or her ability to focus attention may be compromised, and his or her belief in the automatic thoughts may be heightened. Anxiety may increase as time passes, because the client is likely to become more and more concerned about the upcoming in-session exposure.

Therapists must attempt to balance two simultaneously present but contradictory goals—to help the client examine his or her automatic thoughts in sufficient detail to be useful and to help the client keep his or her anxiety in check by keeping this portion of the procedure as brief as possible. **Consistent use of brief focused questions is probably the best therapeutic approach.** These will help the client remain attentive to the task at hand but not overburden his or her response capacities during a time of potentially high anxiety. If the therapists do too much talking, the client will tune them out. If they ask questions that are too general, the client's responses will miss the mark, and the dialogue may become tangential.

It is also important to exercise care in the selection of automatic thoughts for attention. Not all automatic thoughts are created equal! Some automatic thoughts are too closely held by the client, and he or she may not be a willing participant in attempts to change them. In terms of cognitive-behavioral theory, some thoughts are central to a person's self-schema. If a specific belief forms the "bed-rock" of the person's cognitive structure, there are likely to be too many other re-lated beliefs supporting it, and change in that belief is unlikely to occur early in treatment.

Early in treatment, it is better to select an automatic thought that is some-what peripheral to the hypothesized cognitive structure, as it will be less closely held by the client and less supported by other parts of the client's belief system. Change in this and related automatic thoughts then serves to undermine the support structure of the more central beliefs, and they may come tumbling down!

An example of this situation is the client described later in this chapter who feared that other people would see his anxiety in public-speaking situations, that they would judge him negatively, and that his career would suffer as a result. He originally presented several ATs to his group, thoughts that concerned his ner-vousness, others' perception of it, their negative judgments, and the short- and long-term consequences of their judgments. In cognitive restructuring, we could start at the beginning and question his prediction that he would be nervous the next time he had to speak. However, this strategy would be quite unproductive. The client's belief that he would be anxious was simply too strong. He was cer-tain of its accuracy, and there was little room for movement. Clients are unlikely to be as convinced of the consequences of their nervousness as they are about be-ing nervous in the first place (because anxiety in social situations is often part of their basic self-definition). As a result, we focused on whether other people could see his anxiety, whether they would judge him so negatively, and so forth. Under-mining these thoughts chips away at the structure that supports more central be-liefs about the self. As this client learned to be less concerned about the conse-quences of his anxiety, he had less to be anxious about!

It is not necessary that the client emerge from cognitive restructuring firmly believing the rational response. In fact, this is very unlikely. All that is necessary is for the client to keep an open mind, to consider the viability of the rational response, and to be willing to evaluate it in light of what transpires in the in-session exposure. Therapists should *never* argue with clients that the rational response is the right re-sponse. The use of belief ratings in this context is discussed later in this chapter.

"I WON'T BE ABLE TO THINK OF ANYTHING TO SAY."

This automatic thought is extremely common in anticipation of social interac-tions, especially when the situation calls for making small talk with an unfamiliar person. It may be even more strongly endorsed when the person is a potential romantic interest. It is often associated with the (mistaken) notions that the superficial topics common to casual conversation are unacceptable or that the client needs to come up with truly elegant conversation topics in order to be accepted, to avoid boring the other person, and so forth. Thus the client may think of a number of things to talk about but quickly disqualify them.

Consider the single male client who must attend various social events in order to meet women. In disputing this AT, the client may be asked, "What evidence do you have that you won't be able to think of anything to say?" and the following dialogue might ensue:

CLIENT (C): I never can. My mind is always a blank.

THERAPIST (T): I question whether you can *never* think of anything to say, although it may often seem that way. Are there times when you *can* think of things to say?

C: Well, it's not too bad when I talk to people I know pretty well.

T: So at least with those people, you can think of things to say. What kinds of things do you talk about with the people you know pretty well?

C: Oh, I don't know, the weather, the news, sports, whatever's going on with them.

T: Could you talk about these things with a woman you meet at a party?

C: No! She'd think I was so superficial!

T: Group, what do you think about what C is saying here?

SECOND CLIENT (C2): What else can he talk about? He just met her. They have to talk about superficial things.

THIRD CLIENT (C3): Yeah, it's too quick to talk about anything important.

T: C, what do you think? They seem to be telling you that these superficial things are the very things you "should" be talking about.

C: I guess I can talk about more important things when I get to know her a bit, huh?

T: Sounds good to me. Now can we put this together into a rational response that you can use to help yourself? What is the most important point to come out of this discussion?

C: Well, I guess the point is it's all right to talk about mundane things. How's that?

T: Do you think you can use that as a rational response in your in-session exposure?

C: Yeah. (*T records rational response on easel for use in the ensuing exposure exercise.*)

Another approach to the automatic thought, "I won't be able to think of anything to say," is to attack other thoughts associated with it. A common concern is that there will be long silences in the conversation and that the client will not be able to break a silence once it has begun. Clients may be helped to question the frequency with which silences of more than a few seconds actually occur, and this can be measured during in-session exposures. When silences do occur, they may be asked to estimate the length of time the silences last. Clients will routinely overestimate the length of silences, and this probably has much to do with why silences appear so frightening. Additionally, clients who are concerned about silences seem to view conversations as a one-sided affair. They think that conversations exist so that the other person can judge them. There is often little concept that conversations exist so that two people can get to know each other a bit and make *mutual* judgments or that both parties in a conversation have equal responsibility for keeping up their end. Consider the following interchange between a therapist and a client who would soon go to a make-believe cocktail party as part of an in-session exposure. His assignment in the in-session exposure was to make conversation with a woman he knew from work.

T: C, you listed "I won't be able to think of anything to say" as one of your automatic thoughts for this situation. Tell us about it.

C: It'll be awful!

T: Specifics, please. What do you think will happen?

C: I won't be able to come up with anything, I'll just go blank, there won't be any conversation. We'll just stand there and stare at each other. She'll think I'm from another planet!

T: You know there are lots of silences that occur in every conversation, right?

C: Yeah, but once these are started. . . .

T: How long do you think a silence like this would last?

C: (*stated with great certainty*) Oh, maybe 3 minutes.

T: (*ignoring the behavioral improbability of a 3-minute silence*) Do you think any 3-minute silences would occur during the in-session exposure?

C: Yes.

T: If the in-session exposure lasts 15 minutes, how many 3-minute silences would there be?

C: 2 or 3.

T: OK, you are making a hypothesis that there will be two or three 3-minute silences during your in-session exposure. Let's be scientists and check it out during the in-session exposure. But before we get to that, let's talk about something else. Why do silences happen?

C: Because nobody talks. What are you getting at?

T: Right, because nobody talks. How many people are there?

C: Two, me and her.

T: Right, again. How many people have to be quiet at the same time for there to be a major silence?

C: Two ... oh, I get you. She has to be silent, too, not just me.

T: Yes, she has to be silent, too. Does she have as much responsibility as you to keep the conversation going, or is it all on your shoulders?

This line of questioning is based on a rather egalitarian view. It can be argued that if you initiate a conversation with another person, its maintenance is more than half your responsibility. However, because the client is likely to be engaging in all-or-nothing thinking and assuming that he has 100% responsibility, there is plenty of "wiggle room." Even if the client were to decide that a 70–30 split is most appropriate, he would probably experience a degree of relief.

C: She has just as much responsibility as me.

T: So if there's a silence ... ?

C: It's not all my fault!

T: You got it! One more thing. Why do you think she might be silent?

C: Well, she might be shy herself or maybe she's uncomfortable at these awful cocktail parties.

If the concept that the other person might be anxious had been brought up earlier in the dialogue, it is likely that the client would have been more contrary. At this point, however, he was excited about what he had learned in the previous few minutes and thinking quite positively. Extremely schema-incongruent ideas (e.g., part of the problem may belong to someone other than the client) are best brought up later in the discussion, after a client has already demonstrated acceptance of other less central concepts.

T: What can we pull together here that you can use as a rational response?

C: Well, you seem to think that silences won't happen as much as I do. Anyway, if they do, it's as much her responsibility as mine. I don't have to carry all the weight or all the guilt! (*T summarizes and records rational response on easel.*)

"I'LL MESS UP."

A related automatic thought is that the client will fail to perform well enough to achieve whatever goal is at hand. This may occur in social interaction, as in the previous examples, or in any number of other situations that are more explicitly evaluative, such as making presentations or being interviewed for a job. In one of our groups, a male client who was dissatisfied with his current job had avoided trying to get a new one because he believed he could not interview well enough to be hired. Before an in-session exposure on this theme, the client reported the following automatic thoughts: "I'll mess up the interview"; "I'll get flustered"; "I'll make a fool of myself"; "I won't get hired"; and "Unless I do it perfectly, I won't get the job." All of these automatic thoughts are examples of fortune telling. The following dialogue demonstrates how these thoughts were addressed:

T: C, let's focus on two of the automatic thoughts you report, "I'll mess up the interview" and "Unless I do it perfectly, I won't get the job." What do you mean when you say "mess up the interview"?

C: I'll mess it up. I'll be so nervous, I won't be able to express myself. I won't be able to answer questions or ask any, either.

T: What evidence do you have to support that?

C: I know I'll be nervous.

T: But does being nervous mean you won't be able to answer or ask questions? Is it possible that you could do so even if you are nervous?

Note that the therapists must always select an aspect of an AT for attention. In this circumstance, T focused on the consequences of C's anxiety and chooses not to question whether C will be anxious or whether C views the experience of anxiety in all-or-nothing terms.

C: I guess I could, but I won't come off well.

T: What do you mean?

C: The interviewer will see that I'm nervous and think something is wrong with me. [See the next section for a more detailed intervention strategy for this type of automatic thought.]

T: Aren't people often nervous in job interviews? Wouldn't the interviewer expect you to be nervous?

Again the therapist purposefully does not engage the discussion of just how nervous the client might be, as that might contribute to the client's catastrophic thinking.

C: I suppose.

T: So the question here is really whether or not you can say at least some of the things you want to while you are nervous.

C: Yeah.

T: You believe you are qualified for this job, don't you?

C: No question, I can do the job if I can get it.

T: You have all the required skills and experience?

C: And then some.

T: You'll spend time before the interview preparing your case, won't you, just like we asked you to do for tonight's exposure?

C: Yes.

T: If you are prepared, will you be able to make most of your points?

C: Yes, I suppose I will.

T: Well, you'll have a chance to test that in the exposure. What if you can't get to all the points you want to make?

C: I suppose I'll be able to make enough of them.

T: Good! You know you just disputed that last automatic thought, that you'll have to do it perfectly to get the job.

C: I guess I did.

T: Can you pull this all together into a rational response or two?

C: How about "If I prepare, I'll be able to make my points" or "I don't have to be perfect to be hired"?

T: Those are two very fine rational responses. Let's also keep in mind that this is only your first interview. What happens if you don't get this job despite all your efforts?

C: I guess I can try for another.

T: Right. And isn't that another rational response you can use? "This is only one job." (*Records rational responses on easel. After further discussion, the cli-*

ent selected "I don't have to be perfect to be hired" as the one rational response on which he would focus in the upcoming in-session exposure.)

"MY ANXIETY WILL SHOW AND PEOPLE WILL JUDGE ME NEGATIVELY": THE PIE CHART TECHNIQUE

This is probably the most common set of ATs presented to us by our clients. Thus we have attempted several strategies to deal with them. In this section, we present a disputational strategy we call the "Pie Chart Technique." Pie charts, just like the ones our teachers used in elementary school, can be powerful tools for cognitive restructuring. Here we describe the use of a pie chart as part of an intervention with a client who feared his anxiety would be visible to others in a public-speaking situation.

The client had to give a presentation to an audience of 10 to 15 people at his workplace. This situation served as the basis for his in-session exposure, and he reported a series of automatic thoughts, including the following:

"I will be anxious."
"My voice will quiver."
"My hands will shake."
"Others will see my anxiety."
"They will think there is something wrong with me."
"They won't take me seriously."
"I won't get ahead in my career because of it."

We conceded that the client would be anxious. Although he was engaging in all-or-nothing thinking, the client was unlikely to accept the proposition that he might have been less than totally overwhelmed with anxiety. Instead, we engaged him in the following dialogue as a means of disputing a number of his ATs:

T: Let's consider for a moment that you give this presentation a number of times, enough so that one hundred persons might be able to see it, OK?

C: Uh, yes. (*Shudders at the prospect.*)

T: Well, I'm going to draw a circle on the easel. (*Draws circle.*) This circle represents those one hundred people. Now, you are going to give your talk. What happens?

C: I'll be really anxious, my hands will shake, my voice will quiver. It'll be horrible. Everyone will see.

T: Let's accept for now that you will be anxious. That may not always be the case, but we'll assume it's true this time. You will be anxious, your hands will shake, and your voice will quiver. Of the one hundred people, how many people will notice?

Now we begin the actual intervention. The main goal of this exercise is to undermine the client's idea that *everyone* will detect his anxiety and that they will *all* draw negative conclusions. The main strategy is to question at every possible point whether there are any persons who might react differently, thereby reducing each time the percentage of persons who will ultimately draw the feared conclusion.

C: Everybody will.

T: Let's not be so sure. Can you think of any reasons why someone might not notice your anxiety? Group members, can you help us out here?

When constructing a pie chart, it is very important to involve the other group members to the greatest extent possible. They will join in, contributing additional reasons why the feared consequence is less likely than C believes. Each alternative that is generated by the group is put to C, who must then respond with the number of persons out of 100 who will react in a particular manner. Because of the social demand inherent in this situation, C is unlikely to offer the response of 0% to any query. Therefore, the more alternatives (and the more involvement of group members), the better.

C: Well . . .

T: What are some possible reasons that someone might not notice your anxiety?

C2: How about . . . they might not be paying attention?

T: Good! Why might they not be paying attention?

C3: They might be daydreaming. They might be tired because they were up too late the night before.

C2: They might hate their job so they don't pay attention.

C: They might be talking to the person they are sitting next to rather than paying attention.

T: Good and good again! So there are a lot of reasons why they might not be paying much attention to you, right?

C: (*hesitantly*) Right.

T: OK, now let's go back and review all these reasons why they might not be paying attention to you. First, they might be daydreaming. Out of one hundred people, how many daydreamers might there be?

C: Oh, maybe five.

The therapists accept whatever C offers. It is not important that C be accurate in his estimates, only that he acknowledge that there are some people who might not be paying attention for some of the reasons.

T: OK, five people might have been daydreaming and fail to detect your anxiety because of it. (*Turns back to the easel.*) I'm going to cross out a sliver of this "pie," OK? (*Does so. Marks out a portion of the circle roughly equal to 5/100 of the total area of the circle.*) It represents the people we don't have to worry about! Now, how many people might be tired because they were up too late the night before?

C: Oh, I don't know. Maybe two or three.

C3: I don't know where you work, but my office is a bunch of party animals. They're always nodding off in meetings!

C: OK, maybe four or five.

T: Let's be conservative and say four. (*Marks off another 4%.*) Now, how many people might not be paying attention because they are talking to the person they are sitting next to?

C: Oh, I guess there would be some of those. Maybe a half dozen or so.

T: Six more people. (*Marks off another 6%.*) How many people would just not listen because they don't like their jobs and don't want to be there?

C: Well, I do work for the state, and there's a lot of dead wood. Another five?

T: OK, another five. Let's see that's five + four + six + five. That adds up to twenty people out of one hundred who wouldn't notice your anxiety because they weren't paying attention. Well, you seem to have disproved the idea that *everybody* would notice your anxiety and cause you a problem! Let me add another question. Is it possible that someone could be paying attention and still not notice your anxiety?

C: No, how could they miss it?

T: I know what you're saying, but I've been a therapist for a long time, and I tell you people are *lousy* observers of other people's behavior. Has it ever happened to you that you're feeling a certain way, say angry or frustrated, and other people didn't seem to have a clue?

C2: Yeah, I know what you mean. My wife says she knows me pretty well but she never knows when I'm upset.

C3: And my husband never knows when I feel stressed out from work.

T: And those are people who know you well. What about other people, co-workers or casual acquaintances, who don't know you so well? Would they always be able to tell when you are anxious?

C: I get your point. I guess not. So maybe ten people wouldn't notice even if they were looking!

T: (*Marks off another 10%.*) Now we're down to seventy. Let's ask another question. Seventy people might be paying attention and notice that your hands are shaking and your voice quivers. Do you believe that all seventy of these people would think badly of you?

C: Yes.

T: So you believe everyone who would notice your anxiety symptoms would come to a negative conclusion. OK, group, what are some things that people might think if they saw that C's hands shook and his voice quivered when he gave his presentation?

C2: They might think he wasn't feeling well. Maybe he was sick or something.

T: They could think that, you're right. If they did think that, would they think badly of him?

C2: No, they'd probably just hope he felt better soon and think he was pretty cool for talking when he doesn't feel well.

T: What else could they think?

C3: They might think he had too much coffee to drink.

T: True, anything else?

C: They might think I was nervous!

T: True again, but would they have to think badly of you because of it? Could they maybe not care?

C: I don't know about that.

T: Could they maybe be sympathetic? Could they maybe think you are pretty cool for doing this even if you are nervous? What do you think? What do the rest of you think?

C3: Yeah, I bet a lot of them couldn't care less.

C2: And there are a lot of people who hate to do that stuff. I bet they think, "Better you than me!"

T: Can you buy any of this, C?

C: Yeah, a little.

T: OK, let's review then? Some people won't notice because they're not paying attention. Others won't notice because they wouldn't see it if you took out an ad in the *New York Times*. Others might see it, but they could come to a number of different conclusions, right?

C: Right.

T: Let's work with our chart a little bit. How many of the seventy people would think you were sick or had too much coffee?

C: Ten?

T: OK, sixty left. (*Marks off another section.*) How many would think you were nervous but would not care?

C: Well, there are a lot of people at these meetings who I don't know. I don't see them often because they work in other offices. Maybe twenty.

T: We're really cooking now! Only forty left! (*Marks off another slice.*) How many would be sympathetic or at least know what you are going through?

C: Probably a bunch. Maybe another twenty!

T: (*as he marks off another large slice*) Down to twenty. Now, C, out of those twenty, how many are people who really matter? Even if they thought badly of you, how much of a difference would they make?

C: I see what you're getting at. Well, most are peers or less. Some I don't care for. Maybe just two or three!

T: So two or three people out of one hundred. Is that enough to get worked up about?

C: I guess not!

The results of this intervention are displayed in Figure 12.2. To review, the Pie Chart Technique involves the repeated and persistent questioning of the target client's predictions about other people's reactions to his or her anxiety experience. It emphasizes alternative points of view each small step along the way. It is not important that the client's statements about the number of people who will respond in a particular way are accurate because the simple admission that people react in a number of different ways is a major step. Also, the effort to actively involve other members of the group is an important component of the Pie Chart Technique because it adds a substantial dose of social influence to the therapeutic mix. The

Original Belief: Of 100 people, all would notice his anxiety and view him negatively as a result.

Conclusion: Of 100 people, only 3% might react as he feared.

Completed Pie Chart:

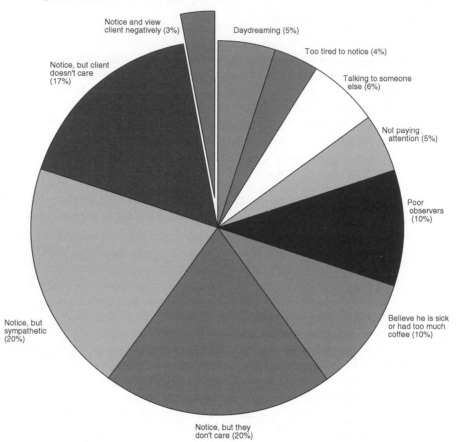

FIGURE 12.2. The Pie-Chart Technique: A completed pie chart for a client with a fear that his anxiety would be visible to others and lead to negative consequences.

client will be hesitant to say that no one holds an alternative point of view, because the other group members are unlikely to accept this. The Pie Chart Technique can be a powerful mix of cognitive restructuring and benevolent social pressure that may facilitate a change in negative thinking.

Automatic Thoughts about the Inappropriateness of Behavior

We have now worked with a number of clients who have dysfunctional beliefs about the inappropriateness of certain specific behaviors. For instance, one client believed that it was inappropriate to maintain eye contact with others because to do so would be to invade their privacy. He also believed that blinking was an indication of personal weakness and of having something to hide. Obviously, he was not able to totally inhibit blinking, but his attempts to do so resulted in significant physical pain and an unusual facial expression. In social interactions, he was withdrawn, avoided eye contact, and tried even harder than usual not to blink. He was constantly worried that others would think he was invading their space or that he had something to hide. A second client spoke with such a low voice that he could barely be heard. He was a big man with the capacity for a big voice, but he believed that it was bad to speak loudly. He believed that, if he raised his voice, others would think he was shouting, wonder what was wrong with him, and reject him. Not so surprisingly, these clients appeared to be very socially un-skilled and in need of social skills training. However, on closer examination, they were quite capable of executing the target behaviors. They simply would not let themselves do so.

The first client did not reveal to the group his beliefs about eye contact and blinking until several sessions into treatment. Early attempts at in-session expo-sures or homework assignments were quite unsuccessful as a result. When he did tell the group about his beliefs, an in-session exposure was designed for him in which he was prompted at regular intervals to engage in the two target behaviors, blinking and eye contact, while repeating a rational response designed to help him do so. Predictably, he reported the following automatic thoughts before the in-session exposure:

"I shouldn't blink."
"I'll be vulnerable."
"Others will think I'm covering up something."

The therapist then initiated a discussion to dispute these automatic thoughts. The portion of dialogue presented below focuses on the client's thoughts about blinking.

T: C, let's look at your automatic thought, "I shouldn't blink." Why shouldn't you?

C: Because people will think I'm hiding something, that I'm weak.

T: Why would they think that?

C: Because I keep them from looking into my soul when I blink.

T: How's that? (*Clearly surprised at these unusual thoughts.*)

C: When I blink, people can't look into my eyes and see what I'm made of, what kind of a person I am. If I blink, people will think I'm doing it on purpose to hide something about me.

Note that these thoughts are inconsistent with the client's ideas that keeping eye contact invades others' privacy. However, the therapist decided that that inconsistency was best confronted at another time.

T: Do most people think that?

C: Yeah. Doesn't everyone?

T: I don't know. Why don't we ask some of the other folks? (*Gestures that C should query other members of the group.*)

C: (*turning to another client*) C2, what do you think?

C2: I think people blink because their eyes need the water. It has nothing to do with your soul!

C: C3?

C3: I don't think it matters why people blink. It's just something that people do.

C: C4?

C4: It's involuntary. People blink because that's how God made us.

C: (*Queries other group members and gets similar reactions.*)

T: So C, what do you make of this?

C: I guess people are telling me that I'm way off base! I don't know what to think.

T: They're telling you even more than that. They are saying, "people should blink," aren't they?

C: Yeah.

T: Do you buy it?

C: I don't know. It feels really strange and uncomfortable. It's just so different.

T: You don't have to believe it all at once. As we go to your in-session exposure, will you entertain the idea of letting yourself blink some?

C: Uh, yeah.

T: Can you pull some of this discussion together into a rational response?

C: "It's natural to blink. It's what people are supposed to do." Is that OK?

T: It should do nicely.

Clients who endorse maladaptive beliefs about specific behaviors, such as eye contact, voice volume, or blinking, or those who believe they have nothing to talk about may cause the therapist to straddle the line between CBGT and social skills training. For extremely skill-deficient clients, a more focused skills-oriented approach may be indicated. However, for many of our clients, the degree of skill deficit may be small compared with the interference produced by their belief systems. A cognitive-behavioral approach in which their maladaptive beliefs are examined and in which they give themselves instructions to engage in or prepare themselves for the anxiety-provoking behavior (e.g., maintaining eye contact or generating a list of topics for casual conversations) is often successful and compatible with CBGT.

Discussion of concerns about the appropriateness or inappropriateness of specific behaviors is greatly complicated if there are cultural or racial differences involved. It is important for the therapists to be mindful of the different expectations that different cultures have for various behaviors or for the same behavior when performed by men or by women—for example, eye contact, interpersonal distance, specific forms of address, and so forth. These issues may influence the goals that clients from different cultural or subcultural backgrounds may set for specific in-session exposures or homework assignments. Cultural, ethnic, or other differences between the client and the other person in a problematic situation may, in fact, be major contributors to the client's anxious thoughts about that situation. These differences may also feature prominently in the anxiety experience of persons who are new to the culture in which the CBGT group is conducted. Sensitivity to these issues is a very important goal for any therapist working with socially anxious clients.

Rating Clients' Degree of Belief in Automatic Thoughts and Rational Responses

To help clients move toward greater acceptance of the newly formulated rational response, it is helpful to ask them to rate the degree of their belief in the ATs of most importance to the exposure situation and the rational responses on 0–100 scales before the exposure begins. The AT will probably be more strongly endorsed than the rational response prior to the exposure. The belief ratings need not be a focus of discussion before the exposure but should be recorded for later discussion.

Goal Setting

The final step in cognitive preparation for in-session exposures is the definition of successful performance by the target client. An attempt is made to agree on a level of performance that the client may find acceptable but that is not tainted by perfectionistic standards or unrealistic expectations.

The client is simply asked, *"What's your goal?"* The response to this question provides an intriguing window into the thinking of persons with social phobia, as it is invariably extreme or unattainable. The person with public-speaking phobia will want to give her talk without showing her nervousness or stumbling over a single word, the man with a fear of asking women for dates will want to sweep her off her feet, the person with writing-in-public fears will want to sign the check without shaking, and most clients will want to accomplish whatever it is without getting anxious. In each of these examples, the clients set unrealistic standards for themselves (or portray their belief that others hold extreme standards for them), and when they are unable to reach these standards, they will see themselves as having failed, proved their incompetence, humiliated themselves, and so on. This process of unrealistic goal setting and harsh self-criticism may be central to clients' failures in their previous self-exposure efforts.

Clients' goals for in-session exposures not only may be unrealistic but also may have several other critical characteristics. Goals may be stated in a general way so that assessment of goal attainment is difficult. For instance, the client may simply state that he or she wants to do well. Of course, but what does "well" mean? This may be a veiled perfectionistic goal, as "well" might actually mean "perfectly." Alternately, "well" may simply be a word with an imprecise operational definition, and the client may have a difficult time determining whether he or she has done well. In this situation, the client's negative cognitive biases will almost always lead him or her to believe he or she has failed. Thus, **goals should be stated in terms of concrete and specific events that can be easily monitored by the client**.

Goals may also be stated in such a way that the desired outcome is not under the control of the client. The date-anxious male client who requires that a woman accept his invitation for dinner is potentially entrapped because the woman may be unavailable, committed, uninterested, and so forth. She may refuse his overtures despite the fact that he has initiated a contact, maintained a conversation, and extended the invitation with consummate skill and grace. Similarly, the boss may not consent to the requested raise in pay, and the obnoxious upstairs neighbor may not turn down his stereo just because they were asked, even if they were asked well. Thus **the client's goal needs to be stated in terms of his or her own behavior, rather than the behavior of another person or the outcome of the situation**.

Clients often appear to prefer goals that are stated in terms of their affective states. Most commonly, a client will say that he or she wants to behave in a certain way without becoming nervous. Despite the fact that the client's overriding goal in treatment is to achieve anxiety reduction, the application of this goal to specific situations is insidious and self-defeating. First, it contains within it the thinking error of all-or-nothing thinking—the client views the situation as one in which he or she will either become anxious or remain relaxed but does not acknowledge that there are several points in between. Thus any experience of anxiety can be equated with failure. Second, this approach to goal setting focuses the client on his or her physiological arousal as an indicator of success/failure. However, arousal is only loosely related to overt behavior and is often invisible to others. An elegant presentation made by someone who is nervous is, nonetheless, elegant. It is much more important to help the client learn that he or she is capable of functioning in the presence of anxiety than to try to eliminate it completely. Thus **goals should be construed in terms of overt behavior rather than affective state**.

To summarize, goals should be stated in terms that are

- Realistically attainable by the client.
- Concrete and specific.
- Behavioral rather than affective.
- Under the control of the client.

In practice, goals are often suggested to the client (and later in treatment, suggested by the client) in terms of the performance of a specific number of behavioral acts or performance for a specified period of time, *regardless of the client's anxiety level.*

Examples of goals for in-session exposures include the following:

- Share three pieces of information about yourself with a person you are meeting for the first time.
- Ask five questions of someone you would like to know better.
- Answer seven questions from the audience on the topic of your presentation.
- Speak on a prearranged topic for six minutes.

- Take five bites of food while conversing with someone on a date.
- Make small talk for five minutes and then ask the other person to go to the concert with you.
- Look up from your notes and make eye contact with your audience on five different occasions during your presentation.

Two additional goals are added by the therapists as a matter of standard practice:

- Hang in there despite your anxiety.
- Use your cognitive coping skills.

During an In-Session Exposure: SUDS Ratings and Rational Responses

Every 60 seconds or so, clients are requested to give a SUDS rating (see Chapter 11, section on SUDS Recording). SUDS ratings can also be requested at other times if the SUDS recorder notices a meaningful change in the client's anxiety and wants to mark it for later examination in the postprocessing of the in-session exposure.[1] It may be useful, for example, to ask a client, "At the time when you asked your neighbor to shovel his walkway after last night's snowstorm, your SUDS increased from 40 to 65. What was going through your mind right then?" Similarly, a different lesson can be taught by asking, "Your anxiety dropped from 80 to 30 after the conversation turned to discussing your kids. What was going through your mind at that point?"

As noted previously, the rational responses developed prior to the in-session exposure have been recorded on the easel, and the easel is now placed where the client can see it. The client can use the rational responses to answer ATs that occur during the in-session exposure. Even with this obvious visual aid, however, clients often reported that they became too anxious to remember to use their rational responses or to cope with their automatic thoughts in any way. Therefore, we have incorporated rational responses into our procedures in a more systematic way.

Because the flow of the in-session exposure is briefly interrupted by the SUDS procedure, the opportunity exists to focus the client on his or her rational response(s). After the client gives a rating in response to "SUDS?" the SUDS recorder may simply say, "rational response?" The client is asked to read the rational response(s) aloud, thereby forcing himself or herself to momentarily focus on its coping content. In addition, the client is asked to answer automatic thoughts as they occur during the in-session exposure by using the rational response(s) and to maintain focus on the agreed-on behavioral goals.

The client may treat the reading of the rational response as an assigned duty rather than a coping response. Similarly, he or she may view it as a distraction that may preclude him or her from completing whatever tasks are involved in the in-session exposure and rush through it. Therapists should be aware of these attitudes and intervene when necessary. If the reading of the rational response is viewed as a burden, it will not be helpful, simply because the client is unlikely to consider its meaning or implications. Clients should be encouraged to read the rational response aloud and "with feeling."

Variations on the basic procedure are possible. For instance, the client may not only read the rational response aloud but also attempt to voice at least one implication of the rational response. A client might develop the rational response, "I can always talk about the weather or other trivial topics" to the automatic thought, "I won't be able to think of anything to say." When asked for a SUDS rating, he or she could read the rational response and state an implication, for example, "That means I don't have to worry about silences." In another variation, as clients begin to make progress in treatment, an attempt can be made to fade instructional control and put the client more in charge. After the first couple of SUDS probes, which are conducted as described previously, the easel may be covered and the client asked to repeat the rational response aloud from memory. After a few more SUDS probes, the client may repeat the rational response silently to himself or herself.

After an In-Session Exposure: The Cognitive Debriefing

After the completion of an in-session exposure, there is much cognitive restructuring work to do. We allow therapists a fair degree of latitude in choosing how to conduct this "cognitive debriefing" or "postprocessing" of the in-session exposure, but there are a number of interventions that should be considered. These are listed in Figure 12.1 and reviewed in the following.

Assessment of Goal Attainment

Before the in-session exposure, goals were agreed on by the participants. However, the client may have agreed to these goals halfheartedly, and he or she may persist in evaluating his or her performance on the basis of less adaptive (often unstated) goals. To help the client stay focused on attainment of adaptive goals, therapists should ask *"Did you accomplish your goal(s)?"* rather than more general questions such as, "How did you do?"[2] The client may equivocate or state that he or she failed because he or she was anxious during the in-session exposure. Therapists should then restate the agreed-on goals and evaluate whether or not these goals were met, regardless of the client's state of arousal. With careful goal setting before the in-session exposure, it is extremely likely that the goals will have been attained, and the therapists and group members should strongly reinforce the notion that the target client was able to behave in a functional manner despite the presence of anxiety.

A client's tendency to cling to maladaptive goals will typically reveal a series of automatic thoughts related to themes of perfectionism, such as, "If I make a mistake, it will be a total disaster" or "People won't accept me unless I am perfect." These automatic thoughts can be addressed in the same manner as described in the section, "The Process of Disputation of Automatic Thoughts and Development of Rational Responses." These automatic thoughts should also be recorded by the therapists for possible attention during the goal-setting portion of the client's next in-session exposure.

During the in-session exposure, it is generally a good idea for the SUDS recorder or one of the therapists to actively track the client's progress toward the stated goals (these may be recorded on the In-Session Exposure Recording Form, Figure 11.1). By noting the occurrence of specific goal behaviors or the number of times these behaviors occur, it is possible to reinforce the client's fragile sense of goal attainment. A client in a recent group, for instance, agreed to the goals of sharing three pieces of personal information and asking three questions during an in-session exposure of conversing with an attractive other at a local pub. The client was hesitant to agree to these goals because she was uncertain that she would be able to meet the challenge. A therapist who kept a careful count during the 10-minute role play reported to the client's extreme amazement that she had stated 9 points of personal information and asked 12 questions!

Review of Occurrence of Automatic Thoughts and Use of Rational Responses

After goal review, the client should be asked whether the ATs listed before the in-session exposure actually occurred. If so, did the client employ his or her rational responses? It is important, especially early in treatment, to convey the strong expectation that clients actively confront their ATs rather than simply accept them. If the client did not use the specific rational response(s) developed during the preexposure period but used other means of active coping, these should be examined. If the client's strategy was an adaptive one, it may be very powerful because it was entirely self-generated.

Review of Evidence in Support of Automatic Thoughts versus Rational Responses

Next, the client's ATs and rational responses should be closely examined in light of the exposure experience. The primary question here is whether the negative predictions about the client's ability to perform or the reactions of others were realized in the in-session exposure or whether the events were better accounted for by the message of the rational response. The specific questions to ask will depend on the specific events that unfolded during the exposure. However, questions like those presented in Figure 12.3 should facilitate this effort. Basically, this is a return to the process of disputation of ATs used before the exposure, but now evidence from the exposure must be incorporated.

Therapists should select several of the most important ATs and ask the client whether each AT was supported by the events of the in-session exposure (or use other questions from Figure 12.3 if they are more appropriate to the specific AT). For example, a therapist might ask, "Brian, your thought was 'I will look stupid.' Do you think you looked stupid?" After the client responds, it is useful to ask the role player(s) to weigh in on the matter (e.g., "Susan, did Brian look stupid to you?"). Then the reactions of the other group members can be surveyed. This order of questioning may be important, because clients who are upset with their performances may be reluctant to contradict therapists, other group members, or the role player(s) because of their social anxiety or a desire to just get the whole thing over with. Additionally, hearing the specifics of the client's own reaction lets the others provide more specific feedback (especially if the thought was relatively specific, e.g., "I will mumble"). Questioning thoughts one by one is much superior to asking in a more general way whether any of the client's ATs turned out to be true.

As is apparent from the preceding example, feedback from role players may be an important part of postexposure cognitive restructuring, and a few points about this process need to be made. It is wise to brief role players about the kind of feedback they may be expected to provide. For example, if the likely question is whether the target client's anxiety will be visible to others during the exposure, role players may worry what to say if the client is visibly anxious. They should be instructed to provide accurate feedback, but to do so gently. If no anxiety is evident, they should say so, but otherwise they might say something like, "You sounded a bit anxious before your speech, but I didn't find it at all distracting. I think your speech was very interesting and I really enjoyed listening to it." It is important to communicate to clients that it is OK to appear anxious. Telling them they seemed so calm when they did not sends precisely the opposite message.

Occurrence of Other Automatic Thoughts

It is important to determine whether any automatic thoughts that had not been previously discussed occurred to the client during the in-session exposure. If so,

1. Were you concerned that _____ would occur during the exposure?

2. Did _____ occur during the exposure?

3. How did you cope with _____ when it happened?

4. Did you use your rational response(s) to help yourself cope when _____ happened? Was it helpful to you to do so?

5. Was _____ as difficult (or horrible) as you expected it would be?

6. If _____ happened to you in real life, could you cope with it?

7. What evidence do you have that your automatic thought was true?

8. What evidence do you have that your automatic thought was in error?

9. What evidence do you have that your rational response may be true?

FIGURE 12.3. List of questions for evaluating the evidence after completion of in-session exposures.

what was their nature? How did the client cope with them? If some unanticipated automatic thoughts did occur to the client, the therapists may choose to work on them at that moment (if they were extremely distressing or grabbed most of the client's attention) or, otherwise, record them for attention before the client's next in-session exposure.

Examination of the Pattern of SUDS Ratings

SUDS ratings were collected about every 60 seconds during the in-session exposure, and these ratings reveal much about the client's experience. It may be helpful to draw a rough graph of the client's SUDS ratings on the easel, but the primary goal is to discuss with clients what happened to their anxiety when they experienced certain automatic thoughts, when they used their rational responses or alternative coping statements, or when certain behavioral events occurred during the in-session exposure. This step is very important and should be included in the processing of most in-session exposures. SUDS ratings may fall into a number of different patterns (see the next section), but most clients will reveal an uneven pattern in which anxiety moves up and down over the course of the in-session exposure.

Whenever there is a clear increase in SUDS, the client should be asked whether any automatic thoughts occurred. Whenever there is a decrease, the client should be asked if this coincided with an active attempt to use a rational response or to otherwise dispute an automatic thought. By so doing, therapists communicate to the clients that they can affect their anxiety experience by constructively attending to their own cognitive processes.

POSSIBLE PATTERNS OF SUDS RATINGS

As mentioned, clients' SUDS ratings may fall into a number of patterns. However, the number of patterns is not infinite. They fall into five general categories that have different implications for cognitive interventions. These are presented in Figure 12.4.

First is the pattern we call the *spike*. The client's SUDS ratings move up and down over the course of the in-session exposure, producing a series of peaks and valleys. The preferred cognitive intervention is that described previously, looking for ATs that are associated with increased anxiety and rational responses or other coping attempts that are associated with reduced anxiety. It is also important to note here that different behaviors required of the client during the in-session exposure may contribute to the spiked pattern. For instance, a client with a fear of public speaking may give a speech that is punctuated with audience questions, and his or her anxiety response may be different when giving the talk as compared with answering questions or interacting with the audience. Similarly, a dating-anxious client may experience a rise in anxiety as the time to ask for a date approaches and a drop in anxiety after he or she has taken that risk. This is an important piece of learning for the client with social phobia, who may view anxiety in all-or-nothing terms.

A second pattern is one we call the *steady decline*. In this pattern, the client's anxiety is elevated at the beginning of the in-session exposure but shows a consistent, more or less linear downward trend. At the end of the in-session exposure, the client may be considerably less anxious than he or she was at the beginning. This pattern is most common among clients who experience a high degree of anticipatory anxiety. The high initial SUDS ratings represent their catastrophic expectations of what might occur during the in-session exposure, but their SUDS start to decrease as they see themselves able to handle the situation and as they do not see their catastrophic predictions confirmed. Of course, this experience is itself a potently rewarding one for the client. However, he or she is likely to remain afraid of the initial burst of anxiety. Cognitive interventions may be oriented toward helping the client see that he or she was able to perform despite the initial anxiety and that the anxiety experience was a temporary one. The client can develop a rational response for future in-session exposures or homework assignments that resembles, "hang in there and the anxiety will go away." Of course, this rational response should be reintroduced to the client during the preparation for the next in-session exposure.

Another common pattern is the *habituation curve*. In this pattern, the client begins with a moderate level of anxiety and experiences an initial rise in SUDS ratings, but then the anxiety begins to decline. Like the steady decline, this pattern involves a time of considerable anxiety, but the anxiety experience does not last. However, the habituation curve is different in that the client will see his or her anxiety escalate and may become afraid that it will continue to rise unabated until it is out of control. Cognitive interventions for the habituation curve may in-

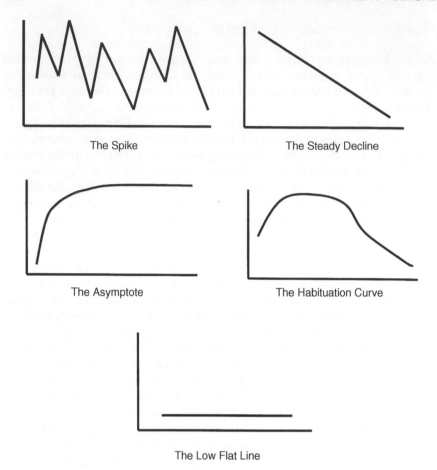

The Spike

The Steady Decline

The Asymptote

The Habituation Curve

The Low Flat Line

FIGURE 12.4. Possible patterns of SUDS ratings during in-session exposures.

clude several components. First, it is important to examine the client's automatic thoughts early in the in-session exposure, as these are likely to contribute to the early rise in anxiety. It is likely that the client is not actively using rational responses during this interval and may feel that he or she is at the mercy of the anxiety. Second, the therapist should emphasize to the client that the anxiety experience is temporary and reemphasize the client's role in reducing anxiety by using rational responses. Third, the therapist should note that the client continued to perform and met his or her goals (if this was the case) despite the high anxiety. Fourth, the notion that continued practice will bring the anxiety down should be reinforced.

A fourth pattern is the *asymptote*, which involves a moderate level of initial anxiety, followed by an increase in anxiety to near-maximal levels. Unlike the other patterns, the client's SUDS ratings remain high until the end of the in-session exposure. This is a very difficult situation, and one that will inevitably be viewed as a failure by the client, whether or not he or she met the preestablished behavioral goals. When an asymptote occurs, it is important to acknowledge the client's difficulty but to also communicate to the client that the therapists believe that this pattern will not continue forever. Continued practice and use of rational responses will result in reduction of anxiety over time. Furthermore, the client may have been able to perform quite reasonably and have done so in the face of extreme anxiety. With continued coping, things can only get better, and the client has already coped with the worst. In addition, the therapists should carefully consider whether or not the chosen in-session exposure was simply too difficult for the client at this time in treatment and whether the next in-session exposure should revolve around a more manageable situation.

The final pattern to be discussed is the *low flat line*. In this situation, the client reports very little anxious arousal during the in-session exposure. The low flat line may occur for a variety of reasons, and the therapists should carefully investigate the reasons for its occurrence. It may happen because the client confronted a difficult situation but coped with it so well that anxiety was never experienced. If so, the client may view this as a big step forward. However, it may also occur for other reasons that are less positive. It may happen because the primary anxiety-evoking stimulus was not properly incorporated into the in-session exposure. If so, this stimulus needs to be identified and incorporated into future efforts. It may occur because the client has engaged in some form of cognitive avoidance. He or she may have forced himself or herself to think about something else or may have repeatedly told himself or herself that the in-session exposure was not real so there was no cause to be anxious. These avoidance strategies will generally come to light during postprocessing of the in-session exposure, and the therapists will need to encourage the client to become more meaningfully involved.

Rerating of Belief in Automatic Thoughts and Rational Responses

After the evidence for and against the ATs and rational responses has been discussed, the client should be asked to rerate his or her belief in each, using the same 0–100 scale. When exposure exercises have provided evidence to counter the client's negative beliefs, there should be a shift toward increased belief in the rational response. The client should also be asked if the rational response should be adjusted in some way based on the outcome of the in-session exposure and postprocessing.

The Final Summary

The last step in the debriefing of an in-session exposure is the client's summary. Many things happen in a brief period before, during, and after an in-session exposure, and the client may come away from it with his or her head spinning. Similarly, it is possible that the client may have failed to understand or accept the lessons of an in-session exposure. It is a useful assessment and aid to generalization to ask the target client to summarize what he or she learned from the in-session exposure.

At the end of the cognitive debriefing, the client should be asked to consider and thoughtfully answer the following question: *"What did you learn from your in-session exposure? How can you take this lesson and apply it to your everyday life?"*

Behavioral Experiments

A. T. Beck and his colleagues (A. T. Beck et al., 1979; A. T. Beck et al., 1985) have often referred to the *behavioral experiment*, that is, a situation in which the client may actively do something that will provide a test of his or her dysfunctional beliefs. ATs are treated as hypotheses to be tested rather than facts to be accepted, relevant data are collected, and the hypotheses are then evaluated in light of the data. In a very real sense, each in-session exposure is a behavioral experiment, and the cognitive restructuring activities that surround them are attempts to undermine clients' faith in the "scientific validity" of their maladaptive hypotheses. In this section, however, we share with you some behavioral experiments that we have used frequently to examine two specific automatic thoughts: (1) "Everyone can see my anxiety," and (2) "Nobody likes me."

"Everyone Can See My Anxiety."

This automatic thought is so common among clients with social phobia that we deal with it almost every session. As a result, a variety of interventions are required for its modification, so that therapists can avoid being repetitious or stereotypic in response to clients' concerns. Here we describe a behavioral experiment that can be used after an in-session exposure to test the client's hypothesis that his or her anxiety is visible to others.

SILENT SUDS

Recall again the female client described in Chapter 10 and earlier in this chapter who presented with fears of interacting with men she found to be physically attractive and who reported the automatic thought, "He'll be able to tell I'm nervous" when she thought about having conversations with any of these men.

The Pie Chart Technique may have been a very appropriate intervention for her beliefs about what would happen as a result of the detection of her anxiety, but another strategy was helpful in getting her to realize that her anxiety simply was not that apparent. The following simple strategy worked very well with this client and may be very useful for any client whose anxiety is not as apparent as he or she believes. The client participated in an in-session exposure in which she was to initiate a conversation with an attractive man she happened to meet in a grocery store. She reported that she would be overwhelmed with anxiety—she would tremble, she would be unable to maintain eye contact, she would not be able to think of anything to say, and when she did speak, her voice would crack. With so many visible symptoms of her anxiety, how could the man fail to notice? After some cognitive restructuring activities, the in-session exposure took place. The conversation, in fact, went very smoothly. Although she reported being extremely anxious, the only visible sign was a moderate reduction in the amount of eye contact. However, she remained convinced that her anxiety was there for all to see.

She was asked to rate the visibility of her anxiety on a 0–100 scale that was similar to the SUDS scale that she was quite familiar with. However, she was asked to write down her rating rather than say it aloud. Simultaneously (and without knowledge of the client's self-rating), the other group members and therapists also wrote down their ratings of the client's anxiety *as it appeared to them* on the same 0–100 scale. No one was permitted to show their rating to anyone else. In a sense, the client's rating was a representation of her hypothesis about the visibility of her anxiety, and the other persons' ratings were the data in this behavioral experiment. After all ratings were completed, the participants simultaneously revealed their ratings. The client's self-rating was a 90. The other participants' ratings were all in the 20s! The client left this exercise with her belief in the visibility of her anxiety visibly shaken.

A similar behavioral experiment was incorporated into an in-session exposure for a male client with a fear of speaking in public. The client had to chair meetings and conduct training seminars regularly as part of his job. He feared that he would become overwhelmingly anxious during one of his talks, that his anxiety would be clearly visible to others, and that as a result they would question his competence or the appropriateness of his holding a position of leadership. However, a pretreatment behavior test revealed that he was an effective, elegant speaker whose anxiety had no external referents. For his in-session exposure, the client presented materials that he would use in an upcoming workshop. During the in-session exposure, whenever he was requested to give a SUDS rating, he wrote it on the easel, which was positioned at his right hand but out of the view of the other group members, rather than stating it aloud. When he did so, the other group members and therapists also wrote down their 0–100 ratings of the client's anxiety as it appeared to them. At the end of the in-session exposure, a wealth of data had been generated—10 ratings by the client and 70 ratings by the other participants. The fact that these ratings were made on a minute-to-minute basis during the in-session exposure rather than retrospectively determined appeared to add to the potency of the behavioral experiment. In this case, the client rated himself in the 70s, whereas the others rated him between 5 and 10![3]

VIDEO FEEDBACK

Another intervention that is very useful for concerns about the visibility of anxiety (as well as other concerns about the adequacy of one's performance or the way one appears to others) is video feedback. In fact, video feedback can be such a useful tool that we have considered making it a part of every in-session exposure. However, we choose to leave the decision to use video equipment to the therapists of each CBGT group, as it may not be universally available.

As described in Chapter 3, Rapee and Hayman (1996) demonstrated that socially anxious persons rated their speech performances less negatively when they saw a videotape than they did from memory. Furthermore, when asked to give a second speech, those who rated their first speech from the video were more positive about the second speech than those who rated their first speech from memory. Videotape feedback may be a potent source of disconfirmatory feedback for persons with social phobia.

Therapists may wish to use video feedback as an adjunct to in-session exposures. In that case, it is reasonable to ask the client what he or she expects to see when the tape is viewed and to treat the response as an automatic thought that may be confronted just like any other AT. What does the client expect to see in terms of observed behavior, mannerisms, or appearance? How would therapists or other group members know if the client appeared on tape the way he or she expects to appear? Specificity here should make later evaluation of the client's prediction easier to accomplish. After the exposure is completed, but before the tape is viewed, the client might be asked whether he or she expects to appear as originally predicted, better, or worse and to specify the reasons for any shift of opinion. After viewing the tape, the client should examine in detail any differences between the predicted performance and the performance as viewed on tape and to address possible reasons for the discrepancy, should there be one. This approach is similar to one recently outlined by Harvey, Clark, Ehlers, and Rapee (2000). It may be obvious that video feedback is best not used when clients' behavior or appearance is objectively problematic or if the client's mental set is so negative that the video feedback might be difficult for the client to incorporate.

"Nobody Likes Me."

In Chapter 11, we described a male client who was afraid that no one would like him if they found out what he was "really" like. Of course, this fear led him to avoid most social interactions and to limit himself to superficial conversation at all other times. He was not willing to talk to others about personally meaningful material. An in-session exposure was designed for him in which he would speak to the group for 3 minutes about his superficial characteristics, 3 minutes about his daily activities, and 3 minutes about his personal goals and dreams (see Chapter 11). Each topic was more threatening than the last. Whereas he believed he could talk to others about his superficial characteristics without alienating them, he feared that they would come to dislike him when he spoke on the latter two topics, especially his goals and dreams. During the in-session exposure, minute-by-minute SUDS ratings were replaced by ratings of "likeability," which were completed in writing by both the client and the other participants. The client predicted that his likeability ratings would decline steeply (and they would not be that high to begin with) when he began to speak on more personal topics. In fact, the ratings of the other participants revealed the *opposite* pattern—as he spoke about more meaningful material, they liked him better!

Cognitive Restructuring from Beginning to End

We have described cognitive restructuring methods for use before, during, and after in-session exposures. In this section, we demonstrate how these activities may be put together in a clinical case example. You may wish to refer to Figure 12.1 as you follow the dialogue presented below. Salient points are highlighted in text boxes throughout the dialogue.

The client is a clinician in a community mental health agency who has to make presentations of intake evaluations to a treatment team consisting of social workers, a psychologist, and a psychiatrist. Although she has made these presentations weekly for the past 2 years, she has always had extreme anticipatory anxiety and substantial anxiety during the presentations. She has used Xanax (alprazolam) to control symptoms, but it has not worked well, and she dislikes taking medication. Physiological symptoms include increased heart rate, shortness of breath, and sweating.

T: C, one of your more difficult situations is the weekly case presentation you have to do for work.

C: Yeah, those are really hard. I get so anxious that I was thinking about quitting my job.

T: Let's work on that situation this week. Could you tell me a little bit about it?

C: Well, I have to make a presentation to the treatment team on each intake I do each week. That's the other social workers, the psychologist, and the psychiatrist.

T: OK, I would like you to think about that situation. Put yourself into the situation and tell me what automatic thoughts come into your mind as you think about making a presentation to the treatment team. [Identification of automatic thoughts]

C: I'll get anxious. I always worry about getting anxious.

T: "I'll get anxious." Let's put that one down. (*Records thought on easel.*)

C: I won't do a good presentation.

T: OK. (*Records thought on easel.*) What else? What would happen if you really got anxious?

Here T prompts C to think beyond the immediately apparent aspects of the situation and attempts to elicit thoughts about the consequences of anxiety and poor performance, which C has not yet specified.

C: That's what I worry about. If I get really anxious, I'll just fall apart. That would be horrible.

T: (*Records thought on easel.*) What do you mean by "fall apart"?

T does not allow C to move further until C has defined what it means to "fall apart." This is the beginning of T's effort to move C's vague and nonoperationalized horrors into the daylight where they can be more easily examined.

C: I won't be able to talk, I'll start shaking, maybe pass out, or have to run out of the room.

T: (*Records thoughts on easel.*) So "falling apart" means not being able to talk at all, shaking, passing out or having to leave. What is the worst of those? The one that would be worst if it happened?

An important and subtle aspect of cognitive-behavioral treatment is demonstrated here when C states her horrific thoughts and T responds calmly. This nonverbal proclamation that T is less concerned about these consequences than C is critical to success. If T were to show concern at the possibility of the consequences C fears, C's fears would be bolstered.

C: Having to run out. I'd be so humiliated I could never go back. I get nervous just thinking about it.

T: Let's work with that thought: "I'll get so anxious, I'll have to run out of the room." Looking at your list of thinking errors, how would you classify that thought? [Identification of thinking errors]

Not only does T start the formal process of cognitive restructuring here by asking C to identify errors in her ATs, but T also makes a decision to focus cognitive preparation for the exposure on one specific AT. This is a very efficient means of conducting cognitive restructuring and may often be preferred to more broad-ranging cognitive analyses that consume additional group time.

C: It could be fortune telling, predicting something bad before it actually happens.

T: Good. Let's go with that. Let's see if we can step back and try to look at that thought a little more logically so we can come up with a rational response to help you combat it.

This AT also contains aspects of emotional reasoning and all-or-nothing thinking. T decides that the fortune telling aspects of the thought will provide sufficient grist for cognitive work and moves on.

C: OK.

T: Looking at your list of disputing questions, how would you question that fortune-telling thought? [Disputation of automatic thought]

T succinctly summarizes what C should do (dispute the AT) and why (because it contains a thinking error, fortune telling, that may be harmful to C).

C: Do I know for certain that I will get so anxious that I will have to run out of the room?

T: And how would you answer that?

C: Well, I don't know for certain it will happen this time. But if it is a bad day and I get really anxious, I'll have to leave.

T: Look at another one of the disputing questions. Does getting extremely anxious have to lead to running out of the room? [Disputation of automatic thought]

> T reinforces the notion that cognitive restructuring of automatic thoughts is
> a process and leads C to bring multiple disputing questions to bear on this
> AT.

C: Well . . . maybe not.

T: Have you had times in the past when you were extremely anxious?
Times that have been particularly bad?

C: Yes. Just before I started treatment was one of the worst. My heart was
pounding so hard I could hardly think (*referring to an individualized behavioral
test during pretreatment assessment in which she was required to give a report at
a mock-up of a staff meeting*).

T: So you were extremely anxious that time. Did you run out of the room?

C: No.

T: Have you ever run out of the room in the middle of your presentation?

C: No, but I have thought about doing it.

T: So, even at times when you have been extremely anxious, you have been
able to stay in the room and finish your case presentation?

C: I guess so.

T: So let's look at another disputing question. What evidence do you have
that, if you get extremely anxious, you will have to run out of the room? [Dispu-
tation of automatic thought]

C: None. I guess I just worry about it but it has never happened.

T: That's true. You do worry about it but it has never happened. Let's try
and turn the ideas we have been talking about into a rational response that you
can use to help combat the thought, "I'll get so anxious, I'll have to run out of the
room," when it comes up. [Development of rational response]

C: Even if I get really anxious I probably won't have to run out of the
room?

> C's initial attempt is not bad, but it is offered meekly and with a look to T
> for approval. T reinforces the attempt but keeps C in the driver's seat as the
> process continues . . .

T: Let's review what we've learned about this AT. First, you learned that it
is an example of the fortune-telling error. What else did you learn?

C: Well, I don't know for certain that I'll get so anxious that I'll have to run
out.

T: Good. What else? What about your behavior test?

C: I got totally anxious there and did not run away.

T: Right. In fact, you said that you have never left a presentation in the middle *no matter how much you worried that you would*. So how can we put all this together for you?

C: How about, "I'll probably be able to stick it out this time. I always have before"?

T: That's great. Now, let's use our 100-point scale of belief. How much do you believe, "I'll get so anxious, I'll have to run out of the room"? [Assessment in belief of AT]

C: It still bothers me a lot, maybe 70.

T: How much do you believe, "I'll probably be able to stick it out this time. I always have before"? [Assessment of belief in rational response]

C: I know it's right, but . . . maybe 30-ish.

T asks for belief ratings but does not get into a discussion about them at this time. Instead T chooses to rely on data provided by the in-session exposure to contribute to the restructuring of C's beliefs.

T: OK, let's set up the exposure. You brought the case notes I had asked you to bring last time?

Note that the details of set-up of the in-session exposure have been omitted.

T: Let's set a goal for the exposure—what do you have to do to call it a success? [Goal setting]

C: I don't want to get anxious. How about not getting anxious as the goal?

T: That's a good long-term goal. That's where we would like you to be eventually, but we should set a smaller goal for this exposure. How about something related to the automatic thought we worked on?

T makes the case that goal setting should not be tied to anxiety goals but instead refocuses goal setting on the specifics of the prior discussion.

C: Like not falling apart or leaving or something?

The Client's Automatic Thoughts

- "I'll get anxious."
- "I won't do a good presentation."
- "If I get really anxious, I'll just fall apart."
- "If I get really anxious, I won't be able to talk."
- "If I get really anxious, I'll start shaking."
- "If I get really anxious, I may pass out."
- "If I get really anxious, I'll have to run out of the room."

Targeted Automatic Thought

- "I'll get so anxious, I'll have to run out of the room." (Belief rating 70)

Rational Response

- "I'll probably be able to stick it out this time. I always have before." (Belief rating 30)

Goals

- Stay in the room for the length of the in-session exposure.
- Use rational responses to combat automatic thoughts.

FIGURE 12.5. Summary of cognitive restructuring activities prior to an in-session exposure in which the client fears presenting intake assessments at staff meetings.

T: Something like that, but remember that we don't want to use terms that set you off, like "falling apart." How about staying in the room for your whole presentation—and also remember the part that we always add—to use your rational response to cope with your ATs and anxiety during the exposure.

C: OK.

A summary of the cognitive restructuring activity that preceded the in-session exposure is provided in Figure 12.5. Figure 12.6 displays the client's SUDS ratings given during the in-session exposure. We resume the dialogue at the conclusion of the in-session exposure.

T: OK, C, did you make your goals?

C: I got really anxious. It was hard.

T: Did you make your goals? [Assessment of goal attainment]

C: No, I didn't do too well. I got really anxious. My heart was pounding.

T: That wasn't your goal, though. What was the goal we set?

C: Oh. To stay in the room and use my rational response.

T: Did you do that?

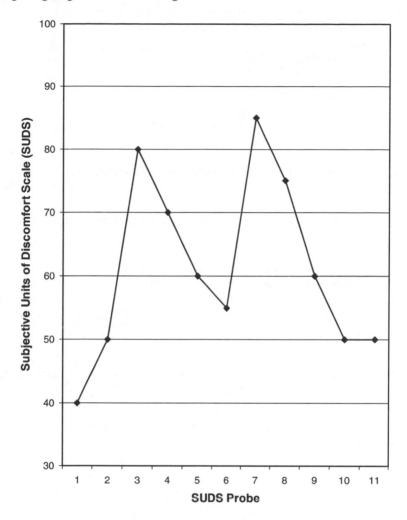

FIGURE 12.6. SUDS ratings during the in-session exposure of presenting an intake assessment at a staff meeting.

C: I guess so.

T: Yes, you did. Even though you were extremely anxious, you hung in there. That's great. It looks like you have even more evidence to support your rational response.

C: That's true. I was anxious, and even though I wanted to leave, I didn't.

T: What about some of the other things you were concerned about . . . that you would start shaking, pass out, not be able to talk? Did these happen the way you thought they would? [Assessment of evidence regarding ATs]

C: I got pretty shaky, but I didn't pass out, did I?

T: No, you didn't, and it's great to see that you're on top of that. Now, let's look at the SUDS pattern. You went up to 80, then it started to come back down, and then it spiked up again to 85. What happened there? [Examination of the pattern of SUDS ratings]

C: I looked up and saw someone who looked bored, so I thought I must not have been doing a very good job. Then I got really anxious and that is when I wanted to leave.

T: So it sounds like there is another automatic thought in there . . . "If they are bored, I must not be doing a very good job." [Identification of unanticipated automatic thought]

C: Yeah.

T: That's one we'll have to save for next time. What happened that made your anxiety come down again? [Examination of the pattern of SUDS ratings]

C: When you asked me for the SUDS rating, I read my rational response. That helped a little, then as I started to feel a little more comfortable, I thought I could probably make it through. [Assessment of use of rational response during in-session exposure]

T: Good. That's great that you were able to use the rational response to manage your anxiety in the situation. Now that we've discussed how things went, let's return to your belief ratings. After the exposure, how much do you now believe, "I'll get so anxious, I'll have to run out of the room"? [Rerating of belief in AT]

C: Much less, maybe 20.

T: How much do you believe, "I'll probably be able to stick it out this time. I always have before"?

C: A lot more, 75! [Rerating of belief in rational response]

T: Excellent. Finally, the big question . . . What did you learn and what can you take from this that you can use when you have to make a presentation this week? (*Asks for client's final summary.*)

C: I learned a lot. I learned that I could stay in the room. Even if I do get anxious, there's really no reason to think I'll have to run out. And I learned my anxiety comes down!

Group Involvement in Cognitive Restructuring

Many of the activities described in this chapter focus on the interaction of the therapist(s) with a single client. Other group members may be easily involved, however, and the benefits of this involvement are substantial for everyone involved. Increasing the involvement of all group members will result in additional input that the target client must consider during cognitive restructuring before in-session exposures and additional feedback about his or her performance after-ward. Because clients with social phobia can always look at other clients' thoughts more rationally than they can look at their own, clients will become po-tent agents of cognitive intervention for their peers. Furthermore, their input is less likely to be discounted by the target client than input from the therapists. In addition, all group members will benefit from involvement in the work of other clients. They will receive direct treatment whenever they are the target, but they will receive a large additional dose of vicarious treatment through their participa-tion in the treatment of other clients. For all these reasons, therapists should be continuously aware of the need to involve clients in as many aspects of the CBGT group as possible. Clients may play roles in other clients' in-session exposures, they may help to question and probe automatic thoughts, they may share their ex-periences that may help dispute other clients' automatic thoughts, and they may lean on other clients just hard enough that the others are compelled to entertain additional points of view. Once the first few sessions are passed, facilitating group participation is not a difficult matter.

Notes

1. Although the procedure for collecting minute-by-minute SUDS ratings should be em-ployed in most instances, there are a few circumstances in which therapists may choose to suspend it. The most obvious of these are the client who gives chronically high SUDS ratings or one whose SUDS reports seem to routinely underestimate the amount of anxiety that is communicated through nonverbal channels. In these cases, the therapists should continue the minute-by-minute focus on rational responses dis-cussed in this section.
2. It is usually the case that asking "How did you do?" will elicit the client's less adaptive goal strivings. Therefore, it is generally best to avoid this phrasing. However, if the therapists wish to assess the degree to which the client has truly adopted the more adaptive approach to goal setting, this question can be usefully put forth.
3. Although it did not occur in the context of CBGT, another approach to testing out be-liefs about the consequences of visible anxiety symptoms was shared by David M. Clark at a recent meeting of the Association for Advancement of Behavior Therapy. He told the story of a client who feared that people would notice his profuse sweating. So he and the client both used water to make big, huge wet spots under their arms and went into the store to buy batteries. Dr. Clark went first and had the client observe as he pointed to batteries and asked their prices with his wet armpit in full view of the clerk. The client was absolutely shocked to realize that the clerk seemed to pay no at-tention to Dr. Clark's armpits! This is a wonderful example of using humor to show the client that his or her most catastrophic expectations are not so likely to come true.

13

Homework Procedures

Throughout treatment therapists stress that clients must learn new skills and new ways of viewing anxiety-provoking situations. They further emphasize that the only way to be certain that these new skills will have a meaningful impact on clients' everyday existence is to apply them outside the treatment setting. In order to facilitate this effort, assignments are routinely given for the practice or application of new skills to real-life situations.

Homework assignments for the first two sessions (described earlier) are designed to help clients learn to identify automatic thoughts as they occur, to tie their occurrence to the experience of untoward emotions, to identify the cognitive errors contained in automatic thoughts, to examine their automatic thoughts objectively, and to develop rational responses to them. Homework assignments given in later sessions are individualized and tied as directly as possible to the content of each client's in-session exposures and overall treatment goals. Although specific assignments are given to each client each week, it is also important to encourage clients to adopt a **HOMEWORK ATTITUDE**. That is, they will make the most of treatment if they look for every opportunity to practice their skills and try to do something each and every day, large or small, to confront their anxiety. To underscore this point, we tell our clients they will benefit most from **DOING IT DAILY**.

Examples of "doing it daily" (Hope et al., 2000, p. 138)[1] include:

- Say hello and one other thing to a person you do not normally speak with.
- Make a phone call that you would rather put off because you are anxious about it.

- Give someone a compliment when you normally would not say anything.
- Speak up one extra time in a group of people or at a meeting.
- Ask someone a question that will help you get to know the person a little better.
- Make an effort to do some small task when others may be observing, such as pouring someone's coffee, putting change in a vending machine, unlocking a door, driving with someone in the car, writing a check rather than paying cash, and so forth.

At the end of each session, a homework assignment for the coming week is discussed with each client. These assignments are negotiated with, rather than imposed on, the client, and the client's agreement is considered a necessary part of the negotiation process. The client will typically be asked to do in real life whatever it is that he or she has done in his or her most recent in-session exposure and to do it as many times during the coming week as seems possible or practical. Specific goals for each homework assignment are also discussed and agreed on in the same manner as described for in-session exposures (see Chapter 12, the subsection on goal setting). In early sessions, the therapists should propose homework assignments and negotiate their exact nature with each client. In later sessions, therapists should have proposals for possible homework assignments for each client in mind but should be able to begin the discussion of homework by asking, "What do you think would be a good idea for you to work on this week for homework?" Clients who have embraced the treatment will often come up with assignments that are more challenging, creative, or personally meaningful than those envisioned by the therapists.

When agreement is reached on an assignment, a therapist records the assignment and goals on NCR (no carbon required) paper, giving one copy to the client and retaining the other for the clinical record. Rational responses that the client found helpful during the in-session exposure should also be recorded to help the client remember to use them during the homework exposure.

Before Attempting a Homework Assignment

Clients are not encouraged simply to enter feared situations and endure the pain. Rather, they are encouraged to take an active, coping approach to their homework assignments. Before they actually attempt assignments, they should be asked to set aside a brief period of time (usually 30 minutes or less) for cognitive preparation. In so doing, each client should conduct a self-administered version of the cognitive restructuring procedures described in Chapter 12 (see the section titled "Before an In-Session Exposure" and Figure 12.1). This effort will be greatly facilitated by the use of the first portion of the Be Your Own Cognitive Therapist (BYOCT) Worksheet, originally developed by and modified from Hope et al. (2000)[2], which is presented in Figure 13.1. The client should:

1. Imagine the assigned situation and bring it clearly to mind.
2. Record the automatic thoughts that occur to him or her in anticipation of the event and rate his or her degree of belief in each AT (as well as the emotions they arouse) on the BYOCT Worksheet.
3. Examine and identify the thinking errors in the automatic thoughts. (Several thinking errors are noted on the BYOCT Worksheet, but the client should probably keep a copy of the List of Thinking Errors, Figure 10.1, handy.)
4. Challenge these ATs with disputing questions and record the answers. (Several disputing questions are noted on the BYOCT Worksheet, but the client should probably keep a copy of the List of Disputing Questions, Figure 10.3, handy.)
5. Derive rational responses to the automatic thoughts based on this process (or apply rational responses that were developed during in-session exposures to the target situation).
6. Review and record the behavioral goals that were agreed on as part of the original discussion of the homework assignment.

As clients complete these cognitive coping procedures before doing their homework, they facilitate the learning and generalization of these skills, teach themselves to think productively about situations rather than engaging in unstructured catastrophizing, and increase the chances that homework assignments will have productive outcomes.

The Behavioral Assignment

After completion of these cognitive exercises, the client should then attempt the homework task. Clients are encouraged to keep in mind that completing an assignment means to do the tasks agreed on in session while practicing their cognitive coping skills. Specifically, successful completion of homework assignments includes the following:

1. Conducting the cognitive preparation for the assigned task.
2. Entering the feared situation and completing the assigned task.
3. Tolerating anxiety and staying in the situation until the task is completed.

4. Using cognitive coping skills as practiced in the group and in preparation for the homework task during the situation.

Successful completion of a homework assignment does not require high levels of behavioral performance at low levels of anxiety.

After the Assignment Is Completed

After the assigned homework task is done, it is time to return to self-administered cognitive restructuring activities. Just as described for cognitive restructuring after in-session exposures in Chapter 12, clients are asked to debrief the homework assignment in a way that can help them better manage their social anxiety. Clients should:

1. Ask themselves whether or not they met the agreed-on goals for the homework assignment, being very careful to *maintain a focus on assigned goals rather than desired goals*. Goal attainment should be viewed as a cause for great celebration, and clients should be encouraged to do nice things for themselves when they reach their goals.

2. Examine the validity of the ATs they had in anticipation of the situation. For this purpose, clients should select the one AT that was most distressing or important to them as they prepared to do their homework task. Clients should evaluate the evidence in support of the AT that they derived from the exposure task and record it on the BYOCT Worksheet. They should do the same for evidence derived from the exposure task that refutes the AT. Then the evidence for and against the AT should be carefully considered and the belief in the AT rerated.

3. Record their rational responses on the "Debriefing After the Exposure" portion of the BYOCT Worksheet. Clients should then check whether or not they used the rational responses and record the evidence in support of the rational responses in the proper space on the worksheet. After consideration of this evidence, they should rerate the degree of belief in the rational response. The BYOCT Worksheet also provides space for editing rational responses on the basis of the exposure experience.

4. Determine whether automatic thoughts occurred that were not anticipated. If so, the clients should write them down. If they were able to adequately deal with them using their cognitive coping skills, this is a positive sign of the generalization of cognitive coping skills to automatic thoughts that differ from the ones confronted in the group. If the clients had trouble responding to unexpected ATs during the exposure, they should address them at this time.

Be Your Own Cognitive Therapist (BYOCT) Worksheet

DATE	NAME

PREPARATION BEFORE THE EXPOSURE

1. **Situation** (*Briefly describe the anxiety-provoking situation.*)

2. **Automatic Thoughts** (*List the ATs you have about this situation and rate how strongly you believe each to be true on a 0–100 scale.*)	3. **Thinking Errors** (*see list below*)
EMOTIONS YOU FEEL AS YOU THINK THESE THOUGHTS (circle all that apply) anxious/nervous, angry, frustrated, sad, irritated, embarrassed, ashamed, hateful, other: _____	*THINKING ERRORS: All-or-Nothing Thinking, Overgeneralization, Mental Filter, Disqualifying the Positive, Mind Reading, Fortune Telling, Catastrophizing, Emotional Reasoning, "Should" Statements, Labeling, Maladaptive Thoughts*

4. **Challenges** (*Use the Disputing Questions below or others you prefer. Challenge the most important AT(s) you listed above. Be sure to answer the question raised by the Disputing Question.*)

DISPUTING QUESTIONS: Do I know for certain that _____ ? Am I 100% sure that _____ ? What evidence do I have that _____ ? What is the worst that could happen? How bad is that? Do I have a crystal ball? Is there another explanation for _____ ? Does _____ have to lead to or equal _____ ? Is there another point of view? What does _____ mean? Does _____ really mean that I am a(n) _____ ?

5. **Rational response(s)** (*Summarize the challenges into a rational statement to use to combat each AT. Rate the degree of your belief in the rational response(s) on a 0–100 scale*)

6. **Achievable behavioral goal** (*Something that you can do and that can be seen by others*)

DEBRIEFING AFTER THE EXPOSURE
7. Did you achieve your goal? (Watch out for Disqualifying the Positive! Give yourself credit.) *Check one:* Yes_____ No_____   If you did not meet your goal, describe what prevented you from doing so in the space below.
8. Which AT was most distressing or seemed most important as you prepared for the exposure? Write it in the space below.
What evidence do you have <u>from your exposure experience</u> that this AT was true? How valid is this evidence?   What evidence do you have <u>from your exposure experience</u> that this AT was in error? How valid is this evidence?   Rerate the degree of belief that you have in the AT on the 0–100 scale.   Has your belief in the AT decreased? (*check one*)   Yes_____ No_____ Current belief _____
9. What was your rational response?
Did you use it to combat these ATs? (*check one*) Yes_____ No_____   What evidence do you have <u>from your exposure experience</u> that your rational response may be true? Write it in the space below.   Rerate the degree of belief that you have in your rational response on the 0–100 scale.   Has your belief in the rational response increased? (*check one*)   Yes_____ No_____ Current belief _____   Was there any aspect of the rational response(s) that missed the mark? Do you need to revise it? Do so in the space below.
10. Did you have any unexpected ATs? Have you had any troublesome ATs about the exposure since it ended? (Challenge these ATs and develop rational responses for use with them)
11. **What Did You Learn?** (Summarize one or two main points you learned from this exposure that you can use in the future.)
Congratulate yourself for working hard to help yourself. Well done.

FIGURE 13.1. The Be Your Own Cognitive Therapist (BYOCT) Worksheet. Adapted from *Managing Social Anxiety: A Cognitive-Behavioral Therapy Approach* (Client Workbook) (Figure 7.1, pp. 125–126), by D. A. Hope, R. G. Heimberg, H. R. Juster, and C. L. Turk, 2000. Copyright 2000 by Graywind Publications. Adapted by permission.

5. Determine whether additional automatic thoughts occurred after the homework assignment was fully completed. These thoughts are likely to have a negative self-evaluative flavor and may involve the thinking errors of labeling ("I was such a jerk") or disqualifying the positive ("The conversation was OK, but I bet she won't be as nice the next time"). These thoughts are unlikely to have been anticipated by clients because their earlier imagining of the situation would be more likely to reveal anticipatory concerns. However, they may be quite important because clients may react to them by turning success into failure, trivializing goal attainment, and reducing their beliefs that they can successfully meet their goals. These ATs should also be addressed as part of the debriefing of the homework experience.

6. In the final section of the BYOCT Worksheet, clients should summarize their homework experience, attempting to derive one or two main points that they learned that can be applied to similar situations in the future.

Summary of Homework Procedures

The structure of homework assignments is consistent with the overall philosophy of CBGT, that cognitive and behavioral techniques are most effective when they are fully integrated with each other and when the techniques ultimately come to rest in the hands of the clients. However, clients are asked to complete a number of complex tasks, as well as to engage in potentially anxiety-provoking behaviors. As a means of helping clients remember the several steps of CBGT homework assignments, the Steps for Overcoming Social Anxiety with Exposure and Cognitive Restructuring form (Figure 13.2) should be distributed to each client in Session 3. When this form is distributed, clients should also be given extra copies of the List of Thinking Errors (Figure 10.1), the List of Disputing Questions (Figure 10.3), and the BYOCT Worksheet (Figure 13.1).

Sample Homework Tasks

In this section, we share a number of tasks that have been used by clients in our groups or in our broader experience in treating clients with social phobia. In most circumstances, specific homework tasks are derived from the needs of the specific client in relation to the requirements of his or her everyday life. Therapists should be careful to leave sufficient time for the discussion of homework tasks with clients (see Chapter 14 for a discussion of partitioning time in CBGT sessions). Because homework tasks are sometimes difficult to generate, suggested homework tasks are presented here for the major categories of concerns presented by clients with social phobia. Many of these suggestions are from Hope et al. (2000).[3]

**Steps for Overcoming Social Anxiety
with Exposure and Cognitive Restructuring**

Record responses on the BYOCT Worksheet for Homework Exposures.

Before entering the exposure situation . . .

1. Imagine yourself in the anxiety-provoking situation that you will work on.
2. Identify the automatic thoughts (ATs) you experience. Rate the degree of your belief in each AT on the 0–100 scale, and indicate the emotions related to your ATs.
3. Identify the Thinking Errors in each of your ATs.
4. Challenge one or two of the ATs that are most distressing to you with Disputing Questions. Be sure to answer the questions.
5. Summarize your answers to the Disputing Questions into a rational response.
6. Pick an achievable behavioral goal (or focus on the one that was agreed on in the group).

Enter the exposure situation . . .

Complete the exposure task, using your rational responses to help control your anxiety. Stay in the situation until it reaches a natural conclusion or until your anxiety decreases. Stay focused on your specific goals for this situation. Keep your eyes open so that you can learn the largest amount from your efforts.

After the exposure is over, debrief the experience . . .

7. Ask yourself whether you achieved your goal.
8. Refocus on the ATs you challenged before the exposure. Pick the one you found most distressing or that seemed most important as you prepared for the exposure. Evaluate the evidence for and against this AT. Rerate your belief in the AT on the 0–100 scale. Did it decrease?
9. Focus on your rational response. Evaluate the evidence that it is true. Rerate your belief in your rational response on the 0–100 scale. Did it increase? Does your rational response need any fine tuning? If so, take a moment to do so now.
10. Did you have any unexpected ATs? Take a moment to challenge them now. Also, have you had any distressing ATs since you finished the exposure task? Take a moment to challenge them now. Do not allow them to interfere with your success.
11. What is your final summary? Summarize what you can take from this experience that you can use in similar situations in the future.
12. Relax and reward yourself for your efforts. Remember to bring your written work to the next session.

FIGURE 13.2. Steps for Overcoming Social Anxiety with Exposure and Cognitive Restructuring. Adapted from *Managing Social Anxiety: A Cognitive-Behavioral Therapy Approach* (Client Workbook) (Figure 8.1, p. 132), by D. A. Hope, R. G. Heimberg, H. R. Juster, and C. L. Turk, 2000. Copyright 2000 by Graywind Publications. Adapted by permission.

It is recommended that clients read Chapters 7 and 8 in the Client Workbook, which address the first homework exposure and issues that arise in doing *in vivo* exposures during the rest of the group. Chapter 7 also includes a detailed example of a client's homework exposure and his completed efforts on an earlier version of the BYOCT Worksheet. Chapters 9 through 11 of the Client Workbook are content-specific and should be assigned to clients with fears of being observed or making mistakes in front of others (Chapter 9), fears of social interaction (Chapter 10), or fears of public speaking (Chapter 11).

Getting Started

- Make a list of what parts of your life reflect who you are and what parts reflect your social anxiety symptoms.
- Make a list of organizations that you would be interested in joining in order to meet new people.
- Look at the schedule of classes at local colleges or adult education facilities for offerings that might provide an opportunity for public speaking.
- Find out the meeting times and location of the local Toastmasters meeting and the name of the contact person.

Fear of Social Interaction

- Each day say hello to someone in your neighborhood or at your job.
- Talk to someone every Monday about what they did over the weekend.
- Talk to someone in the latter part of the week about their plans for the weekend.
- Invite someone to join you to do something that you enjoy doing on your own.
- Set a goal to start a conversation with at least one new person each week.
- Join an exercise club. Go. Say something to someone each day.
- Join a social club. Attend some of its functions. Talk to someone when you do.
- Join a charitable organization and participate in its functions.
- Join a church, synagogue, or other religious institution of your choice. Go.
- Invite someone to lunch. Do not hide behind work.
- Invite someone whom you find interesting to join you for dinner, a drink, or a show.
- Attend social evenings at local museums, free lectures, and concerts put on by local organizations.

Fear of Public Speaking

- Volunteer to be the person to present updates on projects at meetings.
- Express an opinion at a meeting when you would normally say nothing.
- Ask a question during or after a presentation or lecture.
- Serve as the chairperson for a committee at work or for a community organization.
- Read scriptures or a prayer aloud in front of the congregation at a religious service.
- Speak up at a self-help group or twelve-step meeting.
- Teach a class or lead a training with a group of people.
- Tell a joke or story to a group of people at a social gathering.

Eating in Front of Others

- Dine inside the fast-food restaurant rather than using the drive-through window.
- Eat at a deli rather than picking up something to take home.
- Invite coworkers, relatives, or friends to join you for lunch, dinner, or Sunday brunch either to your home or at a restaurant.
- Invite coworkers or friends to Happy Hour and have hors d'oeuvres.
- Choose items to eat that you find more anxiety provoking.
- Eat with chopsticks at Asian restaurants.
- Have at least a little bit of food whenever it is offered if it involves eating with others.
- Create extra opportunities for eating with others by bringing food to share with coworkers, family, or friends at occasions at which food would be appropriate but not necessarily present.
- Go to restaurants at times when they are more or less crowded, whichever is more difficult for you.

Drinking in Front of Others

- Carry something to drink with you whenever possible. Take any opportunity to drink when others are present.
- Stop at a fast-food restaurant or coffee shop and have your drink inside rather than getting something to go.
- If you are a member of a church, try to take communion whenever possible.
- Remove the straw from a drink (or use one if that is more anxiety provoking).

- Pick beverages (or types of containers) that you find more difficult to drink (or drink from) whenever possible.
- Invite coworkers, friends, or family to join you at events at which beverages will be served, such as meals, Happy Hour, and so forth.
- Take breaks at work with others and drink something.
- Be sure to order extra beverages when dining out, such as a beverage and water with the dinner and coffee after dinner, to provide more opportunities to practice.

Writing in Front of Others

- Write a check or use a credit card rather than paying cash.
- Do not start writing the check until it is your turn to check out at a store. Be sure to fill out the complete check and all of the details in your check register in front of everyone.
- Go inside the bank rather than using the drive-through window or the automatic teller.
- Go to banks and stores at the busiest time.
- Volunteer to take minutes at a meeting.
- Volunteer to write on the chalkboard or easel during a meeting or class.
- If you are making a presentation, try to write on a chalkboard or easel whenever possible.
- If there is more than one place to pay for items in a store, pay for part of your items in each place, using a check or credit card each time.
- Do your grocery shopping by purchasing a few items at several different stores, writing a check each time.
- Use a gas station at which you can pay by credit card to a cashier rather than just swiping your card at the pump.

Fears of Making Mistakes in Front of Others

- Take up a new hobby or sport and take a class. Some possibilities include instrumental or vocal music lessons, sports lessons (tennis, golf, etc.), dance classes, drawing or painting classes, arts and crafts classes, and woodworking classes.
- Take your dog to obedience classes. Even if you do everything right, your pet is likely to refuse your direction from time to time!
- Join a community sports team.
- Make harmless mistakes on purpose. Volunteer to read something aloud in a meeting and stumble over your words occasionally, pay for something with "exact change" but be over or under by a few cents, and so forth.

- Play games in which you are likely to make mistakes, such as trivia games or charades.
- If you are worried about spilling things, have a friend or family member help you by holding a glass while you pour in water. Deliberately pour in too much water so the glass overflows.
- Using water from a companion's glass in a restaurant, deliberately pour extra water into your own glass so it is difficult to drink without spilling a little. Repeatedly take a drink.

Homework Review and Assignment

The final homework question is, How does it fit into the flow of CBGT sessions? Therapists should bring their NCR copies of each client's assignment to the session so that each element of each client's assignment can be reviewed. If therapists rely only on their memories of multiple homework assignments to six different clients, they are likely to forget portions of one or more clients' homework assignments. They will then miss an opportunity to publicly recognize and support the client's courageous effort to confront anxiety or fail to help the client deal with a situation that resulted in avoidance rather than approach during the previous week. Each session begins with a period devoted to homework review. Each client who is not slated to be the target of an in-session exposure that evening is asked to tell the group what his or her homework assignment was and how it went. His or her account should include a description of the assignment, the goal, the things he or she learned in the cognitive preparation period, the behavioral outcome, and the results of the cognitive debriefing. With practice, CBGT therapists can train clients to give their accounting in 10 minutes or less (per client). Other clients report on their homework as they begin preparations for their in-session exposures. In most cases, the homework review should be considered a time for rewarding effort and focusing positive attention on the client rather than becoming involved in detailed cognitive restructuring activities. It is our experience that it is more difficult to do cognitive work that focuses on homework assignments than it is to do work that focuses on an in-session exposure (possibly because the client's view of the situation is more difficult to refute). When homework assignments do not go well, however, it is important to establish why, and this may lead into cognitive work.

It is generally a good idea for therapists to collect the clients' written homework assignments. Most important, clients' knowledge that therapists will examine their written homework may motivate them to complete these assignments and to do so with increased effort. Examination of clients' written work also provides important information about their depth of understanding of cognitive-behavioral concepts and the need for some individual tutorial on these concepts or other aspects of homework completion that may not have been well understood. Furthermore, clients may be more forthright about their ATs on paper than they may be in verbal interaction during the group. Armed with the information clients provide in this manner, therapists can guide discussion of clients' concerns so that the most important aspects are emphasized. Homework sheets should be returned to the clients for their future reference, but photocopies of their written work may be usefully retained.

At the end of the group session, 20 minutes should be devoted to speaking briefly with each client and negotiating a new homework assignment. Thereafter, the group meeting is adjourned.

We return to the topic of homework assignments again in the latter portion of Chapter 14, which presents a discussion of problems that may arise in the conduct of various aspects of CBGT and what to do about them.

Notes

1. From *Managing Social Anxiety: A Cognitive-Behavioral Therapy Approach* (Client Workbook) (p. 138), by D. A. Hope, R. G. Heimberg, H. R. Juster, and C. L. Turk, 2000. Copyright 2000 by Graywind Publications. Reprinted by permission.
2. The Be Your Own Cognitive Therapist Worksheet (Figure 13.1) and the Steps for Overcoming Social Anxiety with Exposure and Cognitive Restructuring (Figure 13.2) were adapted from the Client Workbook by Hope et al. (2000). Changes from the figures originally presented by Hope et al. are intended to increase their utility. However, if the Client Workbook is used as an adjunct to treatment with CBGT, these differences may be confusing to clients and should be brought to their attention.
3. From *Managing Social Anxiety: A Cognitive-Behavioral Therapy Approach* (Client Workbook) (pp. 153–155, 171–172), by D. A. Hope, R. G. Heimberg, H. R. Juster, and C. L. Turk, 2000. Copyright 2000 by Graywind Publications. Reprinted by permission.

14

Sessions 3–12: Putting It All Together and Troubleshooting Cognitive-Behavioral Group Therapy

In this chapter, we discuss several important topics. First, we discuss the review of homework and the introduction of in-session exposures in Session 3 and provide a list of needed materials for Session 3 and beyond. Second, we describe the partitioning of session time between in-session exposures and other activities in the remaining sessions of CBGT. Third, we discuss issues specific to the final session of CBGT. Fourth, we discuss the importance of posttreatment assessment and the potential need for future treatment planning. Fifth, we discuss the utility of booster sessions. Sixth, we discuss the process of advance planning for CBGT sessions. Next, we discuss in some detail the things that can go wrong in the conduct of CBGT and what to do about them. Finally, we provide a list of additional resources about various aspects of CBGT.

MATERIALS FOR SESSION 3 AND BEYOND

- Copies of the Brief Fear of Negative Evaluation Scale (Figure 6.4)
- Clipboards and pens
- Tape recorder and audiotapes
- Easel or chalkboard with markers or chalk
- Blank NCR sheets for new homework assignments
- Completed NCR sheets of homework assignments from last session
- Copies of the List of Thinking Errors (Figure 10.1)
- Copies of the List of Disputing Questions (Figure 10.3)

- Copies of the Be Your Own Cognitive Therapist Worksheet (Figure 13.1)
- Copies of Steps for Overcoming Social Anxiety with Exposure and Cognitive Restructuring (Figure 13.2)
- Copies of the Cognitive Restructuring Practice Form (Figure 10.4) (for use in Sessions 3–4 only)

It is a good idea to keep extra copies of these forms available throughout treatment.

TASKS FOR SESSIONS 3–11

- Assessment of Fear of Negative Evaluation
- Review of Homework Assignments
- In-Session Exposures
  - Cognitive Preparation
  - In-Session Exposure
  - Cognitive Debriefing
- Assignment of Homework for the Following Week

Reviewing Homework and Introducing In-Session Exposures in Session 3

The primary activity in Session 3 is the initiation of in-session exposures, but there are three prior tasks. First, clients should complete the BFNE as usual. Second, therapists and clients should debrief the homework assignment given at the end of Session 2. Clients were instructed to practice using the Cognitive Restructuring Practice Form (Figure 10.4) to identify the thinking errors in ATs they experienced during the week and to challenge a selected AT, culminating in the development of a rational response. They may also have been asked to read Chapter 6 from the Client Workbook. Clients' reaction to this assignment should be discussed and difficulties with the procedure addressed. When this has been achieved, therapists should introduce in-session exposures.

Hope et al. (2000) provide a summary of points for clients to keep in mind as they begin in-session exposures. The clients have the power to make the in-session exposures very positive and useful experiences for themselves or to reduce their impact.

Therapists should provide an outline of an in-session exposure (e.g., that a target situation will be selected, that the client will provide a list of ATs that will be the focus of disputation and cognitive restructuring efforts, that the client will be asked to repeat his or her Rational Response and provide Subjective Units of Discomfort Scale [SUDS] ratings at regular intervals, and that there will be further cognitive restructuring activity after the exposure is completed). Therapists and clients should then discuss Hope et al.'s (2000) list of *Do's and Don'ts for Exposures,*[1] which includes:

- DO throw yourself into the exposure as completely as possible.
- DON'T try to avoid the anxiety by interrupting the exposure or making it less realistic.
- DO say your rational response to yourself as ATs come up.
- DO repeat your rational response aloud when you give a SUDS rating.
- DO give SUDS ratings quickly without worrying about being too precise. Trying to be too precise can be a subtle way to avoid fully participating in the exposure.
- DO stay in role until your therapist says it is time to stop.
- DON'T be discouraged if it does not go as well as you would like. Remember it usually takes repeated exposures to fully conquer one's fears.

Therapists should make every attempt to keep things moving at a brisk pace in this session, as clients may be quite anxious in anticipation of the in-session exposures. It is critical that one in-session exposure take place in this session. A second should be attempted if time permits. When exposures are concluded for the session, targeted clients should receive homework assignments related to their in-session exposures, and the use of the Be Your Own Cognitive Therapist Worksheet should be described (see Chapter 13). The Steps for Overcoming Social Anxiety with Exposure and Cognitive Restructuring form (Figure 13.2) should be distributed, and clients should be instructed to refer to this form when completing the BYOCT Worksheet. Extra copies of the List of Thinking Errors and List of Disputing Questions should be distributed as needed. Clients who do not have an exposure in this session should repeat the assignment that they were given at the end of the previous session, using the Cognitive Restructuring Practice Form. Assignments may also be made from the Client Workbook, most notably Chapter 7, which includes examples of the use of an earlier form of the BYOCT Worksheet.

Partitioning Session Time

Time management is a potentially significant problem in the conduct of CBGT. Therefore, it is important to keep an eye on time and make sure that the session is moving along. As mentioned earlier, CBGT groups should last about 2½ hours per session. During Sessions 4–11 (presuming a 12-session group), therapists should attempt to adhere to the following schedule:

1. Before session: Administration and review of BFNEs.
2. 30 minutes: Review homework assignments for clients who are not scheduled for in-session exposure during the session.
3. 100 minutes: Conduct three in-session exposures, including homework review for the targeted clients (brief homework review followed by approximately 10 minutes of cognitive preparation, 10 minutes of in-session exposure, and 10 minutes of cognitive debriefing for each).
4. 20 minutes: Develop homework assignments for the next week.

This schedule is deceptively simple. It requires that there be little wasted time or discussion of tangential topics. Furthermore, it is quite important that therapists make every effort to conduct three in-session exposures in most sessions. Unless this goal is attained, it is unlikely that the clients will have received a sufficient "dose" of the active ingredients of CBGT. A form that we use to schedule in-session activities is reproduced in Figure 14.1. Many of the issues discussed later in the section on troubleshooting have to do with issues of time management.

Session 12: Consolidation of Gains and Looking to the Future

TASKS FOR SESSION 12

- Assessment of Fear of Negative Evaluation
- Review of Homework Assignments
- In-Session Exposures
- Identification of Clients' Accomplishments and Remaining Anxieties
- Setting of Future Goals for Each Client
- Identification of Methods to Accomplish Clients' Goals
- Recording and Distribution of Written Copies of Client Goals
- Final Good-byes

The twelfth session is important because it is the last one. Therapists may plan to conduct one or two in-session exposures in Session 12, but these should be devoted to preparing clients for real-life situations that will occur soon after the end of the group or to working on themes that have been addressed in previous in-session exposures. The final session is not a good time to introduce in-session exposures for situations that have not been previously addressed. The most important task in Session 12 is preparing the clients for life after CBGT.

At this time, clients will have reached different stages of relief from their social phobias. Few clients will have made no improvement, but it is the unusual client who is totally free of social anxiety, and every client will be faced with anxiety-provoking situations in the future. Therefore, CBGT therapists should attempt to instill the notions that further anxiety will be encountered and that the

CBGT In-Session Schedule

Date _____ Group # _____ Session # _____

Time	Activity	Clients	Therapists
_____	Homework Review #1	_____	_____
_____	Homework Review #2	_____	_____
_____	Homework Review #3	_____	_____
_____	Homework Review #4	_____	_____
_____	Set-up for Exposure #1	_____	_____
_____	Exposure	_____	_____
_____	Debriefing	_____	_____
_____	Homework Review #5	_____	_____
_____	Set-up for Exposure #2	_____	_____
_____	Exposure	_____	_____
_____	Debriefing	_____	_____
_____	Homework Review #6	_____	_____
_____	Set-up for Exposure #3	_____	_____
_____	Exposure	_____	_____
_____	Debriefing	_____	_____
_____	Assignment of Homework for the Coming Week	All	_____
_____	End of Session		

FIGURE 14.1. CBGT In-Session Schedule.

clients should maintain the same coping attitude toward future anxieties that they have learned during treatment. In a very real sense, clients should look at future anxiety-provoking situations as if each situation were a newly developed homework assignment. They should be encouraged to take the time to use their cognitive coping skills to confront these situations. Just as described in Chapter 13, they should devote time to cognitive preparations, do the anxiety-provoking deed, and conduct a cognitive debriefing.

Clients should read Chapter 13 of the Client Workbook in anticipation of
Session 12.

During the final session, each client should be asked to respond to a series of
questions:

- What have they accomplished during their treatment for social anxiety?
  - What anxieties have they learned to manage?
  - What new skills have they learned?
  - What changes have they made in their lives?
  - In what ways are they more self-confident?
  - What things have they done that they had not done before (or that they
    had not done for a long time)?
- What was the most important thing that they learned in CBGT that con-
  tributed to anxiety reduction?
- What disputing questions and rational responses were the most meaning-
  ful for them?
- What anxieties remain?
- What specific situations do they need to confront to overcome remaining
  anxieties?
- What specific goals can they set for themselves to help them combat
  these remaining anxieties?

Each client should be asked to set a specific goal that he or she will attempt
to accomplish within the next month. This goal should be written up as a
homework assignment and a copy provided to the client.

- Are there specific automatic thoughts that continue to bother them as they
  think about these goals and situations? What can they do to generate data
  that can undermine these automatic thoughts?

Therapists should strongly reinforce the progress that each client has made
and convey their belief that continued use of cognitive coping skills will lead to
continued anxiety reduction. It is useful to share with clients that this is, in
fact, what we have seen with many clients who have gone before. Therapists
should also indicate their willingness to serve as consultants to clients who are
faced with difficult situations in the future, as discussed in the following
section.

Finally, we have routinely observed that clients are often loath to leave the
final CBGT session. They will often hang around, talking to therapists and other

clients for extended periods of time, not wanting to make final good-byes. As a means of formally recognizing this desire, we make refreshments available and encourage clients to stay for awhile, to chat, and to take their leave as they wish.

Termination Issues

Of course, termination issues arise in all types of psychotherapy, and CBGT is no exception. Many of these issues are well addressed in the topics discussed in Session 12. However, it is wise to raise the time-limited nature of the group earlier in treatment. For instance, we mention at the beginning of Session 7 that we are now entering the second half of the group. Clients are encouraged to take a more active role in designing their in-session exposures and homework assignments and in conducting their own cognitive restructuring. They are also encouraged to make sure that the topics that are most important to them are raised for attention in the remaining sessions. The upcoming end of group sessions may also generate a number of automatic thoughts—it is not uncommon for clients to worry that they will not be able to sustain their momentum or that they may lose their hard-fought gains after therapy sessions have concluded or when they will no longer have regular contact with one or both of the therapists. These ATs should be addressed as any others that have come up over the course of treatment. It is not necessary to wait until Session 12 to discuss these topics.

Posttreatment Assessment

In Chapter 6, we outlined an approach to the assessment of clients' presenting concerns. We would like to make a strong pitch for the importance of repeating the assessment at the conclusion of the group. We recommend that this assessment include at least one instrument from each of the primary domains of assessment, that is, a clinician-administered scale such as the Liebowitz Social Anxiety Scale, a self-report scale such as the Social Interaction Anxiety Scale, and a behavioral assessment of the clients' specific situation(s) of concern. The BFNE from the last session should also be available as a measure of change in the cognitive arena, and a measure of general functioning such as the Quality of Life Inventory is also quite useful. It is our experience that clients often have a tendency to minimize or disqualify the changes they have made in the absence of cold hard data.

Each CBGT client should have an individual exit interview with one of the group therapists, and this interview should include a discussion of the posttreatment assessment data and a broader discussion of the client's progress toward important personal goals. Clients who have made relatively less progress will especially benefit from this, as their remaining anxieties and the need for (and type of) additional treatment can be thoroughly discussed. If medication is to be considered as a possible future option, the therapist and client might consult Chapter 14 of the Client Workbook, which focuses on pharmacotherapy for social anxiety.

Additional Sessions

It should be standard practice to make available to clients the opportunity to return to treatment in the future. This may be an additional trial of CBGT or individual cognitive-behavioral therapy in cases in which there is significant return of anxiety or, more commonly, a brief series of individual sessions (usually only two or three) when the client is confronted with an upcoming event that he or she finds overwhelming. It is not uncommon for clients who have done very well in CBGT to continue to progress but then to hit a stumbling block. Curiously, the difficult situation may be one they would never have confronted prior to treatment. For instance, many socially avoidant clients may have come to treatment with no history of significant sexual relationships. Many may never have dated at all. After treatment, however, a client may have significantly reduced this anxiety and may have started to date regularly. He or she develops a meaningful relationship with another person, and all appears to be going well. Then, for whatever reasons, the other person decides the relationship is not right for them. These events happen every day, but they are new and shocking for many persons with social phobia, and they may signal the occurrence of extreme distress and the return of anxiety and self-doubt. Without intervention, this client may be at increased risk for relapse, but if he or she has an open invitation for a brief set of individual booster sessions, this outcome may be averted. These sessions should be true to the format of CBGT, including a slimmed-down version of in-session exposures with the therapist as role player and focusing on the new situation as a homework assignment to be confronted.

In our research, we have sometimes conducted booster sessions for CBGT groups. After 12 weeks of standard treatment, groups have continued to meet for an additional six to seven sessions at monthly intervals. This strategy *may* promote stabilization of gains and reduce risk for relapse, but our studies have not yielded clear data in this regard.

Another version of "booster sessions" was introduced to us by one of our own CBGT groups. This particular group of clients responded very well to treatment. Although several group members were virtually asymptomatic, they did not feel ready to abandon CBGT, regular meetings, or each other. They chose, quite on their own, to continue regular meetings at a restaurant across the street from the clinic. Since that time, we have encouraged other groups to do so as well.

Session Planning in Cognitive-Behavioral Group Therapy

In this section, we want to share with you a bit about our approach to session planning in CBGT. It is our standard practice to meet weekly, after reviewing the session tape if possible, to discuss issues that arose in the previous session and to prepare for the upcoming one. We pay special attention to in-session exposures or homework assignments that did not go as well as planned, looking either to improve the structure so that it is easier for the client to comply or to reorient the client to focus on specific automatic thoughts that may have arisen during the exposures or homework assignments. Many of these activities are discussed in the next section.

At each planning meeting, we also develop a blueprint for the upcoming session using the form provided in Figure 14.1. We anticipate which clients, in what order, will be targeted for in-session exposures. Specific topics for these exposures are generated, although clients will be given the choice of the generated topic or other topics that seem more important at the moment. We also generate topics for clients for whom an in-session exposure may not be planned, in order to protect against unannounced absences of targeted group members. A similar approach is taken to generate a list of potential homework assignments for relevant clients.

In constructing in-session exposures, the need to recruit additional personnel or obtain specific props is determined. Specific instructions to be given to recruited role players are developed if necessary. Furthermore, it is useful to anticipate how each targeted client might react to his or her exposure topic. How anxious might the client become? What ATs is he or she likely to experience? How might the restructuring of those ATs be approached? Advance planning of this nature allows the therapists to use their time most efficiently in session.

Troubleshooting Cognitive-Behavioral Group Therapy

Problems that may arise in CBGT are many and varied. In this section, we address difficulties relating to in-session exposures, cognitive restructuring activities, and homework assignments.

In-Session Exposures

We previously mentioned the potential problem that the target client may experience no anxiety during the in-session exposure. Of course, this is not automatically a problem. The client may have expected to be anxious, may have participated fully in the in-session exposure, and may have coped so well that anxiety was never experienced. However, this does not happen as often as we would like!

When no anxiety is reported, the reason is likely to stem from one of three sources. First, the client may be anxious but unwilling to report it. Second, the key anxiety-evoking aspects of the feared situation may not have been incorporated into the in-session exposure. Third, the client may have engaged in some sort of disqualification of the in-session exposure experience, thinking to himself or herself that the in-session exposure is not real, that it does not matter anyway, and so forth. Each of these problems requires a unique solution.

If the client does not report or underreports anxiety that he or she has experienced, the reason is probably that he or she has the automatic thought that admission of anxiety equals failure, reflects badly on his or her competence, or will lead to rejection by the group. In this situation, it is likely that the client will exhibit behavioral signs of anxiety that are inconsistent with his or her self-report. Gently and supportively pointing this out to the client may lead to an examination of automatic thoughts related to reporting anxiety. Generally, this problem disappears after the first few in-session exposures, as the client sees other clients report anxiety without the feared consequences.

If the client reports that the in-session exposure simply did not provoke anxiety, the structure of the in-session exposure itself must be examined. As noted in Chapter 11, it is possible that the specific ingredient that the client fears was not included in the exposure or was not sufficiently prominent. The key feature may have been overlooked in the original planning of the in-session exposure, or the other role players may simply not have executed their roles well enough. In the first case, it is back to the drawing board to try to do a better job next time. In the second case, it will be necessary to do a more thorough job of instructing role players on the desired behaviors, to carefully select role players who are more capable of producing the desired effect, or to recruit role players from outside the group who possess the desired characteristics or skills.

If the client reports no anxiety and it appears that he or she has disqualified the experience, further analysis of the reasons will be necessary. The client may have a problem accepting the overall treatment rationale. If the client does not believe that the activities of CBGT will be helpful, there is little reason that he or she should expose himself or herself to additional anxiety. Alternately, the selected situation may simply be too difficult or frightening for the client, and the therapists should consider a less anxiety-provoking situation for the next in-session exposure. It must be stressed to the client, however, that cognitive avoidance will lead only to a diminution of treatment gains.

Another problem with in-session exposures may arise when group members are selected to serve as role players. Although this is generally a good strategy and should be followed whenever possible, there will be times that it will cause problems. These clients may experience anxiety of their own in the role they are asked to play, and as a result, they may become inhibited in the role play. As previously stated, other group members with fears similar to those of the target client should generally not be selected as role players unless the in-session exposure is construed as a combined exercise targeting multiple clients. For example, a woman with fears of men is a poor selection for an in-session exposure for a male client with fears of women, and vice versa. Alternately, clients may be overly concerned about causing anxiety for the target client and may tend to make the in-session exposure too easy for him or her. For instance, if silences are feared by the target client in an in-session exposure of a heterosocial interaction, the other client may tend to jump in and break silences prematurely. It is important to thoroughly discuss these issues with the role-playing client before the in-session exposure begins. The in-session exposure can be stopped and started again if the role-playing client's behavior is problematic.

In-session exposures may turn out badly if the target client's worst fears do come true. This is best avoided by having the client attempt less difficult situations before more difficult ones. However, it will never be totally avoided. If this occurs, the therapists should adopt an attitude of support and encouragement, the client should examine whether the feared event was in fact as awful as he or she predicted, and, if it was, the group should talk about what the client may do in future in-session exposures to reduce the chances of this outcome. It is often the result of the target client's unbending focus on the possibility of the negative outcome and represents a self-fulfilling prophecy.

Cognitive Restructuring

Problems in conducting cognitive restructuring can be broadly categorized into two groups, those presented by clients and those arising from the behavior of therapists.

CLIENT PROBLEMS

A very common problem is the client who reports no thoughts about a specific situation despite the presence of high anxiety. Clients often experience a number of automatic thoughts about anxiety-provoking situations but conceptualize them as feelings or reactions rather than thoughts. This may become quickly apparent if therapists follow a report of no thoughts with such questions as, "What did you think might happen in that situation?" or "What were you worried about?" Clients who staunchly report that "I don't think, I just get anxious" typically respond to these questions with a torrent of automatic thoughts. In general, it is best to avoid arguing with clients that, of course, they think.

Early in the treatment process, clients may not recognize or accept the notion that their thoughts are distorted or irrational. Even if there are clear logical errors in clients' reported thoughts, persuasion or argument is unlikely to open their minds. It may be more successful to focus, as Persons (1989) suggests, on the notion of maladaptive thoughts. Whether or not a thought is irrational, it may not be in the client's best interest to focus on it (see Chapter 10). Therapists can also suggest to the client that they design a behavioral experiment to test the client's predictions. The results of the behavioral experiment may carry more weight than arm twisting.

A small number of clients do not grasp the central concepts of CBGT. Although this is not a frequent problem, every therapist will confront it sooner or later. CBGT is sufficiently flexible that several options are available. First, therapists may simply deemphasize the cognitive portion of CBGT and focus more heavily on repeated exposure. Second, the therapists may reduce the complexity of cognitive restructuring tasks for the client who is overly concrete in his or her thinking. Following this strategy, CBGT becomes "repeated exposure with self-statement substitution." That is, it is possible to work with the client to develop a specific set of self-instructions that they will apply in anxiety-provoking situations. The concrete-thinking client will be likely to repeat these self-instructions verbatim when anxious, but we have seen several benefit with this procedure.

THERAPIST PROBLEMS

First and foremost among therapist problems is poor time management. As noted earlier, it is important to stay focused on the business of CBGT in order to complete three in-session exposures per session. Therapists can seriously reduce their chances of accomplishing this goal by allowing clients to tell long and detailed stories about their anxious experiences, and this should be avoided. Clients may give long-winded presentations because they are unsure of the aspects that are most important for discussion, and they should be aided in this selection by therapists' questions. Clients may also learn that long accounts of homework or of situations that are troubling them may allow them to put off the beginning of an in-session exposure and the anxiety that goes with it.

Therapists may make other decisions that will result in poor time management and otherwise undermine the effectiveness of CBGT. They may be overly complete in their solicitation of automatic thoughts before an in-session exposure. Similarly, they may attempt to dispute too many automatic thoughts at that time. However, it serves little purpose to generate 10 or 12 automatic thoughts, attempt to identify the thinking errors in each one of them, and dispute each one. To do so simply generates more information than a client can retain, and it will be of little use to him or her during in-session exposures or homework assignments. Clients may also find it difficult to keep their attention focused on cognitive restructuring activities for the extended period required for exhaustive analysis of several automatic thoughts and may find themselves either drifting off topic or becoming focused on the anxiety-provoking aspects of the upcoming in-scssion exposure. As suggested in Chapter 13, it is far better to focus on a smaller sample of ATs—one or two is plenty—and do a thorough job with them.

Therapists should exercise care in the selection of automatic thoughts for attention during cognitive restructuring. It is a frequent mistake of beginning CBGT therapists to question thoughts that are unlikely to lead to productive change. As in the example provided in Chapter 12, it is unlikely to be productive to challenge thoughts such as "I'll be anxious" in the early part of treatment. Because the client has plenty of history with the situation in which he or she *has* been anxious or because he or she has had plenty of time to catastrophize about it, the client is unlikely to yield. Also, as long as the client holds distorted beliefs about the negative consequences of his or her behavior in the situation, the client's prediction of anxiety is not entirely incorrect. It matters little that "I'll be anxious" may represent all-or-nothing thinking or fortune telling. On the other hand, thoughts about the specific negative consequences may be more open for modification, and successful change in these beliefs may undermine the reasons that the client predicts anxiety in the first place. Therapists should select automatic thoughts for attention based on their representation of the client's cognitive structure and how specific automatic thoughts relate to it. Attack the cognitive structure from the periphery rather than the center.

The "peripheral versus central" distinction is an important one to keep in mind. Especially early in treatment, ATs that are reflections of a client's most closely held and distorted core beliefs are unlikely to yield to cognitive restructuring efforts. These thoughts (e.g., "I am incompetent" or "I am unlovable") represent ideas about themselves that clients hold as absolute truths if they have reflected on them at all. Intermediate beliefs such as "If I prepare for hours and hours for my presentation, then I may not humiliate myself" are somewhat more amenable to change because of their conditional, if–then nature. However, thoughts that focus on specific, observable, or verifiable outcomes of specific situations will be most amenable to change because the accuracy or inaccuracy of the thought can ultimately be examined or made the focus of a behavioral experiment. It is much easier to evaluate the accuracy of the expectation that the audience will laugh at the client if he loses his train of thought than it is to evaluate whether he will be found competent or acceptable at judgment day.

Because automatic thoughts are embedded in a cognitive structure, even the most peripheral automatic thoughts do not change easily. Therefore, therapists should expect clients to reject their efforts to help them think more rationally. Supportive persistence on the part of therapists is an absolute requirement for the conduct of CBGT. Impatient therapists are likely to argue with clients that their thoughts are distorted and may even tell the client what the "correct" thoughts are. There is hardly a less effective strategy available to the CBGT therapist than this!

Therapists may make a similar mistake because of time-management concerns or simply because they have not developed an effective strategy for using directive questioning. They may tell the client what his or her automatic thoughts are, what thinking errors they contain, and what a good rational response might be. The therapists may not come across in an argumentative fashion, but their behavior is still poorly considered. Clients need to do most of their own work in order to learn the skills necessary for long-lasting change. By the end of treatment, they need to know that they can do "it" without the therapists' assistance. Therapists must lead them through it, but therapists must not do it for them!

Another common error is to act as if all cognitive restructuring work must be completed before the exposure begins. This irrational therapist belief will result in drawn-out episodes of cognitive restructuring that degenerate into arguments between therapists and client or into overt agreement by the client to something he or she does not really accept. It is important to lead the client through the prescribed steps of cognitive restructuring before the exposure, but the client need not thoroughly believe the alternatives to his or her automatic thoughts before they have been put to the test. Therapists should never forget that *the in-session exposure is their most effective cognitive restructuring weapon*. If a client does not see something in discussion, he or she might very well see it in exposure. Don't get bogged down in unproductive cognitive restructuring activities. Move on to the in-session exposure, and get on with it!

Homework Assignments Gone Awry

Several difficulties may arise in the development or conduct of homework assignments. Problems that occur with homework completion (i.e., the application of cognitive coping skills in personally relevant anxiety-provoking situations) are a major reason for failures in CBGT. These problems demand the attention of therapists and their creative efforts to solve them.

The first problem is that it may simply be difficult to come up with an appropriate homework assignment. Some clients may experience extreme anxiety, but only in situations that occur infrequently. Consider, for example, the socially anxious college professor who is fearful of speaking in front of others but whose anxiety is only intrusive when presenting a paper at a meeting of an academic society. However, the opportunities to attend conferences are limited by his or her department's travel budget. He or she may discount other speaking opportunities because the audience does not have the relevant expertise and therefore may not have the capacity to pass negative judgment on his or her work.

Similarly, clients may have made choices to avoid situations that are anxiety provoking. The person who is generally fearful of others and has worked for years as a night watchman may have few opportunities to interact with others. The person who fears giving presentations in graduate school is unlikely to be enrolled when he or she seeks treatment. In general, clients may be too fearful to make dramatic steps to avail themselves of opportunities to be anxious! However, they must be encouraged to do so. With clients who have little opportunity for relevant homework assignments as they enter treatment, the first few assignments may be oriented toward the creation of homework opportunities. The socially isolated person may be encouraged to join a health club or a social organization that will provide opportunities for social interaction. The student with public-speaking fears may be encouraged to enroll in a course on public speaking. The college professor may be encouraged to present his or her work at brown-bag symposia or departmental colloquia or to take advantage of organizations such as Toastmasters International, in which he or she can learn much about public speaking and can address audiences with a broad range of expertise. As a clearly second-best solution, but one that may have to be utilized with clients who are afraid to make these steps early in treatment, the client may be asked to complete the portions of homework assignments that do not involve behavioral performance. That is, he or she may be asked to visualize the target situation and list, categorize, and dispute the automatic thoughts that occur to him or her during the visualization.

Once a homework assignment has been devised, numerous problems may still arise. Of course, one of these is that the client simply does not complete the assignment. It is important here to avoid the implication that the client is "bad" for not doing his or her homework, both because this is moralistic and paternalistic and because clients with social phobia may react poorly to perceived negative evaluation by the therapists. At the same time, it is necessary to determine the reasons for the failure. One possibility is that the therapists did not involve the client in the selection and design of the homework assignment and that the client did not accept it. Because many clients with social phobia have problems with assertive behavior, it is unlikely that the client would have complained about this in the group session. Although it is important for therapists to obtain the cooperation of clients in carrying out homework assignments, they must also be certain that the client's assent is honest. Another reason for the failure to complete homework is procrastination or avoidance. The client may decide that the assignment can be completed tomorrow, or the next day, or the next day. Before he or she knows it, the week is over. Alternately, the client may have avoided the assignment because it was simply too scary. It may not have seemed so tough during the group meeting, but when it came time to do the homework, it was overwhelming. In this case, the therapists can assign specific cognitive restructuring homework in which the client is asked to assess the true dangerousness of the homework situation; they can assign a situation that is less difficult; or they can assign a "buddy," another client whom the first client can call for a dose of support and encouragement before the homework assignment is attempted.

Clients often come to the group meeting and report that they did not complete their homework assignment but that the reasons for their failure to do so were beyond their control. In fact, there is often some truth to what the clients are saying. When a client is assigned the task of stating an opinion at a once-a-week staff meeting, he or she may be left high and dry if the meeting is cancelled because the boss is sick. The client assigned to call a female acquaintance and ask her out may call several times only to find out that she is away on vacation. The client who must confront a professor about a course grade will find it hard to do so when the professor is off at a professional meeting. It is important to ascertain whether the client is telling the truth or attempting to cover up avoidance and save face, as we found in the recent case of a client who was assigned the task of going to a grocery store during a busy time and making conversation with the other people in the checkout line. He reported to us that he went to the grocery store every day after work (a typically busy time), but there was never anyone in line. Of course there was, but the client was not one of them! However, the important point is this: If the client is unable to complete a homework assignment as agreed on in the group because of an unexpected circumstance, he or she needs to think of other ways to capture the spirit of the assignment. The first client described above may look for other arenas in which he might express a contrary opinion; the second client might consider calling someone else; the third might consider talking to another authority figure if one is available; and so forth. Clients should be encouraged to do whatever they can whenever possible to help themselves overcome anxiety. This is the "homework attitude" described previously.

Of course, the client may complete a homework assignment in ways that are problematic. One common problem is that clients do not take the time to do the necessary cognitive preparations. These steps are often arduous and involve thinking about something that is unpleasant and anxiety provoking. However, failure to do cognitive preparations may increase the probability of an unsatisfactory homework outcome, and clients should be strongly encouraged to complete the preparations. There are also times when clients, even when well prepared, find it hard to utilize cognitive coping skills in the actual homework situation. The situation itself may overwhelm the client and capture his or her attention so that it is hard to focus on anything else. In this case, we have found it useful to recommend that the client visualize the situation, imagining himself or herself actually practicing the coping self-statements that were derived in the group or in earlier homework preparations. These cognitive rehearsals appear to render rational responses more available to clients when they are in the heat of anxious battle.

Clients may attempt homework assignments and, in fact, complete them successfully. However, it is not unusual for a client to appear quite upset over what seems to be a positive outcome. In these situations, it is almost a certainty that the client has somehow disqualified his or her success. It is likely that the client, although agreeing to a specific behavioral goal, has not truly embraced it. Instead, he or she may still maintain that the only acceptable goal is flawless performance without anxiety. Of course, this perfectionistic goal is as pernicious in homework as it is in in-session exposures. Alternatively, the client may recognize his or her successful performance but trivialize it (disqualifying the positive). He may decide that it wasn't that hard to begin with, that she doesn't know what she was getting so worked up about, or that the successful performance was a result of the other person's generosity rather than the client's efforts. These types of thinking errors about homework performance need to be addressed in the same way as any other thinking errors that might arise during group.

Finally, the client may attempt a homework assignment, and it may turn out badly. The other person may have a negative reaction to the client, the client may enter the situation and freeze, and so forth. Homework failures may decrease the client's sense of self-efficacy and increase his or her desire to avoid difficult situations. It is important, although not easy, to help the client adopt a problem-solving set about the homework failure. What went wrong? What can be learned from it that may help the client in future situations? Depending on the circumstances, it may even be useful to ask the client whether the experience was as horrible as he or she expected it to be. Often, it is not!

Additional Source Materials for Cognitive-Behavioral Group Therapy

In this final section, we provide source material on other aspects of CBGT for social phobia that could not be covered in this book. Following is a list of articles and chapters that describe (1) the specifics of the clinical treatment of clients who participated in CBGT, (2) the outcomes of studies of the clinical efficacy of CBGT in comparison with control groups, exposure therapy, and pharmacotherapy, and (3) the findings of studies regarding both person and process factors that may influence the outcome of CBGT. The last group is a list of selected papers that review, either qualitatively or with meta-analytic methods, the efficacy of cognitive-behavioral approaches to the treatment of social phobia, not specifically limited to CBGT. These papers are not listed in the reference section of this book unless they were cited in other chapters.

Clinical Reports of Individuals Treated with CBGT

Gruber, K., & Heimberg, R. G. (1997). A cognitive-behavioral treatment package for social anxiety. In W. T. Roth (Ed.), *Treatments for anxiety disorders* (pp. 245–279). San Francisco: Jossey-Bass.

Heimberg, R. G., & Juster, H. R. (1994). Treatment of social phobia in cognitive behavioral groups. *Journal of Clinical Psychiatry, 55*(6, Suppl.), 38–46.

Heimberg, R. G., Juster, H. R., Hope, D. A., & Mattia, J. I. (1995). Cognitive behavioral group treatment for social phobia: Description, case presentation and empirical support. In M. B. Stein (Ed.), *Social phobia: Clinical and research perspectives* (pp. 293–321). Washington, DC: American Psychiatric Press.

Hope, D. A., & Heimberg, R. G. (1990). Dating anxiety. In H. Leitenberg (Ed.), *Handbook of social and evaluative anxiety* (pp. 217–246). New York: Plenum Press.

Hope, D. A., & Heimberg, R. G. (1993). Social phobia and social anxiety. In D. H. Barlow (Ed.), *Clinical handbook of psychological disorders: A step-by-step treatment manual* (2nd ed., pp. 99–136). New York: Guilford Press.

Hope, D. A., & Heimberg, R. G. (1994). Social phobia. In. C. Last & M. Hersen (Eds.), *Adult behavior therapy casebook* (pp. 125–138). New York: Plenum Press.

Turk, C. L., Heimberg, R. G., & Hope, D. A. (2001). Social anxiety disorder. In D. H. Barlow (Ed.), *Clinical handbook of psychological disorders: A step-by-step treatment manual* (3rd ed., pp. 114–153). New York: Guilford Press.

Empirical Studies of the Efficacy of CBGT

Gelernter, C. S., Uhde, T. W., Cimbolic, P., Arnkoff, D. B., Vittone, B. J., Tancer, M. E., & Bartko, J. J. (1991). Cognitive-behavioral and pharmacological treatments for social phobia: A controlled study. *Archives of General Psychiatry, 48,* 938–945.

Heimberg, R. G., Dodge, C. S., Hope, D. A., Kennedy, C. R., Zollo, L., & Becker, R. E. (1990). Cognitive behavioral group treatment of social phobia: Comparison to a credible placebo control. *Cognitive Therapy and Research, 14,* 1–23.

Heimberg, R. G., Liebowitz, M. R., Hope, D. A., Schneier, F. R., Holt, C. S., Welkowitz, L., Juster, H. R., Campeas, R., Bruch, M. A., Cloitre, M., Fallon, B., & Klein, D. F. (1998). Cognitive-behavioral group therapy versus phenelzine in social phobia: 12-week outcome. *Archives of General Psychiatry, 55,* 1133–1141.

Heimberg, R. G., Salzman, D., Holt, C. S., & Blendell, K. (1993). Cognitive behavioral group treatment of social phobia: Effectiveness at 5-year follow-up. *Cognitive Therapy and Research, 17,* 325–339.

Hope, D. A., Heimberg, R. G., & Bruch, M. A. (1995). Dismantling cognitive-behavioral group therapy for social phobia. *Behaviour Research and Therapy, 33,* 637–650.

Liebowitz, M. R., Heimberg, R. G., Schneier, F. R., Hope, D. A., Davies, S., Holt, C. S., Goetz, D., Juster, H. R., Lin, S.-L., Bruch, M. A., Marshall, R., & Klein, D. F. (1999). Cognitive-behavioral group therapy versus phenelzine in social phobia: Long-term outcome. *Depression and Anxiety, 10,* 89–98.

Otto, M. W., Pollack, M. H., Gould, R. A., Worthington, J. J., McArdle, E. T., Rosenbaum, J. F., & Heimberg, R. G. (2000). A comparison of the efficacy of clonazepam and cognitive-behavioral group therapy for the treatment of social phobia. *Journal of Anxiety Disorders, 14,* 345–358.

Factors That May Influence Response to CBGT

Bruch, M. A., Heimberg, R. G., & Hope, D. A. (1991). States of mind model and cognitive change in treated social phobics. *Cognitive Therapy and Research, 15,* 429–441.

Brown, E. J., Heimberg, R. G., & Juster, H. R. (1995). Social phobia subtype and avoidant personality disorder: Effect on severity of social phobia, impairment, and outcome of cognitive-behavioral treatment. *Behavior Therapy, 26,* 467–486.

Chambless, D. L., Tran, G. Q., & Glass, C. R. (1997). Predictors of response to cognitive-behavioral group therapy for social phobia. *Journal of Anxiety Disorders, 11,* 221–240.

Coles, M. E., Hart, T. A., & Heimberg, R. G. (2001). Cognitive-behavioral group treatment for social phobia. In R. Crozier & L. E. Alden (Eds.), *International handbook of social anxiety* (pp. 449–469). Chichester, England: Wiley.

Edelman, R. E., & Chambless, D. L. (1995). Adherence during sessions and homework in cognitive-behavioral group treatment of social phobia. *Behaviour Research and Therapy, 33,* 573–577.

Hope, D. A., Herbert, J. D., & White, C. (1995). Diagnostic subtype, avoidant personality disorder, and efficacy of cognitive behavioral group therapy for social phobia. *Cognitive Therapy and Research, 19,* 399–417.

Leung, A. W., & Heimberg, R. G. (1996). Homework compliance, perceptions of control, and outcome of cognitive-behavioral treatment of social phobia. *Behaviour Research and Therapy, 34,* 423–432.

Safren, S. A., Heimberg, R. G., & Juster, H. R. (1997). Client expectancies and their relationship to pretreatment symptomatology and outcome of cognitive-behavioral group treatment for social phobia. *Journal of Consulting and Clinical Psychology, 65,* 694–698.

Schoenberger, N. E., Kirsch, I., Gearan, P., Montgomery, G., & Pastyrnak, S. (1997). Hypnotic enhancement of cognitive-behavioral treatment for public speaking anxiety. *Behavior Therapy, 28,* 127–140.

Woody, S. R., Chambless, D. L., & Glass, C. R. (1997). Self-focused attention in the treatment of social phobia. *Behaviour Research and Therapy, 35,* 117–129.

Recent Empirical Reviews of Cognitive-Behavioral Therapy for Social Phobia

Federoff, I. C., & Taylor, S. (2001). Psychological and pharmacological treatments for social phobia: A meta-analysis. *Journal of Clinical Psychopharmacology, 21,* 311–324.

Feske, U., & Chambless, D. L. (1995). Cognitive behavioral versus exposure only treatment for social phobia: A meta-analysis. *Behavior Therapy, 26,* 695–720.

Fresco, D. M., Erwin, B. A., Heimberg, R. G., & Turk, C. L. (2000). Social and specific phobias. In M. Gelder, N. Andreasen, & J. Lopez-Ibor (Eds.), *New Oxford textbook of psychiatry* (pp. 794–807). Oxford, England: Oxford University Press.

Gould, R. A., Buckminster, S., Pollack, M. H., Otto, M. W., & Yap, L. (1997). Cognitive-behavioral and pharmacological treatment for social phobia: A meta-analysis. *Clinical Psychology: Science and Practice, 4,* 291–306.

Heimberg, R. G. (2001). Current status of psychotherapeutic interventions for social phobia. *Journal of Clinical Psychiatry, 62*(Suppl.), 36–42.

Juster, H. R., & Heimberg, R. G. (1998). Social phobia. In A. S. Bellack & M. Hersen (Eds.), *Comprehensive clinical psychology* (Vol. 6, pp. 475–498). Oxford, England: Pergamon Press.

Taylor, S. (1996). Meta-analysis of cognitive-behavioral treatments for social phobia. *Journal of Behavior Therapy and Experimental Psychiatry, 27,* 1–9.

Turk, C. L., Coles, M., & Heimberg, R. G. (2002). Psychotherapy for social phobia. In D. J. Stein & E. Hollander (Eds.), *Textbook of anxiety disorders* (pp. 323–339). Washington, DC: American Psychiatric Press.

Turk, C. L., Fresco, D. M., & Heimberg, R. G. (1999). Social phobia: Cognitive behavior therapy. In M. Hersen & A. S. Bellack (Eds.), *Handbook of comparative treatments of adult disorders* (2nd ed., pp. 287–316). New York: Wiley.

Note

1. From *Managing Social Anxiety: A Cognitive-Behavioral Therapy Approach* (Client Workbook) (p. 117), by D. A. Hope, R. G. Heimberg, H. R. Juster, and C. L. Turk, 2000. Copyright 2000 by Graywind Publications. Reprinted by permission.

References

Abramson, L. Y., Seligman, M. E. P., & Teasdale, J. D. (1978). Learned helplessness in humans: Critique and reformulation. *Journal of Abnormal Psychology, 87,* 49–74.

Alden, L. E., & Bieling, P. (1998). Interpersonal consequences of the pursuit of safety. *Behaviour Research and Therapy, 36,* 53–64.

Alden, L. E., Bieling, P., & Wallace, S. T. (1994). Perfectionism in an interpersonal context: A self-regulation analysis of dysphoria and social anxiety. *Cognitive Therapy and Research, 18,* 297–316.

Alden, L. E., & Wallace, S. T. (1991). Social standards and social withdrawal. *Cognitive Therapy and Research, 15,* 85–100.

Alden, L. E., & Wallace, S. T. (1995). Social phobia and social appraisal in successful and unsuccessful social interactions. *Behaviour Research and Therapy, 33,* 497–505.

Alnaes, R., & Torgersen, S. (1988). The relationship between DSM-III symptom disorders (Axis I) and personality disorders (Axis II) in an outpatient population. *Acta Psychiatrica Scandinavica, 78,* 485–492.

American Psychiatric Association. (1980). *Diagnostic and statistical manual of mental disorders* (3rd ed.). Washington, DC: Author.

American Psychiatric Association. (1987). *Diagnostic and statistical manual of mental disorders* (3rd ed., rev.). Washington, DC: Author.

American Psychiatric Association. (1994). *Diagnostic and statistical manual of mental disorders* (4th ed.). Washington, DC: Author.

Amies, P. L., Gelder, M. G., & Shaw, P. M. (1983). Social phobia: A comparative clinical study. *British Journal of Psychiatry, 142,* 174–179.

Amir, N., Foa, E. B., & Coles, M. E. (1998a). Automatic activation and strategic avoidance of threat-relevant information in social phobia. *Journal of Abnormal Psychology, 107,* 285–290.

Amir, N., Foa, E. B., & Coles, M. E. (1998b). Negative interpretation bias in social phobia. *Behaviour Research and Therapy, 36,* 959–970.

Amir, N., Foa, E. B., & Coles, M. E. (2001). Implicit memory bias for threat-relevant information in generalized social phobia. *Journal of Abnormal Psychology, 109,* 713–720.

Amir, N., McNally, R. J., Riemann, B. C., Burns, J., Lorenz, M., & Mullen, J. T. (1996). Suppression of the emotional Stroop effect by increased anxiety in patients with social phobia. *Behaviour Research and Therapy, 34,* 945–948.

Andrews, G., Freed, S., & Teesson, M. (1994). Proximity and anticipation of a negative outcome in phobias. *Behaviour Research and Therapy, 32,* 643–645.

Andrews, G., Stewart, G., Allen, R., & Henderson, A. S. (1990). The genetics of six neurotic disorders: A twin study. *Journal of Affective Disorders, 19,* 23–29.

Antony, M. M., Purdon, C. L., Huta, V., & Swinson, R. P. (1998). Dimensions of perfectionism across the anxiety disorders. *Behaviour Research and Therapy, 36,* 1143–1154.

Arkin, R. M., Appelman, A. J., & Burger, J. M. (1980). Social anxiety, self-presentation, and the self-serving bias in causal attribution. *Journal of Personality and Social Psychology, 38,* 23–35.

Arrindell, W. A., Emmelkamp, P. M. G., Monsma, A., & Brilman, E. (1983). The role of perceived parental rearing practices in the aetiology of phobic disorders: A controlled study. *British Journal of Psychiatry, 143,* 183–187.

Arrindell, W. A., Kwee, M. G. T., Methorst, G. J., van der Ende, J., Pol, E., & Moritz, M. J. M. (1989). Perceived parental rearing styles of agoraphobic and socially phobic in-patients. *British Journal of Psychiatry, 155,* 526–535.

Asmundson, G. J. G., Sandler, L. S., Wilson, K. G., & Walker, J. R. (1992). Selective attention toward physical threat in patients with panic disorder. *Journal of Anxiety Disorders, 6,* 295–303.

Asmundson, G. J. G., & Stein, M. B. (1994). Selective processing of social threat in patients with generalized social phobia: Evaluation using a dot-probe paradigm. *Journal of Anxiety Disorders, 8,* 107–117.

Barlow, D. H. (1994). Comorbidity in social phobia: Implications for cognitive-behavioral treatment. *Bulletin of the Menninger Clinic, 58*(Suppl. 2), A43–A57.

Barlow, D. H. (2002). *Anxiety and its disorders: The nature and treatment of anxiety and panic* (2nd ed.). New York: Guilford Press.

Beck, A. T., Emery, G., & Greenberg, R. (1985). *Anxiety disorders and phobias: A cognitive perspective.* New York: Basic Books.

Beck, A. T., Epstein, N., Brown, G., & Steer, R. A. (1988). An inventory for measuring clinical anxiety: Psychometric properties. *Journal of Consulting and Clinical Psychology, 56,* 893–897.

Beck, A. T., Rush, A. J., Shaw, B. F., & Emery, G. (1979). *Cognitive therapy of depression.* New York: Guilford Press.

Beck, A. T., Steer, R. A., & Brown, G. K. (1996). *Beck Depression Inventory Manual* (2nd ed.). San Antonio, TX: Psychological Corporation.

Beck, A. T., Steer, R. A., & Garbin, M. G. (1988). Psychometric properties of the Beck Depression Inventory: Twenty-five years of evaluation. *Clinical Psychology Review, 8,* 77–100.

Beck, A. T., Ward, C. H., Mendelson, M., Mock, J., & Erbaugh, J. (1961). An inventory for measuring depression. *Archives of General Psychiatry, 4,* 561–571.

Beck, J. G., Stanley, M. A., Averill, P. M., Baldwin, L. E., & Deagle, E. A. (1992). Attention and memory for threat in panic disorder. *Behaviour Research and Therapy, 30,* 619–629.

Beck, J. S. (1995). *Cognitive therapy: Basics and beyond.* New York: Guilford Press.

Becker, C. B., Namour, N., Zayfert, C., & Hegel, M. T. (2001). Specificity of the Social Interaction Self-Statement Test in social phobia. *Cognitive Therapy and Research, 25,* 227–233.

Beidel, D. C., Borden, J. W., Turner, S. M., & Jacob, R. G. (1989a). The Social Phobia and Anxiety Inventory: Concurrent validity with a clinical sample. *Behaviour Research and Therapy, 27,* 573–576.

Beidel, D. C., & Turner, S. M. (1992). Scoring the Social Phobia and Anxiety Inventory: Comments on Herbert et al. (1991). *Journal of Psychopathology and Behavioral Assessment, 14,* 377–379.

Beidel, D. C., Turner, S. M., & Cooley, M. R. (1993). Assessing reliable and clinically significant change in social phobia: Validity of the Social Phobia and Anxiety Inventory. *Behaviour Research and Therapy, 31,* 331–337.

Beidel, D. C., Turner, S. M., & Fink, C. M. (1996). Assessment of childhood social phobia: Construct, convergent, and discriminative validity of the Social Phobia and Anxiety Inventory for Children (SPAI-C). *Psychological Assessment, 8,* 235–240.

Beidel, D. C., Turner, S. M., Jacob, R. G., & Cooley, M. R. (1989b). Assessment of social phobia: Reliability of an impromptu speech task. *Journal of Anxiety Disorders, 3,* 149–158.

Beidel, D. C., Turner, S. M., & Morris, T. L. (1995). A new inventory to assess childhood social anxiety and phobia: Construct, convergent, and discriminative validity of the Social Phobia and Anxiety Inventory for Children. *Psychological Assessment, 7,* 73–79.

Beidel, D. C., Turner, S. M., Stanley, M. A., & Dancu, C. V. (1989c). The Social Phobia and Anxiety Inventory: Concurrent and external validity. *Behavior Therapy, 20,* 417–427.

Biederman, J., Rosenbaum, J. F., Bolduc-Murphy, E. A., Faraone, S. V., Chaloff, J., Hirshfeld, D. R., & Kagan, J. (1993). A 3–year follow-up of children with and without behavioral inhibition. *Journal of the American Academy of Child and Adolescent Psychiatry, 32,* 814–821.

Biederman, J., Rosenbaum, J. F., Hirshfeld, D. R., Faraone, S. V., Bolduc, E. A., Gersten, M., Meminger, S. R., Kagan, J., Snidman, M., & Reznick, J. S. (1990). Psychiatric correlates of behavioral inhibition in young children of parents with and without psychiatric disorders. *Archives of General Psychiatry, 47,* 21–26.

Bieling, P. J., & Alden, L. E. (1997). The consequences of perfectionism for patients with social phobia. *British Journal of Clinical Psychology, 36,* 387–395.

Bieling, P. J., Antony, M. M., & Swinson, R. P. (1998). The State-Trait Anxiety Inventory, Trait version: Structure and content re-examined. *Behaviour Research and Therapy, 36,* 777–788.

Bland, R. C., Orn, H., & Newman, C. S. (1988). Lifetime prevalence of psychiatric disorders in Edmonton. *Acta Psychiatrica Scandinavica, 77*(Suppl. 338), 24–32.

Bond, C. F., Jr., & Omar, A. S. (1990). Social anxiety, state dependence, and the next-in-line effect. *Journal of Experimental Social Psychology, 26,* 185–198.

Borkovec, T. D., & Nau, S. D. (1972). Credibility of analogue therapy rationales. *Journal of Behavior Therapy and Experimental Psychiatry, 3,* 257–260.

Bourdon, K. H., Boyd, J. H., Rae, D. S., Burns, B. J., Thompson, J. W., & Locke, B. Z. (1988). Gender differences in phobias: Results from the ECA community survey. *Journal of Anxiety Disorders, 2,* 227–241.

Bower, G. (1981). Mood and memory. *American Psychologist, 36,* 129–148.

Bower, G. (1987). Commentary on mood and memory. *Behaviour Research and Therapy, 25,* 443–456.

Breck, B. E., & Smith, S. H. (1983). Selective recall of self-descriptive traits by socially anxious and nonanxious females. *Social Behavior and Personality, 11,* 71–76.

Brewin, C. R., Andrews, B., & Gotlib, I. H. (1993). Psychopathology and early experience: A reappraisal of retrospective reports. *Psychological Bulletin, 113,* 82–98.

Brooks, R. B., Baltazar, P. L., & Munjack, D. J. (1989). Co-occurrence of personality disorders with panic disorder, social phobia, and generalized anxiety disorder: A review of the literature. *Journal of Anxiety Disorders, 3,* 259–285.

Brown, E. J., Heimberg, R. G., & Juster, H. R. (1995). Social phobia subtype and avoidant personality disorder: Effect on severity of social phobia, impairment, and outcome of cognitive-behavioral treatment. *Behavior Therapy, 26,* 467–486.

Brown, E. J., Juster, H. R., Heimberg, R. G., & Winning, C. D. (1998). Stressful life events and personality styles: Relation to impairment and treatment outcome in patients with social phobia. *Journal of Anxiety Disorders, 12,* 233–251.

Brown, E. J., Turovsky, J., Heimberg, R. G., Juster, H. R., Brown, T. A., & Barlow, D. H. (1997). Validation of the Social Interaction Anxiety Scale and the Social Phobia Scale across the anxiety disorders. *Psychological Assessment, 9,* 21–27.

Brown, T. A., & Barlow, D. H. (1992). Comorbidity among anxiety disorders: Implications for treatment and DSM-IV. *Journal of Consulting and Clinical Psychology, 60,* 835–844.

Bruce, T. J., Spiegel, D. A., & Hegel, M. T. (1999). Cognitive-behavioral therapy helps prevent relapse and recurrence of panic disorder following alprazolam discontinuation: A long-term follow-up of the Peoria and Dartmouth studies. *Journal of Consulting and Clinical Psychology, 67,* 151–156.

Bruch, M. A., & Heimberg, R. G. (1994). Differences in perceptions of parental and personal characteristics between generalized and nongeneralized social phobics. *Journal of Anxiety Disorders, 8,* 155–168.

Bruch, M. A., Heimberg, R. G., Berger, P., & Collins, T. M. (1989). Social phobia and perceptions of early parental and personal characteristics. *Anxiety Research, 2,* 57–65.

Bruch, M. A., Heimberg, R. G., & Hope, D. A. (1991). States of mind model and cognitive change in treated social phobics. *Cognitive Therapy and Research, 15,* 429–441.

Buss, A. H. (1980). *Self-consciousness and social anxiety.* San Francisco: Freeman.

Buss, A. H. (1986). A theory of shyness. In W. H. Jones, J. M. Cheek, & S. R. Briggs (Eds.), *Shyness: Perspectives on research and treatment* (pp. 39–46). New York: Plenum Press.

Butler, G. (1985). Exposure as a treatment for social phobia: Some instructive difficulties. *Behaviour Research and Therapy, 23,* 651–657.

Butler, G. (1989). Issues in the application of cognitive and behavioral strategies to the treatment of social phobia. *Clinical Psychology Review, 9,* 91–106.

Butler, G., & Mathews, A. (1983). Cognitive processes in anxiety. *Advances in Behaviour Research and Therapy, 5,* 51–62.

Byrne, D. (1961). Interpersonal attraction and attitude similarity. *Journal of Abnormal and Social Psychology, 62,* 713–715.

Byrne, D., & Nelson, D. (1965). Attraction as a linear function of proportion of positive reinforcements. *Journal of Personality and Social Psychology, 1,* 659–663.

Cacioppo, J. T., Glass, C. R., & Merluzzi, T. V. (1979). Self-statements and self-evalua-tions: A cognitive response analysis of heterosocial anxiety. *Cognitive Therapy and Research, 3,* 249–262.

Canino, G. J., Bird, H. R., Shrout, P. E., Rubio-Stipec, M., Bravo, M., Martinez, R., Sesman, M., & Guevara, L. M. (1987). The prevalence of specific psychiatric disor-ders in Puerto Rico. *Archives of General Psychiatry, 44,* 727–735.

Caspi, A., Elder, G. H., Jr., & Bem, D. J. (1988). Moving away from the world: Life-course patterns of shy children. *Developmental Psychology, 24,* 824–831.

Cassiday, K. L., McNally, R. J., & Zeitlin, S. B. (1992). Cognitive processing of trauma cues in rape victims with post-traumatic stress disorder. *Cognitive Therapy and Re-search, 16,* 283–295.

Chambless, D. L., Cherney, J., Caputo, G. C., & Rheinstein, B. J. G. (1987). Anxiety dis-orders and alcoholism: A study with inpatient alcoholics. *Journal of Anxiety Disor-ders, 1,* 29–40.

Chambless, D. L., Tran, G. Q., & Glass, C. R. (1997). Predictors of response to cognitive-behavioral group therapy for social phobia. *Journal of Anxiety Disorders, 11,* 221–240.

Chapman, T. F., Mannuzza, S., & Fyer, A. J. (1995). Epidemiology and family studies of social phobia. In R. G. Heimberg, M. R. Liebowitz, D. A. Hope, & F. R. Schneier (Eds.), *Social phobia: Diagnosis, assessment, and treatment* (pp. 21–40). New York: Guilford Press.

Clark, D. B., Feske, U., Masia, C. L., Spaulding, S. A., Brown, C., Mammen, O., & Shear, M. K. (1997). Systematic assessment of social phobia in clinical practice. *Depres-sion and Anxiety, 6,* 47–61.

Clark, D. B., Turner, S. M., Beidel, D. C., Donovan, J., Kirisci, L., & Jacob, R. (1994). Re-liability and validity of the Social Phobia and Anxiety Inventory for Adolescents. *Psychological Assessment, 6,* 135–140.

Clark, D. M. (1997). Panic disorder and social phobia. In D. M. Clark & C. G. Fairburn (Eds.), *Science and practice of cognitive behaviour therapy* (pp. 119–153). Oxford, England: Oxford University Press.

Clark, D. M., & Wells, A. (1995). A cognitive model of social phobia. In R. G. Heimberg, M. R. Liebowitz, D. A. Hope, & F. R. Schneier (Eds.), *Social phobia: Diagnosis, as-sessment, and treatment* (pp. 69–93). New York: Guilford Press.

Clark, J. V., & Arkowitz, H. (1975). Social anxiety and self-evaluation of interpersonal performance. *Psychological Reports, 36,* 211–221.

Cloitre, M., Cancienne, J., Heimberg, R. G., Holt, C. S., & Liebowitz, M. R. (1995). Mem-ory bias does not generalize across anxiety disorders. *Behaviour Research and Ther-apy, 33,* 305–307.

Cloitre, M., Heimberg, R. G., Holt, C. S., & Liebowitz, M. R. (1992a). Reaction time to threat stimuli in panic disorder and social phobia. *Behaviour Research and Therapy, 30,* 609–617.

Cloitre, M., Heimberg, R. G., Liebowitz, M. R., & Gitow, A. (1992b). Perceptions of con-trol in panic disorder and social phobia. *Cognitive Therapy and Research, 16,* 569–577.

Cloitre, M., & Liebowitz, M. R. (1991). Memory bias in panic disorder: An investigation of the cognitive avoidance hypothesis. *Cognitive Therapy and Research, 15,* 371–386.

Coles, M. E., Gibb, B. E., & Heimberg, R. G. (2001). A psychometric evaluation of the Beck Depression Inventory in adults with social anxiety disorder. *Depression and Anxiety, 14*, 145–148.

Coles, M. E., & Heimberg, R. G. (2000). Patterns of anxious arousal during exposure to feared situations in individuals with social phobia. *Behaviour Research and Therapy, 38*, 405–424.

Coles, M. E., & Heimberg, R. G. (2002). Memory biases in the anxiety disorders: Current status. *Clinical Psychology Review, 22*, 587–627.

Coles, M. E., Turk, C. L., Heimberg, R. G., & Fresco, D. M. (2001). Effects of varying levels of anxiety within social situations: Relationship to memory perspective and attributions in social phobia. *Behaviour Research and Therapy, 39*, 651–665.

Connor, K. M., Davidson, J. R. T., Churchill, L. E., Sherwood, A., Foa, E., & Weisler, R. H. (2000). Psychometric properties of the Social Phobia Inventory (SPIN): A new self-rating scale. *British Journal of Psychiatry, 176*, 379–386.

Cox, B. J., Direnfeld, D. M., Swinson, R. P., & Norton, G. R. (1994). Suicidal ideation and suicide attempts in panic disorder and social phobia. *American Journal of Psychiatry, 151*, 882–887.

Cox, B. J., Ross, L., Swinson, R. P., & Direnfeld, D. M. (1998). A comparison of social phobia outcome measures in cognitive-behavioral group therapy. *Behavior Modification, 22*, 285–297.

Cox, B. J., & Swinson, R. P. (1995). Assessment and measurement. In M. B. Stein (Ed.), *Social phobia: Clinical and research perspectives* (pp. 261–291). Washington, DC: American Psychiatric Press.

Cox, B. J., Swinson, R. P., & Shaw, B. F. (1991). Value of the Fear Questionnaire in differentiating agoraphobia and social phobia. *British Journal of Psychiatry, 159*, 842–845.

Craik, F. I. M., & Tulving, E. (1975). Depth of processing and the retention of words in episodic memory. *Journal of Experimental Psychology: General, 104*, 268–294.

Craske, M. G., & Barlow, D. H. (2000). *Mastery of your anxiety and panic—third edition* (MAP-3; Client Workbook). San Antonio, TX: Psychological Corporation.

Daly, J. A., Vangelisti, A. L., & Lawrence, S. G. (1989). Self-focused attention and public speaking anxiety. *Personality and Individual Differences, 10*, 903–913.

Davidson, J. R. T., Hughes, D. L., George, L. K., & Blazer, D. G. (1993). The epidemiology of social phobia: Findings from the Duke Epidemiological Catchment Area Study. *Psychological Medicine, 23*, 709–718.

Davidson, J. R. T., Miner, C. M., DeVeaughGeiss, J., Tupler, L. A., Colket, J. T., & Potts, N. L. S. (1997). The Brief Social Phobia Scale: A psychometric evaluation. *Psychological Medicine, 27*, 161–166.

Davidson, J. R. T., Potts, N. L. S., Richichi, E. A., Krishnan, R. R., Ford, S. M., Smith, R. D., & Wilson, W. (1991). The Brief Social Phobia Scale. *Journal of Clinical Psychiatry, 52*, 48–51.

de Ruiter, C., & Brosschot, J. F. (1994). The emotional Stroop interference effect in anxiety: Attentional bias or cognitive avoidance? *Behaviour Research and Therapy, 32*, 315–319.

de Ruiter, C., Rijken, H., Garssen, B., van Schaik, A., & Kraaimaat, F. (1989). Comorbidity among the anxiety disorders. *Journal of Anxiety Disorders, 3*, 57–68.

Dilsaver, S. C., Qamar, A. B., & Del Medico, V. J. (1992). Secondary social phobia in patients with major depression. *Psychiatry Research, 44*, 33–40.

DiNardo, P. A., & Barlow, D. H. (1988). *The Anxiety Disorders Interview Schedule—Revised (ADIS-R)*. Albany, NY: Graywind.

Di Nardo, P. A., Brown, T. A., & Barlow, D. H. (1994). *Anxiety Disorders Interview Schedule for DSM-IV—Lifetime Version (ADIS-IV-L)*. San Antonio, TX: Psychological Corporation.

Dodge, C. S., Heimberg, R. G., Nyman, D., & O'Brien, G. T. (1987). Daily heterosocial interactions of high and low socially anxious college students: A diary study. *Behavior Therapy, 18,* 90–96.

Dodge, C. S., Hope, D. A., Heimberg, R. G., & Becker, R. E. (1988). Evaluation of the Social Interaction Self-Statement Test in a social phobic population. *Cognitive Therapy and Research, 12,* 211–222.

Doerfler, L. A., & Aron, J. (1995). Relationship of goal setting, self-efficacy, and self-evaluation in dysphoric and socially anxious women. *Cognitive Therapy and Research, 19,* 725–738.

Eaton, W. W., Holzer, C. E., III,, Von Korff, M., Anthony, J. C., Helzer, J. E., George, L., Burnam, M. A., Boyd, J. H., Kessler, L. G., & Locke, B. Z. (1984). The design of the Epidemiological Catchment Area surveys: The control and measurement of error. *Archives of General Psychiatry, 41,* 942–948.

Eaton, W. W., & Kessler, L. G. (Eds.). (1985). *Epidemiological field methods in psychiatry: The NIMH Epidemiological Catchment Area Program*. Orlando, FL: Academic Press.

Elting, D. T., & Hope, D. A. (1995). Cognitive assessment. In R. G. Heimberg, M. R. Liebowitz, D. A. Hope, & F. R. Schneier (Eds.), *Social phobia: Diagnosis, assessment, and treatment* (pp. 232–258). New York: Guilford Press.

Eng, W., Coles, M. E., Heimberg, R. G., & Safren, S. A. (2001). Quality of life following cognitive behavioral treatment for social anxiety disorder: Preliminary findings. *Depression and Anxiety, 13,* 192–193.

Faravelli, C., Guerrini Degl'Innocenti, B., & Giardinelli, L. (1989). Epidemiology of anxiety disorders in Florence. *Acta Psychiatrica Scandinavica, 79,* 308–312.

Feske, U., Perry, K. J., Chambless, D. L., Renneberg, B., & Goldstein, A. J. (1996). Avoidant personality disorder as a predictor for severity and treatment outcome among generalized social phobics. *Journal of Personality Disorders, 10,* 174–184.

Fischer, J., & Corcoran, K. (2000). *Measures for clinical practice: A source book* (Vol. 2, 3rd ed.). New York: Free Press.

Foa, E. B., Franklin, M. E., Perry, K. J., & Herbert, J. D. (1996). Cognitive biases in generalized social phobia. *Journal of Abnormal Psychology, 105,* 433–439.

Foa, E. B., Gilboa-Schechtman, E., Amir, N., & Freshman, M. (2000). Memory bias in generalized social phobia: Remembering negative emotional expressions. *Journal of Anxiety Disorders, 14,* 501–519.

Foa, E. B., & Kozak, M. J. (1986). Emotional processing of fear: Exposure to corrective information. *Psychological Bulletin, 99,* 20–35.

Frances, A. (1998). Problems in defining clinical significance in epidemiological studies. *Archives of General Psychiatry, 55,* 119.

Frank, M. G., & Gilovich, T. (1989). Effect of memory perspective on retrospective causal attributions. *Journal of Personality and Social Psychology, 57,* 399–403.

Fresco, D. M., Coles, M. E., Heimberg, R. G., Liebowitz, M. R., Hami,S., Stein, M. B., & Goetz, D. (2001). The Liebowitz Social Anxiety Scale: A comparison of the psychometric properties of self-report and clinician-administered formats. *Psychological Medicine, 31,* 1025–1035.

Frisch, M. B. (1994). *Manual and treatment guide for the Quality of Life Inventory.* Minneapolis, MN: National Computer Systems.

Frisch, M. B., Cornell, J., Villanueva, M., & Retzlaff, P. J. (1992). Clinical validation of the Quality of Life Inventory: A measure of life satisfaction for use in treatment planning and outcome assessment. *Psychological Assessment, 4,* 92–101.

Frost, R. O., Marten, P. A., Lahart, C., & Rosenblate, R. (1990). The dimensions of perfectionism. *Cognitive Therapy and Research, 14,* 449–468.

Fydrich, T., Chambless, D. L., Perry, K. J., Buergner, F., & Beazley, M. B. (1998). Behavioral assessment of social performance: A rating system for social phobia. *Behaviour Research and Therapy, 36,* 995–1010.

Fyer, A. J., Mannuzza, S., Chapman, T. F., Liebowitz, M. R., & Klein, D. F. (1993). A direct family interview study of social phobia. *Archives of General Psychiatry, 50,* 286–293.

Fyer, A. J., Mannuzza, S., Chapman, T. F., Lipsitz, J., Martin, L. Y., & Klein, D. F. (1996). Panic disorder and social phobia: Effects of comorbidity on familial transmission. *Anxiety, 2,* 173–178.

Fyer, A. J., Mannuzza, S., Chapman, T. F., Martin, L. Y., & Klein, D. F. (1995). Specificity in familial aggregation of phobic disorders. *Archives of General Psychiatry, 52,* 564–573.

Gelernter, C. S., Stein, M. B., Tancer, M. E., & Uhde, T. W. (1992). An examination of syndromal validity and diagnostic subtypes in social phobia and panic disorder. *Journal of Clinical Psychiatry, 53,* 23–27.

Gerlsma, C., Kramer, J. J., Scholing, A., & Emmelkamp, P. M. G. (1994). The influence of mood on memories of parental rearing practices. *British Journal of Clinical Psychology, 33,* 159–172.

Gernsbacher, M. S., Varner, K. R., & Faust, M. E. (1990). Investigating differences in general comprehension skill. *Journal of Experimental Psychology: Learning, Memory, and Cognition, 16,* 430–445.

Gilboa-Schechtman, E., Foa, E. B., & Amir, N. (1999). Attentional biases for facial expressions in social phobia: The face-in-the-crowd paradigm. *Cognition and Emotion, 13,* 305–318.

Girodo, M., Dotzenroth, S. E., & Stein, S. J. (1981). Causal attribution bias in shy males: Implications for self-esteem and self-confidence. *Cognitive Therapy and Research, 5,* 325–338.

Glasgow, R. E., & Arkowitz, H. (1975). The behavioral assessment of male and female social competence in dyadic heterosexual interactions. *Behavior Therapy, 6,* 488–498.

Glass, C. R., & Furlong, M. (1990). Cognitive assessment of social anxiety: Affective and behavioral correlates. *Cognitive Therapy and Research, 14,* 365–384.

Glass, C. R., Merluzzi, T. V., Biever, J. L., & Larsen, K. H. (1982). Cognitive assessment of social anxiety: Development and validation of a self-statement questionnaire. *Cognitive Therapy and Research, 6,* 37–55.

Greenberg, P. E., Sisitsky, T., Kessler, R. C., Finkelstein, S. N., Berndt, E. R., Davidson, J. R. T., Ballenger, J. C., & Fyer, A. J. (1999). The economic burden of anxiety disorders in the 1990s. *Journal of Clinical Psychiatry, 60,* 427–435.

Habke, A. M., Hewitt, P. L., Norton, G. R., & Asmundson, G. J. G. (1997). The Social

Phobia and Social Interaction Anxiety Scales: An exploration of the dimensions of social anxiety and sex differences in structure and relations with pathology. *Journal of Psychopathology and Behavioral Assessment, 19,* 21–39.

Hackmann, A., Clark, D. M., & McManus, F. (2000). Recurrent images and early memories in social phobia. *Behaviour Research and Therapy, 38,* 601–610.

Hackmann, A., Surawy, C., & Clark, D. M. (1998). Seeing yourself through others' eyes: A study of spontaneously occurring images in social phobia. *Behavioural and Cognitive Psychotherapy, 26,* 3–12.

Hambrick, J., Heimberg, R. G., & Turk, C. L. (2001, March). *Measuring the measuring stick: Psychometric properties of disability measures among patients with social anxiety disorder.* Poster presented at the annual meeting of the Anxiety Disorders Association of America, Atlanta, GA.

Hamilton, M. (1959). The assessment of anxiety states by rating. *British Journal of Psychiatry, 32,* 50–55.

Hamilton, M. (1960). A rating scale for depression. *Journal of Neurology, Neurosurgery, and Psychiatry, 23,* 56–62.

Hansen, C. H., & Hansen, R. D. (1988). Finding the face in the crowd: An anger superiority effect. *Journal of Personality and Social Psychology, 54,* 917–924.

Hart, T. A., Jack, M. S., Turk, C. L., & Heimberg, R. G. (1999). Issues for the measurement of social anxiety disorder (social phobia). In H. G. M. Westenberg & J. A. Den Boer (Eds.), *Focus on psychiatry: Social anxiety disorder* (pp. 133–155). Amsterdam: Syn-Thesis.

Harvey, A. G., Clark, D. M., Ehlers, A., & Rapee, R. M. (2000). Social anxiety and self-impression: Cognitive preparation enhances the beneficial effects of video feedback following a stressful social task. *Behaviour Research and Therapy, 38,* 1183–1192.

Hazen, A. L., & Stein, M. B. (1995). Clinical phenomenology and comorbidity. In M. B. Stein (Ed.), *Social phobia: Clinical and research perspectives* (pp. 3–41). Washington, DC: American Psychiatric Press.

Heckelman, L. R,, & Schneier, F. R. (1995). Diagnostic issues. In R. G. Heimberg, M. R. Liebowitz, D. A. Hope, & F. R. Schneier (Eds.), *Social phobia: Diagnosis, assessment, and treatment* (pp. 3–20). New York: Guilford Press.

Heimberg, R. G. (1989). Cognitive and behavioral treatments for social phobia: A critical analysis. *Clinical Psychology Review, 9,* 107–128.

Heimberg, R. G. (1994). Cognitive assessment strategies and the measurement of outcome of treatment for social phobia. *Behaviour Research and Therapy, 32,* 269–280.

Heimberg, R. G. (1996). Social phobia, avoidant personality disorder, and the multiaxial conceptualization of interpersonal anxiety. In P. Salkovskis (Ed.), *Trends in cognitive and behavioural therapies* (pp. 43–61). Sussex, England: Wiley.

Heimberg, R. G., Acerra, M. C., & Holstein, A. (1985). Partner similarity mediates interpersonal anxiety. *Cognitive Therapy and Research, 9,* 443–453.

Heimberg, R. G., Bruch, M. A., Hope, D. A., & Dombeck, M. (1990a). Evaluating the States of Mind model: Comparison to an alternative model and effects of method of cognitive assessment. *Cognitive Therapy and Research, 14,* 543–557.

Heimberg, R. G., Dodge, C. S., Hope, D. A., Kennedy, C. R., Zollo, L., & Becker, R. E. (1990b). Cognitive behavioral group treatment of social phobia: Comparison to a credible placebo control. *Cognitive Therapy and Research, 14,* 1–23.

Heimberg, R. G., Holt, C. S., Schneier, F. R., Spitzer, R. L., & Liebowitz, M. R. (1993).

The issue of subtypes in the diagnosis of social phobia. *Journal of Anxiety Disorders, 7,* 249–269.

Heimberg, R. G., Hope, D. A., Dodge, C. S., & Becker, R. E. (1990c). DSM-III-R subtypes of social phobia: Comparison of generalized social phobics and public speaking phobics. *Journal of Nervous and Mental Disease, 173,* 172–179.

Heimberg, R. G., Horner, K. J., Juster, H. R., Safren, S. A., Brown, E. J., Schneier, F. R., & Liebowitz, M. R. (1999). Psychometric properties of the Liebowitz Social Anxiety Scale. *Psychological Medicine, 29,* 199–212.

Heimberg, R. G., & Juster, H. R. (1995). Cognitive-behavioral treatments: Literature review. In R. G. Heimberg, M. R. Liebowitz, D. A. Hope, & F. R. Schneier (Eds.), *Social phobia: Diagnosis, assessment, and treatment* (pp. 261–309). New York: Guilford Press.

Heimberg, R. G., Klosko, J. S., Dodge, C. S., Shadick, R., Becker, R. E., & Barlow, D. H. (1989). Anxiety disorders, depression, and attributional style: A further test of the specificity of depressive attributions. *Cognitive Therapy and Research, 13,* 21–36.

Heimberg, R. G., Liebowitz, M. R., Hope, D. A., Schneier, F. R., Holt, C. S., Welkowitz, L., Juster, H. R., Campeas, R., Bruch, M. A., Cloitre, M., Fallon, B., & Klein, D. F. (1998). Cognitive-behavioral group therapy versus phenelzine in social phobia: 12–week outcome. *Archives of General Psychiatry, 55,* 1133–1141.

Heimberg, R. G., Mueller, G. P., Holt, C. S., Hope, D. A., & Liebowitz, M. R. (1992). Assessment of anxiety in social interaction and being observed by others: The Social Interaction Anxiety Scale and the Social Phobia Scale. *Behavior Therapy, 23,* 53–73.

Heimberg, R. G., Stein, M. B., Hiripi, E., & Kessler, R. C. (2000). Trends in the prevalence of social phobia in the United States: A synthetic cohort analysis of changes over four decades. *European Psychiatry, 15,* 29–37.

Herbert, J. D., Bellack, A. S., & Hope, D. A. (1991). Concurrent validity of the Social Phobia and Anxiety Inventory. *Journal of Psychopathology and Behavioral Assessment, 13,* 357–368.

Herbert, J. D., Bellack, A. S., Hope, D. A., & Mueser, K. T. (1992a). Scoring the Social Phobia and Anxiety Inventory: Reply to Beidel and Turner. *Journal of Psychopathology and Behavioral Assessment, 14,* 381–383.

Herbert, J. D., Hope, D. A., & Bellack, A. S. (1992b). Validity of the distinction between generalized social phobia and avoidant personality disorder. *Journal of Abnormal Psychology, 101,* 332–339.

Hewitt, P. L., & Flett, G. L. (1991). Perfectionism in the self and social contexts: Conceptualization, assessment and association with psychopathology. *Journal of Personality and Social Psychology, 60,* 456–470.

Hirsch, C., & Mathews, A. (1997). Interpretive inferences when reading about emotional events. *Behaviour Research and Therapy, 35,* 1123–1132.

Hirsch, C., & Mathews, A. (2000). Impaired positive inferential bias in social phobia. *Journal of Abnormal Psychology, 109,* 705–712.

Hofmann, S. G. (2000). Self-focused attention before and after treatment of social phobia. *Behaviour Research and Therapy, 38,* 717–725.

Holle, C., Heimberg, R. G., Sweet, R. A., & Holt, C. S. (1995). Alcohol and caffeine use by social phobics: An initial inquiry into drinking patterns and behavior. *Behaviour Research and Therapy, 33,* 561–566.

Holle, C., Neely, J. H., & Heimberg, R. G. (1997). The effects of blocked versus random presentation and semantic relatedness of stimulus words on response to a modified Stroop task among social phobics. *Cognitive Therapy and Research, 21,* 681–697.

Holt, C. S., & Heimberg, R. G. (1990). The Reaction to Treatment Questionnaire: Measuring treatment credibility and outcome expectations. *Behavior Therapist, 13,* 213–214, 222.

Holt, C. S., Heimberg, R. G., & Hope, D. A. (1992a). Avoidant personality disorder and the generalized subtype in social phobia. *Journal of Abnormal Psychology, 101,* 318–325.

Holt, C. S., Heimberg, R. G., Hope, D. A., & Liebowitz, M. R. (1992b). Situational domains of social phobia. *Journal of Anxiety Disorders, 6,* 63–77.

Hope, D. A., & Heimberg, R. G. (1990). Dating anxiety. In H. Leitenberg (Ed.), *Handbook of social and evaluative anxiety* (pp. 217–246). New York: Plenum Press.

Hope, D. A., Heimberg, R. G., & Bruch, M. A. (1995a). Dismantling cognitive-behavioral group therapy for social phobia. *Behaviour Research and Therapy, 33,* 637–650.

Hope, D. A., Heimberg, R. G., Juster, H., & Turk, C. L. (2000). *Managing social anxiety: A cognitive-behavioral therapy approach* (Client Workbook). San Antonio, TX: Psychological Corporation.

Hope, D. A., Heimberg, R. G., & Klein, J. R. (1990a). Social anxiety and the recall of interpersonal information. *Journal of Cognitive Psychotherapy: An International Quarterly, 4,* 185–195.

Hope, D. A., Herbert, J. D., & White, C. (1995b). Diagnostic subtype, avoidant personality disorder, and efficacy of cognitive behavioral group therapy for social phobia. *Cognitive Therapy and Research, 19,* 399–417.

Hope, D. A., Rapee, R. M., Heimberg, R. G., & Dombeck, M. (1990b). Representations of the self in social phobia: Vulnerability to social threat. *Cognitive Therapy and Research, 14,* 177–189.

Hope, D. A., Sigler, K. D., Penn, D. L., & Meier, V. J. (1998). Social anxiety, recall of interpersonal information, and social impact on others. *Journal of Cognitive Psychotherapy: An International Quarterly, 12,* 303–322.

Hope, D. A., Turk, C. L., & Heimberg, R. G. (in press). *Therapist guide for managing social anxiety: A cognitive-behavioral therapy approach* (Client Workbook). San Antonio, TX: Psychological Corporation.

Hudson, J. L., & Rapee, R. M. (2000). The origins of social phobia. *Behavior Modification, 24,* 102–129.

Hwu, H.-G., Yeh, E.-K., & Chang, L.-Y. (1989). Prevalence of psychiatric disorders in Taiwan defined by the Chinese Diagnostic Interview Schedule. *Acta Psychiatrica Scandinavica, 79,* 136–147.

Jack, M. S., Heimberg, R. G., & Mennin, D. S. (1999). Situational panic attacks: Impact on social phobia with and without panic disorder. *Depression and Anxiety 10,* 112–118.

Jacoby, L. L., Allan, L. G., Collins, J. C., & Larwill, L. K. (1988). Memory influences subjective experience: Noise judgment. *Journal of Experimental Psychology: Learning, Memory, and Cognition, 14,* 240–247.

Jacoby, L. L., Toth, J. P., & Yonelinas, A. P. (1993). Separating conscious and unconscious influences of memory: Measuring recollection. *Journal of Experimental Psychology, 122,* 139–154.

Jansen, M. A., Arntz, A., Merckelbach, H., & Mersch, P. P. A. (1994). Personality disorders and features in social phobia and panic disorder. *Journal of Abnormal Psychology, 103,* 391–395.

Johnson, M. R., Turner, S. M., Beidel, D. C., & Lydiard, R. B. (1995). Personality functioning in social phobia. In M. B. Stein (Ed.), *Social phobia: Clinical and research perspectives* (pp. 77–117). Washington, DC: American Psychiatric Press.

Juster, H. R., Brown, E. J., & Heimberg, R. G. (1996a). Sozialphobie (Social phobia). In J. Margraf (Ed.), *Lehrbuch der verhaltenstherapie* [*Textbook of behavior therapy*] (pp. 43–59). Berlin, Germany: Springer-Verlag.

Juster, H. R., Heimberg, R. G., Frost, R. O., Holt, C. S., Mattia, J. I., & Faccenda, K. (1996b). Social phobia and perfectionism. *Personality and Individual Differences, 21,* 403–410.

Kagan, J., Reznick, J. S., & Snidman, N. (1988). Biological bases of childhood shyness. *Science, 240,* 167–171.

Katzelnick, D. J., Kobak, K., Helstad, C., Greist, J., Davidson, J., DeLeire, T., Schneier, F., & Stein, M. (1999, April). *The direct and indirect costs of social phobia in managed care patients.* Paper presented at the meeting of the Anxiety Disorder Association of America, San Diego, CA.

Kendler, K. S. (1996). Parenting: A genetic-epidemiologic perspective. *American Journal of Psychiatry, 153,* 11–20.

Kendler, K. S., Neale, M. C., Kessler, R. C., Heath, A. C., & Eaves, L. J. (1992). The genetic epidemiology of phobias in women: The interrelationship of agoraphobia, social phobia, situational phobia, and simple phobia. *Archives of General Psychiatry, 49,* 273–281.

Kerr, M., Lambert, W. W., & Bem, D. J. (1996). Life course sequelae of childhood shyness in Sweden: Comparison with the United States. *Developmental Psychology, 32,* 1100–1105.

Kessler, R. C., McGonagle, K. A., Zhao, S., Nelson, C. B., Hughes, M., Eshleman, S., Wittchen, H.-U., & Kendler, K. S. (1994). Lifetime and 12–month prevalence of DSM-III-R psychiatric disorders in the United States: Results from the National Comorbidity Survey. *Archives of General Psychiatry, 51,* 8–19.

Kessler, R. C., Stang, P., Wittchen, H.-U., Stein, M., & Walters, E. E. (1999). Lifetime comorbidities between social phobia and mood disorders in the U. S. National Comorbidity Survey. *Psychological Medicine, 29,* 555–567.

Kessler, R. C., Stein, M. B., & Berglund, P. (1998). Social phobia subtypes in the National Comorbidity Survey. *American Journal of Psychiatry, 155,* 613–619.

Kimble, C. E., & Zehr, H. D. (1982). Self-consciousness, information load, self-presentation, and memory in a social situation. *Journal of Social Psychology, 118,* 39–46.

Kushner, M. G., Sher, K. J., & Beitman, B. D. (1990). The relation between alcohol problems and the anxiety disorders. *American Journal of Psychiatry, 146,* 685–695.

Leary, M. R. (1983a). A brief version of the Fear of Negative Evaluation Scale. *Personality and Social Psychology Bulletin, 9,* 371–375.

Leary, M. R. (1983b). *Understanding social anxiety: Social, personality, and clinical perspectives.* Beverly Hills, CA: Sage.

Leary, M. R., Kowalski, R. M., & Campbell, C. D. (1988). Self-presentational concerns and social anxiety: The role of generalized impression expectancies. *Journal of Research in Personality, 22,* 308–321.

Lee, C. K., Kwak, Y. S., Yamamoto, J., Rhee, H., Kim, Y. S., Han, J. H., Choi, J. O., &

Lee, Y. H. (1990a). Psychiatric epidemiology in Korea: I. Gender and age differences in Seoul. *Journal of Nervous and Mental Disease, 178,* 242–246.

Lee, C. K., Kwak, Y. S., Yamamoto, J., Rhee, H., Kim, Y. S., Han, J. H., Choi, J. O., & Lee, Y. H. (1990b). Psychiatric epidemiology in Korea: II. Urban and rural differences. *Journal of Nervous and Mental Disease, 178,* 247–252.

Lelliott, P., McNamee, G., & Marks, I. (1991). Features of agora-, social, and related phobias and validation of the diagnoses. *Journal of Anxiety Disorders, 5,* 313–322.

Lépine, J.-P., & Lellouch, J. (1995). Classification and epidemiology of social phobia. *European Archives of Psychiatry and Clinical Neuroscience, 244,* 290–296.

Leung, A. W., & Heimberg, R. G. (1996). Homework compliance, perceptions of control, and outcome of cognitive-behavioral treatment of social phobia. *Behaviour Research and Therapy, 34,* 423–432.

Leung, A. W., Heimberg, R. G., Holt, C. S., & Bruch, M. A. (1994). Social anxiety and perception of early parenting among American, Chinese American, and social phobic samples. *Anxiety, 1,* 80–89.

Levenson, H. (1973). Multidimensional locus of control in psychiatric patients. *Journal of Consulting and Clinical Psychology, 41,* 397–401.

Levin, A. P., Saoud, J. B., Strauman, T., Gorman, J. M., Fyer, A. J., Crawford, R., & Liebowitz, M. R. (1993). Responses of "generalized" and "discrete" social phobics during public speaking. *Journal of Anxiety Disorders, 7,* 207–221.

Lieb, R., Wittchen, H.-U., Höfler, M., Fuetsch, M., Stein, M. B., & Merikangas, K. R. (2000). Parental psychopathology, parenting styles and the risk of social phobia in offspring. *Archives of General Psychiatry, 57,* 859–866.

Liebowitz, M. R. (1987). Social phobia. *Modern Problems in Pharmacopsychiatry, 22,* 141–173.

Liebowitz, M. R. (2000). Medication treatment of social anxiety. In D. A. Hope, R. G. Heimberg, H. Juster, & C. L. Turk (Eds.), *Managing social anxiety: A cognitive-behavioral therapy approach* (Client Workbook). San Antonio, TX: Psychological Corporation.

Liebowitz, M. R., Gorman, J. M., Fyer, A. J., & Klein, D. F. (1985). Social phobia: Review of a neglected anxiety disorder. *Archives of General Psychiatry, 42,* 729–736.

Liebowitz, M. R., Heimberg, R. G., Fresco, D. M., Travers, J., & Stein, M. B. (2000). Social phobia or social anxiety disorder: What's in a name? *Archives of General Psychiatry, 57,* 191–192.

Lucas, R. A., & Telch, M. J. (1993, November). *Group versus individual treatment of social phobia.* Paper presented at the annual meeting of the Association for Advancement of Behavior Therapy, Atlanta, GA.

Lucock, M. P., & Salkovskis, P. M. (1988). Cognitive factors in social anxiety and its treatment. *Behaviour Research and Therapy, 26,* 297–302.

Lundh, L. G., & Öst, L. G. (1996a). Recognition bias for critical faces in social phobics. *Behaviour Research and Therapy, 34,* 787–794.

Lundh, L. G., & Öst, L. G. (1996b). Stroop interference, self-focus, and perfectionism in social phobics. *Personality and Individual Differences, 20,* 725–731.

Lundh, L. G., & Öst, L. G. (1997). Explicit and implicit memory bias in social phobia: The role of subdiagnostic type. *Behaviour Research and Therapy, 35,* 305–317.

Lundh, L., Thulin, U., Czyzykow, S., & Öst, L. (1998). Recognition bias for safe faces in panic disorder with agoraphobia. *Behaviour Research and Therapy, 36,* 323–337.

MacLeod, C., & Mathews, A. (1988). Anxiety and the allocation of attention to threat. *Quarterly Journal of Experimental Psychology, 40,* 653–670.

MacLeod, C., & Mathews, A. (1991). Biased cognitive operations in anxiety: Accessibility of information or assignment of processing priorities? *Behaviour Research and Therapy, 29,* 599–610.

MacLeod, C., Mathews, A., & Tata, P. (1986). Attentional bias in emotional disorders. *Journal of Abnormal Psychology, 95,* 15–20.

Magee, W. J., Eaton, W. W., Wittchen, H.-U., McGonagle, K. A., & Kessler, R. C. (1996). Agoraphobia, simple phobia, and social phobia in the National Comorbidity Survey. *Archives of General Psychiatry, 53,* 159–168.

Mahone, E. M., Bruch, M. A., & Heimberg, R. G. (1993). Focus of attention and social anxiety: The role of negative self-thoughts and perceived positive attributes of the other. *Cognitive Therapy and Research, 17,* 209–224.

Maidenberg, E., Chen, E., Craske, M., Bohn, P., & Bystritsky, A. (1996). Specificity of attention bias in panic disorder and social phobia. *Journal of Anxiety Disorders, 10,* 529–541.

Mannuzza, S., Fyer, A. J., Liebowitz, M. R., & Klein, D. F. (1990). Delineating the boundaries of social phobia: Its relationship to panic disorder and agoraphobia. *Journal of Anxiety Disorders, 4,* 41–59.

Mannuzza, S., Schneier, F. R., Chapman, T. F., Liebowitz, M. R., Klein, D. F., & Fyer, A. J. (1995). Generalized social phobia: Reliability and validity. *Archives of General Psychiatry, 52,* 230–237.

Mansell, W., Clark, D. M., Ehlers, A., & Chen, Y.-P. (1999). Social anxiety and attention away from emotional faces. *Cognition and Emotion, 13,* 673–690.

Marks, I. M. (1970). The classification of phobic disorders. *British Journal of Psychiatry, 116,* 377–386.

Marks, I. M., & Gelder, M. G. (1966). Different ages of onset in varieties of phobia. *American Journal of Psychiatry, 123,* 218–221.

Marks, I. M., & Mathews, A. M. (1979). Brief standard self-rating for phobic patients. *Behaviour Research and Therapy, 17,* 263–267.

Martin, M., Williams, R. M., & Clark, D. M. (1991). Does anxiety lead to selective processing of threat related information? *Behaviour Research and Therapy, 29,* 147–160.

Mathews, A., & MacLeod, C. (1985). Selective processing of threat cues in anxiety states. *Behaviour Research and Therapy, 23,* 563–569.

Mattia, J. I., Heimberg, R. G., & Hope, D. A. (1993). The Revised Stroop Color-Naming Task in social phobics. *Behaviour Research and Therapy, 31,* 305–313.

Mattick, R. P., & Clarke, J. C. (1998). Development and validation of measures of social phobia scrutiny fear and social interaction anxiety. *Behaviour Research and Therapy, 36,* 455–470.

Mattick, R. P., & Newman, C. R. (1991). Social phobia and avoidant personality disorder. *International Review of Psychiatry, 3,* 163–173.

Mattick, R. P., & Peters, L. (1988). Treatment of severe social phobia: Effects of guided exposure with and without cognitive restructuring. *Journal of Consulting and Clinical Psychology, 56,* 251–260.

Mattick, R. P., Peters, L., & Clarke, J. C. (1989). Exposure and cognitive restructuring for social phobia: A controlled study. *Behavior Therapy, 20,* 3–23.

McManus, F., Clark, D. M., & Hackmann, A. (2000). Specificity of cognitive biases in social phobia and their role in recovery. *Behavioural and Cognitive Psychotherapy, 28,* 201–209.

McNally, R. J., & Foa, E. B. (1987). Cognition and agoraphobia: Bias in the interpretation of threat. *Cognitive Therapy and Research, 11,* 567–588.

McNally, R. J., Foa, E. B., & Donnell, C. D. (1989). Memory bias for anxiety information in patients with panic disorder. *Cognition and Emotion, 3,* 27–44.

McNeil, D. W., Ries, B. J., Taylor, L. J., Boone, M. L., Carter, L. E., Turk, C. L., & Lewin, M. R. (1995a). Comparison of social phobia subtypes using Stroop tests. *Journal of Anxiety Disorders, 9,* 47–57.

McNeil, D. W., Ries, B. J., & Turk, C. L. (1995b). Behavioral assessment: Self-report, physiology, and overt behavior. In R. G. Heimberg, M. R. Liebowitz, D. A. Hope, & F. R. Schneier (Eds.), *Social phobia: Diagnosis, assessment, and treatment* (pp. 202–231). New York: Guilford Press.

Meleshko, K. G. A., & Alden, L. E. (1993). Anxiety and self-disclosure: Toward a motivational model. *Journal of Personality and Social Psychology, 64,* 1000–1009.

Mendlowicz, M. V., & Stein, M. B. (2000). Quality of life in individuals with anxiety disorders. *American Journal of Psychiatry, 157,* 669–682.

Mennin, D. S., Fresco, D. M., & Heimberg, R. G. (1998, November). *Determining subtype of social phobia in session: Validation using a receiver operating characteristic (ROC) analysis.* Poster presented at the annual meeting of the Association for Advancement of Behavior Therapy, Washington, DC.

Mennin, D. S., Fresco, D. M., Heimberg, R. G., Schneier, F. R., Davies, S. O., & Liebowitz, M. R. (in press). Screening for social anxiety disorder in the clinical setting: Using the Liebowitz Social Anxiety Scale. *Journal of Anxiety Disorders.*

Mennin, D., Heimberg, R. G., & Holt, C. S. (2000). Panic, agoraphobia, and generalized anxiety disorder. In A. S. Bellack & M. Hersen (Eds.), *Psychopathology in adulthood* (2nd ed., pp. 169–207). Boston: Allyn & Bacon.

Meyer, T. J., Miller, M. L., Metzger, R. L., & Borkovec, T. D. (1990). Development and validation of the Penn State Worry Questionnaire. *Behaviour Research and Therapy, 28,* 487–495.

Mick, M. A., & Telch, M. J. (1998). Social anxiety and history of behavioral inhibition in young adults. *Journal of Anxiety Disorders, 12,* 1–20.

Mogg, K., Bradley, B. P., Bono, J. D., & Painter, M. (1997). Time course of attentional bias for threatening information in non-clinical anxiety. *Behaviour Research and Therapy, 35,* 297–303.

Mogg, K., & Mathews, A. (1990). Is there a self-referent mood-congruent recall bias in anxiety? *Behaviour Research and Therapy, 28,* 91–92.

Mogg, K., Mathews, A., Eysenck, M., & May, J. (1991). Biased cognitive operations in anxiety: Artifact, processing priorities, or attentional search? *Behaviour Research and Therapy, 29,* 459–467.

Mogg, K., Mathews, A., & Weinman, J. (1987). Memory bias in clinical anxiety. *Journal of Abnormal Psychology, 96,* 94–98.

Molina, S., & Borkovec, T. D. (1994). The Penn State Worry Questionnaire: Psychometric properties and associated characteristics. In G. C. L. Davey & F. Tallis (Eds.), *Worrying: Perspectives on theory, assessment and treatment* (pp. 265–283). Chichester, England: Wiley.

Morgan, H., & Raffle, C. (1999). Does reducing safety behaviours improve treatment response in patients with social phobia? *Australian and New Zealand Journal of Psychiatry, 33,* 503–510.

Mullaney, J. A., & Trippett, C. J. (1979). Alcohol dependence and phobias: Clinical description and relevance. *British Journal of Psychiatry, 135,* 565–573.

Myers, J. K., Weissman, M. M., Tischler, G. I., Holzer, C. E., III, Leaf, P. J., Orvaschel, H., Anthony, J. C., Boyd, J. H., Burke, J. D., Jr., Kramer, M., & Stolzman, R. (1984). Six-month prevalence of psychiatric disorders in three communities: 1980 to 1982. *Archives of General Psychiatry, 41,* 959–967.

Norton, G. R., Cox, B. J., Hewitt, P. L., & McLeod, L. (1997). Personality factors associated with generalized and non-generalized social anxiety. *Personality and Individual Differences, 22,* 655–660.

Nyman, D., & Heimberg, R. G. (1985, November). *Heterosocial anxiety: A reasonable analogue to social phobia?* Paper presented at the meeting of the Association for Advancement of Behavior Therapy, Houston, TX.

O'Banion, K., & Arkowitz, H. (1977). Social anxiety and selective memory for affective information about the self. *Social Behavior and Personality, 5,* 321–328.

Oei, T. P. S., Kenna, D., & Evans, L. (1991a). The reliability and utility of the SAD and FNE scales for anxiety disorder patients. *Personality and Individual Differences, 12,* 111–116.

Oei, T. P. S., Moylan, A., & Evans, L. (1991b). Validity and clinical utility of the Fear Questionnaire for anxiety disorder patients. *Psychological Assessment, 3,* 391–397.

Offord, D. R., Boyle, M. H., Campbell, D., Goering, P., Lin, E., Wong, M., & Racine, Y. A. (1996). One-year prevalence of psychiatric disorder in Ontarians 15 to 64 years of age. *Canadian Journal of Psychiatry, 41,* 559–563.

Öst, L.-G. (1987). Age of onset in different phobias. *Journal of Abnormal Psychology, 96,* 223–229.

Otto, M. W., Pollack, M. H., & Sabatino, S. A. (1996). Maintenance of remission following cognitive behavior therapy for panic disorder: Possible deleterious effects of concurrent medication treatment. *Behavior Therapy, 27,* 473–482.

Otto, M. W., Pollack, M. H., Sachs, G. S., Reiter, S. R., Meltzer-Brody, S., & Rosenbaum, J. F. (1993). Discontinuation of benzodiazepine treatment: Efficacy of cognitive-behavioral therapy for patients with panic disorder. *American Journal of Psychiatry, 150,* 1485–1490.

Parker, G. (1979). Reported parental characteristics of agoraphobics and social phobics. *British Journal of Psychiatry, 135,* 555–560.

Persons, J. B. (1989). *Cognitive therapy in practice: A case formulation approach.* New York: Norton.

Peters, L. (2000). Discriminant validity of the Social Phobia and Anxiety Inventory (SPAI), the Social Phobia Scale (SPS), and the Social Interaction Anxiety Scale (SIAS). *Behaviour Research and Therapy, 38,* 943–950.

Peterson, C., Semmel, A., von Baeyer, C., Abramson, L. Y., Metalsky, G. I., & Seligman, M. E. P. (1982). The Attributional Style Questionnaire. *Cognitive Therapy and Research, 6,* 287–299.

Phillips, K., Fulker, D. W., & Rose, R. J. (1987). Path analysis of seven fear factors in adult twin and sibling pairs and their parents. *Genetic Epidemiology, 4,* 345–355.

Phillips, S. D., & Bruch, M. A. (1988). Shyness and dysfunction in career development. *Journal of Counseling Psychology, 35,* 159–165.

Pollard, C. A., & Henderson, J. G. (1988). Four types of social phobia in a community sample. *Journal of Nervous and Mental Disease, 176,* 440–445.

Pollard, C. A., Henderson, J. G., Frank, M., & Margolis, R. B. (1989). Help-seeking patterns of anxiety-disordered individuals in the general population. *Journal of Anxiety Disorders, 3,* 131–138.

Poulton, R. G., & Andrews, G. (1994). Appraisal of danger and proximity in social phobics. *Behaviour Research and Therapy, 32,* 639–642.

Rachman, S., Grüter-Andrew, J., & Shafran, R. (2000). Post-event processing in social anxiety. *Behaviour Research and Therapy, 38,* 611–617.

Rapee, R. M. (1995). Descriptive psychopathology of social phobia. In R. G. Heimberg, M. R. Liebowitz, D. A. Hope, & F. R. Schneier (Eds.), *Social phobia: Diagnosis, assessment, and treatment* (pp. 41–66). New York: Guilford Press.

Rapee, R. M., & Hayman, K. (1996). The effects of video feedback on the self-evaluation of performance in socially anxious subjects. *Behaviour Research and Therapy, 34,* 315–322.

Rapee, R. M., & Heimberg, R. G. (1997). A cognitive-behavioral model of anxiety in social phobia. *Behaviour Research and Therapy, 35,* 741–756.

Rapee, R. M., & Lim, L. (1992). Discrepancy between self- and observer ratings of performance in social phobics. *Journal of Abnormal Psychology, 101,* 728–731.

Rapee, R. M., McCallum, S. L., Melville, L. F., Ravenscroft, H., & Rodney, J. M. (1994). Memory bias in social phobia. *Behaviour Research and Therapy, 32,* 89–99.

Rapee, R. M., & Melville, L. F. (1997). Recall of family factors in social phobia and panic disorder: Comparison of mother and offspring reports. *Depression and Anxiety, 5,* 7–11.

Regier, D. A., Kaelber, C. T., Rae, D. S., Farmer, M. E., Knauper, B., Kessler, R. C., & Norquist, G. S. (1998). Limitations of diagnostic criteria and assessment instruments for mental disorders: Implications for research and policy. *Archives of General Psychiatry, 55,* 109–115.

Regier, D. A., Myers, J. K., Kramer, M., Robins, L. N., Blazer, D. G., Hough, R. L., Eaton, W. W., & Locke, B. Z. (1984). The NIMH Epidemiological Catchment Area Program: Historical context, major objectives, and study population characteristics. *Archives of General Psychiatry, 41,* 934–941.

Reich, J., Goldenberg, I., Vasile, R., Goisman, R., & Keller, M. (1994). A prospective follow-along study of the course of social phobia. *Psychiatry Research, 54,* 249–258.

Reich, J., Noyes, R., & Yates, W. (1988). Anxiety symptoms distinguishing social phobia from panic and generalized anxiety disorders. *Journal of Nervous and Mental Disease, 176,* 510–513.

Reich, J., & Yates, W. (1988). Family history of psychiatric disorders in social phobia. *Comprehensive Psychiatry, 29,* 72–75.

Reiss, S., Peterson, R. A., Gursky, D. M., & McNally, R. J. (1986). Anxiety sensitivity, anxiety frequency and the prediction of fearfulness. *Behaviour Research and Therapy, 24,* 1–8.

Renneberg, B., Chambless, D. L., & Gracely, E. J. (1992). Prevalence of SCID-diagnosed personality disorders in agoraphobic outpatients. *Journal of Anxiety Disorders, 6,* 111–118.

Reznick, J. S., Hegeman, I. M., Kaufman, E. R., Woods, S. W., & Jacobs, M. (1992). Retrospective and concurrent self-report of behavioral inhibition and their relation to adult mental health. *Development and Psychopathology, 4,* 301–321.

Ries, B. J., McNeil, D. W., Boone, M. L., Turk, C. L., Carter, L. E., & Heimberg, R. G. (1998). Assessment of contemporary social phobia verbal report instruments. *Behaviour Research and Therapy, 36,* 983–994.

Robins, L. N., Helzer, J. E., Croughan, J., & Ratcliff, K. S. (1981). National Institute of Mental Health Diagnostic Interview Schedule: Its history, characteristics, and validity. *Archives of General Psychiatry, 38,* 381–389.

Robins, L. N., Wing, J., Wittchen, H.-U., Helzer, J. E., Babor, T. F., Burke, J., Farmer, A., Jablenski, A., Pickens, R., Regier, D. A., Sartorius, N., & Towle, L. H. (1988). The Composite International Diagnostic Interview: An epidemiologic instrument suitable for use in conjunction with different diagnostic systems and in different cultures. *Archives of General Psychiatry, 45,* 1069–1077.

Rose, R. J., & Ditto, W. B. (1983). A developmental-genetic analysis of common fears from early adolescence to early adulthood. *Child Development, 54,* 361–368.

Rosenbaum, J. F., Biederman, J., Hirshfeld, D. R., Bolduc, E. A., & Chaloff, J. (1991a). Behavioral inhibition in children: A possible precursor to panic disorder and social phobia. *Journal of Clinical Psychiatry, 52*(Suppl. 11), 5–9.

Rosenbaum, J. F., Biederman, J., Hirshfeld, D. R., Bolduc, E. A., Faraone, S. V., Kagan, J., Snidman, N., & Reznick, J. S. (1991b). Further evidence of an association between behavioral inhibition and anxiety disorders: Results from a family study of children from a non-clinical sample. *Journal of Psychiatric Research, 25,* 49–65.

Rosenbaum, J. F., Biederman, J., Pollock, R. A., & Hirshfeld, D. R. (1994). The etiology of social phobia. *Journal of Clinical Psychiatry, 55*(Suppl. 6), 10–16.

Roth, D. A., Antony, M. M., & Swinson, R. P. (2001). Interpretations for anxiety symptoms in social phobia. *Behaviour Research and Therapy, 39,* 129–138.

Roth, D. A., Coles, M. E., & Heimberg, R. G. (in press). The relationship between memories for childhood teasing and anxiety and depression in adulthood. *Journal of Anxiety Disorders.*

Russell, D., Cutrona, C. E., & Jones, W. H. (1986). A trait-situational analysis of shyness. In W. H. Jones, J. M. Cheek, & S. R. Briggs (Eds.), *Shyness: Perspectives on research and treatment* (pp. 239–249). New York: Plenum Press.

Safren, S. A., Heimberg, R. G., Brown, E. J., & Holle, C. (1997a). Quality of life in social phobia. *Depression and Anxiety, 4,* 126–133.

Safren, S. A., Heimberg, R. G., Horner, K. J., Juster, H. R., Schneier, F. R., & Liebowitz, M. R. (1999). Factor structure of social fears: The Liebowitz Social Anxiety Scale. *Journal of Anxiety Disorders, 13,* 253–270.

Safren, S. A., Heimberg, R. G., & Juster, H. R. (1997b). Client expectancies and their relationship to pretreatment symptomatology and outcome of cognitive-behavioral group treatment for social phobia. *Journal of Consulting and Clinical Psychology, 65,* 694–698.

Safren, S. A., Turk, C. L., & Heimberg, R. G. (1998). Factor structure of the Social Interaction Anxiety Scale and the Social Phobia Scale. *Behaviour Research and Therapy, 36,* 443–453.

Sanderson, W. C., DiNardo, P. A., Rapee, R. M., & Barlow, D. H. (1990). Syndrome comorbidity in patients diagnosed with a DSM-III-R anxiety disorder. *Journal of Abnormal Psychology, 99,* 308–312.

Sanderson, W. C., Wetzler, S., Beck, A. T., & Betz, F. (1994). Prevalence of personality disorders among patients with anxiety disorders. *Psychiatry Research, 51,* 167–174.

Sank, L. I., & Shaffer, C. S. (1984). *A therapist's manual for cognitive behavior therapy in groups.* New York: Plenum Press.

Schneier, F. R., Heckelman, L. R., Garfinkel, R., Campeas, R., Fallon, B. A., Gitow, A., Street, L., Del Bene, D., & Liebowitz, M. R. (1994). Functional impairment in social phobia. *Journal of Clinical Psychiatry, 55,* 322–331.

Schneier, F. R., Johnson, J., Hornig, C. D., Liebowitz, M. R., & Weissman, M. M. (1992). Social phobia: Comorbidity and morbidity in an epidemiologic sample. *Archives of General Psychiatry, 49,* 282–288.

Schneier, F. R., Liebowitz, M. R., Beidel, D. C., Fyer, A. J., George, M. S., Heimberg, R. G., Holt, C. S., Klein, A. P., Lydiard, R. B., Mannuzza, S., Martin, L. Y., Nardi, E. G., Roscow, D. B., Spitzer, R. L., Turner, S. M., Uhde, T. W., Vasconcelos, I. L., & Versiani, M. (1996). Social phobia. In T. A. Widiger, A. J. Frances, H. A. Pincus, M. J. First, R. Ross, & W. Davis (Eds.), *DSM-IV source book* (Vol. 2, pp. 507–548). Washington, DC: American Psychiatric Press.

Schneier, F. R., Liebowitz, M. R., Beidel, D. C., Garfinkel, R., Heimberg, R. G., Hornig, C. D., Johnson, J., Juster, H., Law, K., Mannuzza, S., Mattia, J. I., Oberlander, E., Orsillo, S., Turner, S. M., & Weissman, M. M. (1998). MacArthur data reanalysis for DSM-IV: Social phobia. In T. A. Widiger, A. J. Frances, H. A. Pincus, R. Ross, M. J. First, W. Davis, & M. Kline (Eds.), *DSM-IV source book* (Vol. 4, pp. 307–328). Washington, DC: American Psychiatric Press.

Schneier, F. R., Martin, L. Y., Liebowitz, M. R., Gorman, J. M., & Fyer, A. J. (1989). Alcohol abuse in social phobia. *Journal of Anxiety Disorders, 3,* 15–23.

Schneier, F. R., Spitzer, R. L., Gibbon, M., Fyer, A. J., & Liebowitz, M. R. (1991). The relationship of social phobia subtypes and avoidant personality disorder. *Comprehensive Psychiatry, 32,* 1–5.

Schwartz, C. E., Snidman, N., & Kagan, J. (1996). Early temperamental predictors of Stroop interference to threatening information at adolescence. *Journal of Anxiety Disorders, 10,* 89–96.

Schwartz, C. E., Snidman, N., & Kagan, J. (1999). Adolescent social anxiety as an outcome of inhibited temperament in childhood. *Journal of the American Academy of Child and Adolescent Psychiatry, 38,* 1008–1015.

Schwartz, R. M. (1986). The internal dialogue: On the asymmetry between positive and negative coping thoughts. *Cognitive Therapy and Research, 10,* 591–605.

Schwartz, R. M., & Garamoni, G. L. (1989). Cognitive balance and psychopathology: Evaluation of an information processing model of positive and negative states of mind. *Clinical Psychology Review, 9,* 271–294.

Scott, E. L. (2000). *Cognitive-behavioral group therapy for social phobia: Comparing response in individuals with social phobia with and without panic attacks.* Unpublished master's thesis, Temple University, Philadelphia, PA.

Scott, E. L., & Heimberg, R. G. (2000). Social phobia: An update on treatment. *Psychiatric Annals, 30,* 678–686.

Selzer, M. L. (1971). The Michigan Alcoholism Screening Test (MAST): The quest for a new diagnostic instrument. *American Journal of Psychiatry, 127,* 1653–1658.

Smail, P., Stockwell, T., Canter, S., & Hodgson, R. (1984). Alcohol dependence and phobic anxiety states: I. A prevalence study. *British Journal of Psychiatry, 144,* 53–57.

Smith, R. E., & Sarason, I. G. (1975). Social anxiety and the evaluation of negative inter-personal feedback. *Journal of Consulting and Clinical Psychology, 43,* 429.

Smith, T. W., Ingram, R. E., & Brehm, S. S. (1983). Social anxiety, anxious self-preoccu-pation, and recall of self-relevant information. *Journal of Personality and Social Psychology, 44,* 1276–1283.

Solyom, L., Ledwidge, B., & Solyom, C. (1986). Delineating social phobia. *British Jour-nal of Psychiatry, 149,* 464–470.

Spielberger, C. D., Gorsuch, R. L., Lushene, R., Vagg, P. R., & Jacobs, G. A. (1983). *Man-ual for the State-Trait Anxiety Inventory.* Palo Alto, CA: Consulting Psychologists Press.

Spitzer, R. L. (1998). Diagnosis and need for treatment are not the same. *Archives of Gen-eral Psychiatry, 55,* 120.

Spitzer, R. L., & Endicott, J. (1978). *Schedule for Affective Disorders and Schizophrenia— Lifetime Version.* New York: Biometric Research, New York State Psychiatric Insti-tute.

Spitzer, R. L., Endicott, J., & Robins, E. (1978). Research Diagnostic Criteria: Rationale and reliability. *Archives of General Psychiatry, 35,* 773–782.

Spitzer, R. L., Williams, J. B. W., Gibbon, M., & First, M. B. (1990). *Structured Clinical Interview for DSM-III-R Personality Disorders (SCID-II).* Washington, DC: Ameri-can Psychiatric Press.

Stefánsson, J. G., Líndal, E., Björnsson, J. K., & Guðmundsdóttir, Á. (1991). Lifetime prevalence of specific mental disorders among people born in Iceland in 1931. *Acta Psychiatrica Scandinavica, 84,* 142–149.

Stein, M. B., Chartier, M. J., Hazen, A. L., Kozak, M. V., Tancer, M. E., Lander, S., Furer, P., Chubaty, D., & Walker, J. R. (1998). A direct-interview family study of general-ized social phobia. *American Journal of Psychiatry, 155,* 90–97.

Stein, M. B., Fuetsch, M., Müller, N., Höfler, M., Lieb, R., & Wittchen, H.-U. (2001). So-cial anxiety disorder and the risk of depression: A prospective community study of adolescents and young adults. *Archives of General Psychiatry, 58,* 251–256.

Stein, M. B., McQuaid, J. R., Laffaye, C., & McCahill, M. E. (1999). Social phobia in the primary care medical setting. *Journal of Family Practice, 48,* 514–519.

Stein, M. B., Shea, C. A., & Uhde, T. W. (1989). Social phobic symptoms in patients with panic disorder: Practical and theoretical implications. *American Journal of Psychia-try, 146,* 235–238.

Stein, M. B., Tancer, M. E., Gelernter, C. S., Vittone, B. J., & Uhde, T. W. (1990). Major depression in patients with social phobia. *American Journal of Psychiatry, 147,* 637–639.

Stein, M. B., Walker, J. R., & Forde, D. R. (1994). Setting diagnostic thresholds for social phobia: Considerations from a community survey of social anxiety. *American Jour-nal of Psychiatry, 151,* 408–412.

Stein, M. B., Walker, J. R., & Forde, D. R. (1996). Public-speaking fears in a community sample: Prevalence, impact on functioning, and diagnostic classification. *Archives of General Psychiatry, 53,* 169–174.

Stopa, L., & Clark, D. M. (1993). Cognitive processes in social phobia. *Behaviour Re-search and Therapy, 31,* 255–267.

Stopa, L., & Clark, D. M. (2000). Social phobia and interpretation of social events. *Behav-iour Research and Therapy, 38,* 273–283.

Stravynski, A., Elie, R., & Franche, R. L. (1989). Perception of early parenting by patients diagnosed with avoidant personality disorder: A test of the overprotection hypothesis. *Acta Psychiatrica Scandinavica, 80,* 415–420.

Stravynski, A., Lamontagne, Y., & Lavallee, Y. J. (1986). Clinical phobias and avoidant personality disorder among alcoholics admitted to an alcoholism rehabilitation setting. *Canadian Journal of Psychiatry, 31,* 714–719.

Stroop, J. R. (1935). Studies of interference in serial verbal reactions. *Journal of Experimental Psychology, 18,* 643–662.

Taylor, S., Woody, S., McLean, P. D., & Koch, W. J. (1997). Sensitivity of outcome measures for treatments of generalized social phobia. *Assessment, 4,* 181–191.

Teglasi, H., & Hoffman, M. A. (1982). Causal attribution bias in shy subjects. *Journal of Research in Personality, 16,* 376–385.

Thyer, B. A., Parrish, R. T., Curtis, G. C., Nesse, R. M., & Cameron, O. G. (1985). Ages of onset in DSM-III anxiety disorders. *Comprehensive Psychiatry, 26,* 113–122.

Thyer, B. A., Parrish, R. T., Himle, J., Cameron, O. G., Curtis, G. C., & Nesse, R. M. (1986). Alcohol abuse among clinically anxious patients. *Behaviour Research and Therapy, 24,* 357–359.

Torgersen, S. (1979). The nature and origin of common phobic fears. *British Journal of Psychiatry, 134,* 343–351.

Torgersen, S. (1983). Genetic factors in anxiety disorders. *Archives of General Psychiatry, 40,* 1085–1089.

Tran, G. Q., & Chambless, D. L. (1995). Psychopathology of social phobia: Effects of subtype and of avoidant personality disorder. *Journal of Anxiety Disorders, 9,* 489–501.

Turk, C. L., Fresco, D. M., & Heimberg, R. G. (1999). Social phobia: Cognitive behavior therapy. In M. Hersen & A. S. Bellack (Eds.), *Handbook of comparative treatments of adult disorders* (2nd ed., pp. 287–316). New York: Wiley.

Turk, C. L., Heimberg, R. G., Orsillo, S. M., Holt, C. S., Gitow, A., Street, L. L., Schneier, F. R., & Liebowitz, M. R. (1998). An investigation of gender differences in social phobia. *Journal of Anxiety Disorders, 12,* 209–223.

Turk, C. L., Lerner, J., Heimberg, R. G., & Rapee, R. M. (2001). An integrated cognitive-behavioral model of social anxiety. In S. G. Hofmann & P. M. DiBartolo (Eds.), *From social anxiety to social phobia: Multiple perspectives* (pp. 281–303). Needham Heights, MA: Allyn & Bacon.

Turner, R. M. (1987). The effects of personality disorder diagnosis on the outcome of social anxiety symptom reduction. *Journal of Personality Disorders, 1,* 136–143.

Turner, S. M., Beidel, D. C., Borden, J. W., Stanley, M. A., & Jacob, R. G. (1991). Social phobia: Axis I and II correlates. *Journal of Abnormal Psychology, 100,* 102–106.

Turner, S. M., Beidel, D. C., Dancu, C. V., & Keys, D. J. (1986a). Psychopathology of social phobia and comparison to avoidant personality disorder. *Journal of Abnormal Psychology, 95,* 389–394.

Turner, S. M., Beidel, D. C., Dancu, C. V., & Stanley, M. A. (1989a). An empirically derived inventory to measure social fears and anxiety: The Social Phobia and Anxiety Inventory. *Psychological Assessment, 1,* 35–40.

Turner, S. M., Beidel, D. C., & Larkin, K. T. (1986b). Situational determinants of social anxiety in clinic and non-clinic samples: Physiological and cognitive correlates. *Journal of Consulting and Clinical Psychology, 54,* 523–527.

Turner, S. M., Beidel, D. C., & Townsley, R. M. (1990). Social phobia: Relationship to shyness. *Behaviour Research and Therapy, 28,* 497–505.

Turner, S. M., Beidel, D. C., & Townsley, R. M. (1992). Social phobia: A comparison of specific and generalized subtype and avoidant personality disorder. *Journal of Abnormal Psychology, 101,* 326–331.

Turner, S. M., McCanna, M., & Beidel, D. C. (1987). Validity of the Social Avoidance and Distress Scale and the Fear of Negative Evaluation Scale. *Behaviour Research and Therapy, 25,* 113–115.

Turner, S. M., Stanley, M. A., Beidel, D. C., & Bond, L. (1989b). The Social Phobia and Anxiety Inventory: Construct validity. *Journal of Psychopathology and Behavioral Assessment, 11,* 221–234.

Van Ameringen, M., Mancini, C., Styan, G., & Donison, D. (1991). Relationship of social phobia with other psychiatric illness. *Journal of Affective Disorders, 21,* 93–99.

Veljaca, K., & Rapee, R. M. (1998). Detection of negative and positive audience behaviors by socially anxious subjects. *Behaviour Research and Therapy, 36,* 311–321.

Vrana, S. R., Roodman, A., & Beckham, J. C. (1995). Selective processing of trauma-relevant words in post-traumatic stress disorder. *Journal of Anxiety Disorders, 9,* 515–530.

Wacker, H. R., Müllejans, R., Klein, K. H., & Battegay, R. (1992). Identification of cases of anxiety disorders and affective disorders in the community according to ICD-10 and DSM-III-R by using the Composite International Diagnostic Interview (CIDI). *International Journal of Methods in Psychiatric Research, 2,* 91–100.

Walker, J. R., & Stein, M. B. (1995). The epidemiology of social phobia. In M. B. Stein (Ed.), *Social phobia: Clinical and research perspectives* (pp. 43–75). Washington, DC: American Psychiatric Press.

Wallace, S. T., & Alden, L. E. (1991). A comparison of social standards and perceived ability in anxious and nonanxious men. *Cognitive Therapy and Research, 15,* 237–254.

Wallace, S. T., & Alden, L. E. (1995). Social anxiety and standard setting following social success or failure. *Cognitive Therapy and Research, 19,* 613–631.

Wallace, S. T., & Alden, L. E. (1997). Social phobia and positive social events: The price of success. *Journal of Abnormal Psychology, 106,* 416–424.

Watson, D. (1982). The actor and the observer: How are their perceptions of causality different? *Psychological Bulletin, 92,* 682–700.

Watson, D., & Friend, R. (1969). Measurement of social-evaluative anxiety. *Journal of Consulting and Clinical Psychology, 33,* 448–457.

Weiller, E., Bisserbe, J.-C., Boyer, P., Lépine, J.-P., & Lecrubier, Y. (1996). Social phobia in general health care: An unrecognized and undertreated disabling disorder. *British Journal of Psychiatry, 168,* 169–174.

Weissman, M. M., Bland, R. C., Canino, G. J., Greenwald, S., Lee, C.-K., Newman, S. C., Rubio-Stipec, M., & Wickramaratne, P. J. (1996). The cross-national epidemiology of social phobia: A preliminary report. *International Clinical Psychopharmacology, 11*(Suppl. 3), 9–14.

Wells, A., Clark, D. M., & Ahmad, S. (1998). How do I look with my minds eye: Perspective taking in social phobic imagery. *Behaviour Research and Therapy, 36,* 631–634.

Wells, A., Clark, D. M., Salkovskis, P., Ludgate, J., Hackmann, A., & Gelder, M. (1995). Social phobia: The role of in-situation safety behaviors in maintaining anxiety and negative beliefs. *Behavior Therapy, 26,* 153–161.

Wells, A., & Papageorgiou, C. (1999). The observer perspective: Biased imagery in social phobia, agoraphobia, and blood/injury phobia. *Behaviour Research and Therapy, 37,* 653–658.

Wells, J. E., Bushnell, J. A., Hornblow, A. R., Joyce, P. R., & Oakley-Browne, M. A. (1989). Christchurch Psychiatric Epidemiology Study: Part I. Methodology and lifetime prevalence for specific psychiatric disorders. *Australian and New Zealand Journal of Psychiatry, 23,* 315–326.

Wickramaratne, P. J., Weissman, M. M., Leaf, P. J., & Holford, T. R. (1989). Age, period, and cohort effects on the risk of major depression: Results from five United States communities. *Journal of Clinical Epidemiology, 42,* 333–343.

Widiger, T. A. (1992). Generalized social phobia versus avoidant personality disorder: A commentary on three studies. *Journal of Abnormal Psychology, 101,* 340–343.

Williams, J. M. G., Mathews, A., & MacLeod, C. (1996). The emotional Stroop task and psychopathology. *Psychological Bulletin, 120,* 3–24.

Williams, J. M. G., Watts, F. N., MacLeod, C., & Mathews, A. (1997). *Cognitive psychology and emotional disorders* (2nd ed.). Chichester, England: Wiley.

Winton, E. C., Clark, D. M., & Edelmann, R. J. (1995). Social anxiety, fear of negative evaluation, and the detection of negative emotion in others. *Behaviour Research and Therapy, 33,* 193–196.

Wittchen, H.-U., & Beloch, E. (1996). The impact of social phobia on quality of life. *International Clinical Psychopharmacology, 11*(Suppl. 3), 15–23.

Wittchen, H.-U., Stein, M. B., & Kessler, R. C. (1999). Social fears and social phobia in a community sample of adolescents and young adults: Prevalence, risk factors, and comorbidity. *Psychological Medicine, 29,* 309–323.

World Health Organization (1990). *Composite International Diagnostic Interview, Version 1. 0.* Geneva, Switzerland: Author.

Yuen, P. K. (1994). *Social anxiety and the allocation of attention: Evaluation using facial stimuli in a dot-probe paradigm.* Unpublished manuscript, University of Oxford, United Kingdom.

Zweig, D. R., & Brown, D. S. (1985). Psychometric evaluation of a written stimulus presentation format for the Social Interaction Self-Statement Test. *Cognitive Therapy and Research, 9,* 285–295.

Index

"f" indicates a figure; "n" indicates a note; "t" indicates a table

Affective disorder, 43–45
Age at onset, 47, 48*f*
  see also Characteristics
Agoraphobia, 17, 200
  assessment, 112
  comorbidity with, 40–43
  environmental contributions, 22–24
  genetic contributions, 19, 20
  memory bias, 89
  perspective taking, 91–92
  Social Phobia and Anxiety Inventory, 113
Alcoholism
  case example, 94
  cognitive-behavioral group therapy, 140–141
  comorbidity and, 45–46
All-or-nothing thinking, 178*f*, 180–181, 196*f*,
    236, 239, 249, 295
  see also Automatic thoughts; Thinking
    errors
Anxiety
  assessment, 125
  avoidant personality disorder, 37–39
  coping behaviors, 70–71
  explaining components of, 158–161
  three components of, 163
  types of, 6–7
Anxiety disorder, 40–43
  diagnosing, 138–139
  Social Phobia and Anxiety Inventory, 113

Anxiety Disorders Interview Schedule, 136–137
Anxiety response components, 160–161, 162*f*
Assessment
  adjunctive measures, 124–126
  Anxiety Disorders Interview Schedule, 136–
    137
  behavioral testing, 123–124
  clinician-administered, 115–119
  cognitive, 119–123
  cognitive content, 53–55
  cognitive function, 107–108
  posttreatment, 289–290
  self-report, 108–115
Attendance, 151–152
  see also Session one
Attentional bias
  dot-probe paradigm, 80, 81*f*
  research, 83–86, 85*f*
  Stroop color-naming task, 74–80, 76*f*, 78*f*
  task performance, 80–83, 82*f*
Attribution
  perspective taking, 92
  style, 58–59
Automatic thoughts, 292
  see also Rational responses
  belief in, 231–233, 247–248, 257
  case example, 237–239, 262–268, 266*f*
  cognitive restructuring, 165, 168–173
  disrupting, 189–195, 190*f*, 191*f*

Automatic thoughts (*continued*)
  homework, 270, 272, 273, 274*f*–275*f*, 276
  identification of, 177, 178*f*, 179–189, 227–230
  in-session exposure, 250–251
  inappropriateness of behaviors, 245–247
  journaling, 131, 173–175, 174*f*, 177
  making conversation, 233–237
  negative, 104
  occurrence of, 253–254
  regarding being accepted, 260–261
  reviewing, 159, 252–253
  session planning and, 291, 294–295
  session three, 284
  SUDS, 254, 255–256
  supporting, 253, 254*f*
  thought listing, 122
  visible anxiety, 239–245, 244*f*, 258–260
Avoidance, 7–8, 38–39
  see also Avoidant personality disorder; Symptoms
  explaining in treatment, 160–161
Avoidant personality disorder, 5, 34–35, 38*t*
  clinical presentation of, 37–39
  cognitive-behavioral treatment, 39–40
  comorbidity with, 46
  diagnosis, 37
  generalized social phobia and, 35–36, 36*t*, 40
  mood disorders and, 43–44
  threat index, 75, 76*f*, 77
Axis I disorders, 40–43
  alcoholism, 45–46
  depression and suicidality, 43–45
Axis II disorders, 46

B

Behavioral Assessment Tests, 123–124
  see also Assessment
Behavioral components of anxiety, 160–161
  in-session exposure, 163–164
  interaction with other components, 161, 162*f*, 163
Behavioral experiments, 258–261, 294
Behavioral inhibition, 25–28, 27*f*
Behavioral processes, 105–106
Behavioral testing, 107–108
Beliefs, 130, 157, 158, 159
  see also Automatic thoughts
Biased interpretation, 64

Black-and-white thinking. *see* All-or-nothing thinking
Booster sessions, 290
  see also Termination
Brief Fear of Negative Evaluation Scale, 135
Brief Social Phobia Scale, 118–119
  see also Clinician-administered assessment

C

Catastrophizing, 178*f*, 182–184, 196*f*, 295
  see also Automatic thoughts; Thinking errors
  SUDS, 255
Causality attributions, 58–59
Characteristics, 47–51, 48*f*
Child-rearing practices, 22–25
  see also Environmental contributions
Chronicity, 7–8
  see also Symptoms
Circumscribed social phobia, 30
Client characteristics, 133–134, 137–141
Clinician-administered assessment
  see also Assessment
  Brief Social Phobia Scale, 118–119
  Liebowitz Social Anxiety Scale, 115–118, 117*f*
Cognitive assessment, 99*f*, 119–123, 120*f*
  see also Assessment
Cognitive-behavioral group therapy
  see also Cognitive restructuring; Homework; In-session exposure; Session one; Session three and beyond; Session two; Termination
  additional resources, 299–301
  case example, 261–268
  client characteristics, 133–134, 137–141
  goal of, 130
  group size, 133
  homework, 276, 281–282
  medication's effect on, 139–141
  overview, 146, 146–147, 148
  research, 33
  session planning, 291
  specific treatment targets, 143, 145–146
  summarized, 129–130
  termination, 289, 290
  therapist characteristics, 132–133
  time management, 285–286, 287*f*, 294
  troubleshooting, 291–299
Cognitive-behavioral treatment
  see also Cognitive-behavioral group therapy
  avoidant personality disorder, 39–40

following termination, 290
model of, 155–163, 162*f*
self-evaluation, 67
Cognitive component of anxiety
see also Session one
explaining in treatment, 158–161
interaction with other components, 161,
162*f*, 163
Cognitive coping, 231
Cognitive debriefing, 257–258
see also In-session exposure
assessment of goal attainment, 251–252
Cognitive function, 73–74
case example, 105–106
negative context, 53–58, 54*f*, 57*f*
testing, 107–108
Cognitive restructuring, 129, 130
see also Cognitive-behavioral group therapy
automatic thoughts, 173–175, 174*f*, 189–
195, 190*f*, 191*f*, 294–295
case example, 261–268, 264
explaining in treatment, 164
feedback, 253
group involvement in, 268–269
in-session exposure, 131–132, 220, 227, 228*f*
session three, 284
session two homework, 195, 196*f*, 197
termination, 289
training, 131, 165, 168–173
troubleshooting, 293–299
Comorbidity
with alcoholism, 45–46
with anxiety disorders, 40–43
with Axis II disorders, 46
case example, 94
with depression and suicidality, 43–45
employment impairment, 50–51
marital status, 49
in treatment, 138–139, 140–141
Composite International Diagnostic Interview,
11–13
Confidentiality, 152–154, 153*f*
see also Session one
within the group, 147
in-session exposure, 204
Coping behaviors, 70–71, 257
case example, 103
following treatment, 287
Core beliefs, 295
see also Cognitive function
Cultural considerations, 24–25

D
Definition of Social Phobia, 4–5, 8
Depression, 33, 138
alcoholism and, 140–141
assessment of, 124
comorbidity and, 43–45
research, 38–39
Diagnosis
see also DSM-III; DSM-III-R; DSM-IV
avoidant personality disorder, 37
case example, 94
comorbidity, 40–46, 138–139
DSM-III, 4–5
subtypes, 29–34, 32*f*
Diagnostic Interview Schedule, 9–11, 12*t*
see also Diagnosis
Dichotomous thinking. *see* All-or-nothing
thinking
Difference score, 112–114
see also Social Phobia and Anxiety
Inventory
Disability, 125–126
Discrete social phobia, 30
Disqualifying the positive, 178*f*, 184, 196*f*, 276
see also Automatic thoughts; Thinking
errors
Dot-probe paradigm, 80, 81*f*, 84–86
see also Attentional bias
Drinking in public, fear of
see also Feared situations
in-session exposure, 205–206, 218–220
sample homework tasks, 279–280
DSM-III, 4–5
see also Diagnosis
avoidant personality disorder, 34
prevalence research, 9–11, 12*t*
DSM-III-R, 5
see also Diagnosis; Generalized social
phobia
avoidant personality disorder, 34
prevalence research, 11–13, 12*t*, 13*t*
DSM-IV, 5, 6*t*, 29–30
see also Diagnosis
Anxiety Disorders Interview Schedule, 136–
137
avoidant personality disorder, 35*t*
prevalence research, 13–14
Duration, 47–49
see also Characteristics
Dysfunctional beliefs. *see* Automatic thoughts
Dysthymia, 43–45

E

Early Developmental Stages of
    Psychopathology study, 13–14
Eating in public, fear of, 16
    see also Feared situations
    in-session exposure, 205–206, 218–220
    sample homework tasks, 279
Educational impairment, 49–50
    see also Impairment
Emotional reasoning, 178*f*, 184–185, 196*f*
    see also Automatic thoughts; Thinking
        errors
Employment impairment, 50–51
    see also Impairment
Environmental contributions, 22–25
    see also Genetic contributions
    case example, 94, 95–97
    explaining in treatment, 156–157
Epidemiologic Catchment Area Study, 9–10
Etiology, 18
    see also Environmental contributions;
        Genetic contributions
Evaluation
    negative, 102–103
    self, 64–67, 66*f*
    standards of, 68–70
Events
    ambiguous, 63–64
    negative, 59–63, 61*f*, 62*f*
Exposure treatment. *see* In-session exposure

F

Facial expressions
    memory biases for, 88–89
    reactions to, 84–86
Fear Questionnaire, 115
    see also Self-report assessment
Feared situations, 16–18
    see also specific situations
    exposure treatment, 129–130
    sample homework tasks, 276, 278–281
Feedback, 212
    case example, 104
    following in-session exposure, 253
    group, 268–269
    reactions to, 67
    video, 260
Fortune telling, 178*f*, 181–182, 196*f*, 295
    see also Automatic thoughts; Thinking errors
Functional impairment, 47–51
    see also Impairment

G

Gender differences, 14–15, 18
Generalized social phobia
    avoidant personality disorder and, 35–36,
        36*t*, 38*t*, 39, 40
    cognitive-behavioral treatment, 39–40
    comorbidity and, 41
    depression and, 43–45
    DSM-IV, 29
    memory bias, 86–87
    negative interpretations, 63–64
    vs. nongeneralized social phobia, 51–52*n*
    research, 30–34, 32*f*
    Social Phobia and Anxiety Inventory, 113
    Social Phobia Inventory, 114–115
Genetic contributions, 19–20, 21*f*
    see also Environmental contributions
    case example, 94, 95–96
    explaining in treatment, 156
Goal setting, 269*n*
    case example, 265–266
    eating in public phobia, 219
    in-session exposure, 248–250
Goals, 131–132
    case example, 266*f*
    cognitive debriefing, 251–252
    following treatment, 288
    maintaining focus on, 250–251
    reviewing, 273
Group composition
    client characteristics, 133–134, 137–141
    session characteristics, 134–135
    therapist characteristics, 132–133
Group participation, 147, 152
    see also Session one

H

Heart rate reactivity, 31, 32*f*
    see also Physiological responses
History of Social Phobia, 4
Homework, 129, 130
    see also Session one
    alcohol use during, 141
    attitude, 270–271
    automatic thoughts, 131
    client preparation, 148
    completing, 272, 273
    depression, 138
    disqualifying the positive, 184
    following, 273, 276, 287
    making mistakes, 223

preparation for, 152, 164, 271–272, 274*f*–275*f*
procedures, 276, 277*f*
reviewing, 177, 281–282, 284–285
sample tasks for, 276, 278–281
session one, 173–175
session planning and, 291
session two, 195, 196*f*, 197
termination, 289
troubleshooting, 296–299
Homograph paradigm, 83–84, 85*f*
see also Attentional bias

I

Imagery
case example, 105
perspective taking, 90–92
Impairment, 7–8, 47–51
see also Symptoms
In-session exposure, 129–130, 131–132
see also Cognitive-behavioral group therapy
alcohol use during, 141
anxiety during, 212–213
automatic thoughts, 253, 253–254, 254*f*
behavioral experiments, 258–261
brief behaviors, 221–226
case example, 265–268, 267*f*
choosing role players, 210–211
cognitive debriefing, 251–258
cognitive restructuring, 227, 228*f*
defining goals of, 248–250
developing rational responses, 231–233
first exposures, 209–210
group feedback, 268–269
homework follow-up, 271
incorporating feared outcomes, 206–208
introduction to, 163–164, 197–206, 284–285
making conversation, 235
session planning and, 291
vs. social skills training, 211–212
specific examples, 213–221
SUDS, 208–209*f*, 250–251, 254–257, 256*f*
termination, 289
therapist role, 133
troubleshooting, 291–293
In vivo exposure, 129, 278
see also Cognitive-behavioral group
therapy; Homework; In-session exposure
vs. in-session exposures, 199–202
Individualized Fear and Avoidance Hierarchy, 142–143, 144*f*, 145

Interference, 74–80, 76*f*, 78*f*
Internal anxiety cues, 104
Internal dialogue
see also Automatic thoughts
case example, 104
content, 54*f*, 55–58, 57*f*
developing rational responses, 231
negative, 53–55
Interpersonal attraction paradigm, 71–72
see also Romantic involvement, fear of
Interpretations, 63–64
Irrational thoughts. *see* Thinking errors

L

Labeling, 178*f*, 185–186, 196*f*, 276
see also Automatic thoughts; Thinking
errors
Liebowitz Social Anxiety Scale, 115–118, 117*f*, 289
see also Clinician-administered assessment
Limited social phobia, 30

M

Maladaptive thoughts, 178*f*, 188–189, 196*f*
see also Automatic thoughts; Thinking
errors
Marital status, 49
see also Impairment
Memory
bias, 86–90
perceptions affect on, 90–92
Mental filter, 178*f*, 186, 196*f*
see also Automatic thoughts; Thinking
errors
Mental representation, 100–101
Mind reading, 178*f*, 186–187, 196*f*
see also Automatic thoughts; Thinking errors
in vivo exposure, 201
Molar analysis, 123
see also Behavioral Assessment Tests
Molecular analysis, 123
see also Behavioral Assessment Tests
"Must" statements, 178*f*, 187–188, 196*f*
see also Automatic thoughts; Thinking
errors

N

Negative cognitive context, 53–58, 57*f*
cognitive restructuring, 130
thought listing, 122
Negative evaluation, 135

Nongeneralized social phobia
    comorbidity and, 36, 38*t*, 40, 41, 43–45
    vs. generalized social phobia, 51–52*n*
    research, 30–34, 32*f*

O

Obsessive–compulsive disorder
    comorbidity with, 40–43
    negative interpretations, 63–64
Other-oriented perfectionism. *see*
        Perfectionistic thinking
Overgeneralizing, 178*f*, 187, 196*f*
    see also Automatic thoughts; Thinking errors

P

Panic attacks, 42
Panic disorder, 200
    attributions of causality, 59
    avoidant personality disorder and, 36
    cognitive-behavioral group therapy, 138–139
    comorbidity with, 40–43
    duration of, 48–49
    memory bias, 86–87
    perfectionistic thinking, 68
    Social Phobia and Anxiety Inventory, 113–114
Perception
    affects on memory, 90–92
    of an audience, 98–100
Perfectionistic thinking, 68–70
Performance deficits, 63–67
Performing, 16
    see also Feared situations
    self-evaluation of, 64–67, 66*f*, 69–70
    standards, 102
Personality disorders, 46
Pharmacological treatment, 139–141
Physiological responses, 31, 32*f*
    see also Symptoms
    case example, 104, 105–106
    developing rational responses, 232
    explaining in treatment, 160
    goal setting, 249
    in-session exposure, 163–164, 257
    interaction with other components, 161,
        162*f*, 163
Playing in public, fear of, 220
Posttraumatic stress disorder
    comorbidity with, 40–43
    memory bias, 86–87
Predictions, 157, 158, 159
    see also Automatic thoughts

Prevalence, 8, 9–15
Processing tasks, 122–123
    see also Cognitive assessment
Promptness, 152
    see also Session one
Psychometric assessment, 107–108
    see also Assessment
Public rest rooms, fear of, 16
    see also Feared situations
Public speaking, fear of, 16
    see also Feared situations; Nongeneralized
        social phobia
    alcohol use, 46
    assessment, 121
    comorbidity and, 41
    employment impairment, 50–51
    expressing opinions during, 224–225
    in-session exposure, 205, 215–217
    memory disruption, 90
    research, 30–31, 32*f*, 33–34
    sample homework tasks, 279
    self-evaluation of, 64–67, 66*f*
    SUDS, 255
    thinking errors, 186
    threat index, 75, 76*f*, 77

Q

Quality of life
    assessment of, 126
    posttreatment assessment, 289

R

Rapport, 141
Rational responses, 192, 193–195, 254*f*,
        257
    see also Automatic thoughts
    belief in, 247–248, 257
    case example, 265, 266*f*
    developing, 231–233
    homework, 270, 272, 273, 274*f*–275*f*
    in-session exposure, 284–285
    reviewing, 252–253
    SUDS, 250–251, 254, 255–256
Recall
    perspective taking, 90–92
    preferential, 87–89
    thoughts, 230–231
Relationships, 49
    see also Impairment
Relaxation training, 39–40
    see also Cognitive-behavioral treatment

Research, 30–34, 32*f*
Rest rooms, fear of, 16
  see also Feared situations
Role play, 123–124
  see also Behavioral Assessment Tests
  group involvement in, 268–269
  therapist role, 133
  troubleshooting, 292–293
Romantic involvement, fear of
  automatic thoughts, 233–237
  interpersonal attraction paradigm, 71–72
  SUDS, 255

S

Safety behaviors, 70–71, 103
Schemata, 73–74
  see also Cognitive function
Self-evaluative thoughts
  negative, 56, 248
  performing, 64–67, 66*f*
  standards, 68–70
Self-oriented perfectionism. *see* Perfectionistic
  thinking
Self-report assessment
  see also Assessment
  Peer Questionnaire, 115
  Social Interaction Anxiety Scale, 108, 109–
    110*f*, 112
  Social Phobia and Anxiety Inventory, 112–
    114
  Social Phobia Inventory, 114–115
  Social Phobia Scale, 109–110*f*, 112
Self-statements
  content, 54*f*, 55–58, 57*f*
  negative, 53–55
Session characteristics, 134–135
Session one, 131
  assessment, 164–165, 167–168*f*
  cognitive restructuring training, 165, 168–
    173
  discussing treatment, 163–164
  establishing rules, 151–154
  explaining social phobia, 155–163, 162*f*
  homework, 173–175
  introductions, 150–151
  overview, 149–150
  sharing, 154–155
Session three and beyond, 131–132
  materials, 283–284
  termination, 286–290
  time management, 285–286, 287*f*

Session twelve, 132, 286–290
  see also Termination
Session two, 131
  disrupting automatic thoughts, 189–195,
    190*f*, 191*f*
  homework, 195, 196*f*, 197
  identifying thinking errors, 177, 178*f*, 179–
    189
  overview, 176
  preparing for session three, 197–198
  review, 177
"Should" statements, 178*f*, 187–188, 196*f*
  see also Automatic thoughts; Thinking
    errors
Shyness, 6–8
Social adjustment, 38–39
Social events
  ambiguous, 63–64
  negative, 59–63, 61*f*, 62*f*
Social Interaction Anxiety Scale, 108, 109–
  110*f*, 112
  posttreatment assessment, 289
Social Interaction Self-Statement Test, 119–
  121
  see also Cognitive assessment
Social Phobia and Anxiety Inventory, 112–
  114
  see also Self-report assessment
Social Phobia Inventory, 114–115
  see also Self-report assessment
Social Phobia Scale, 108, 110, 111–112*f*
Social skills deficits, 65–67, 104
Social skills training, 245, 247
  see also Feared situations
  avoidant personality disorder, 39–40
  vs. in-session exposure, 211–212
Social threat, 74, 76*f*, 78*f*, 80
  detecting cues of, 80–83, 82*f*
Socially prescribed perfectionism. *see*
  Perfectionistic thinking
Steps for Overcoming Social Anxiety with
  Exposure and Cognitive Restructuring
  form, 276, 277*f*, 285
Stroop color-naming task, 74–80, 76*f*, 78*f*
  see also Attentional bias
  as a clinical assessment, 122–123
  in-session exposure, 223
Subjective costs of negative events, 59–63, 61*f*,
  62*f*
Subjective Units of Discomfort Scale. *see*
  SUDS

SUDS
   case example, 265–268, 267*f*
   discontinuing, 269*n*
   in-session exposure, 225, 250–251, 284–285
   patterns of, 254–257, 256*f*
   silent, 258–260
   treatment orientation interview, 143, 145*f*,
      208
Suicidality, 43–45
Symptoms, 42, 43
   see also Avoidance
   anticipating, 206–208
   case example, 103–104
   depression, 124, 138
   DSM-IV, 6*t*
   measuring, 113–114
   public speaking, 216–217
   sharing in group, 154–155
   vs. shyness, 7–8
Systematic desensitization, 39–40
   see also Cognitive-behavioral treatment

T

Task performance, 80–83, 82*f*
   see also Attentional bias
Temperament, 25–28
   see also Behavioral inhibition
Termination, 132, 286–290
Therapist characteristics, 132–133
Thinking errors, 177, 178*f*, 179–189
   see also specific errors
   case example, 263
   homework, 195, 196*f*, 197, 272, 274*f*–275*f*,
      276
   identification of, 230–231
   session three, 284
   in vivo exposure, 201

Thought listing, 122
   see also Cognitive assessment
Thoughts
   content, 55–58, 57*f*
   frequency, 53–55, 54*f*
   thought listing, 122
Threat index, 74–80, 76*f*, 78*f*
Time management, 285–286, 287*f*, 294
Treatment
   see also Cognitive-behavioral group
      therapy; Cognitive-behavioral treatment
   case example, 105–106
   discussion of, 163–164
   orientation interview, 130–131
   utilizing, 51
Treatment orientation interview, 130–131
   see also Cognitive-behavioral group therapy
   discussing specific fears, 141–142
   Individualized Fear and Avoidance
      Hierarchy, 142–143, 144*f*
   introduction to procedures, 146
   purposes of, 136–137
   SUDS, 143, 145*f*
Treatment targets, 143, 145–146
Twin research, 20
   see also Genetic contributions

V

Vocational impairment, 50–51
   see also Impairment

W

Working in public, fear of, 205–206, 220
Writing in public, fear of, 16
   see also Feared situations
   in-session exposure, 205–206, 218, 221–222
   sample homework tasks, 280